Management of Perioperative Complications in Gynecology

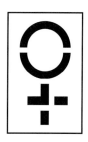

Management of Perioperative Complications in Gynecology

■ ■ ■ ■ ■ ■ ■

Vicki V. Baker, MD

Chief, Division of Gynecologic Oncology
George W. Morley Professor
Department of Obstetrics and Gynecology
University of Michigan Medical Center
Ann Arbor, Michigan

Gunter Deppe, MD

Director, Gynecologic Oncology
Professor, Department of Obstetrics and Gynecology
Wayne State University
School of Medicine
Detroit, Michigan

W.B. SAUNDERS COMPANY
A Division of Harcourt Brace & Company
Philadelphia ■ London ■ Toronto ■ Montreal ■ Sydney ■ Tokyo

W.B. SAUNDERS COMPANY
A Division of Harcourt Brace & Company

The Curtis Center
Independence Square West
Philadelphia, Pennsylvania 19106

Library of Congress Cataloging-in-Publication Data

Management of perioperative complications in gynecology / [edited by]
Vicki V. Baker, Gunter Deppe.

p.   cm.

ISBN 0–7216–5881–4

1. Generative organs, Female—Surgery—Complications.   I. Baker, Vicki V.
II. Deppe, Gunter.   [DNLM: 1. Genital Diseases, Female—surgery.
2. Genital Diseases, Female—therapy.   3. Postoperative Complications.
4. Intraoperative Complications.   5. Preoperative Care.
WP 660 M266 1997]

RG104.2.M36 1997   618. 1′059—dc20

DNLM/DLC   96–15894

MANAGEMENT OF PERIOPERATIVE COMPLICATIONS
IN GYNECOLOGY   ISBN 0–7216–5881–4

Last digit is the print number: 9   8   7   6   5   4   3   2   1

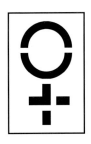

Contributors

■ ■ ■ ■ ■ ■ ■

Vicki V. Baker, MD
Chief, Division of Gynecologic Oncology, and
George W. Morley Professor, Department of
Obstetrics and Gynecology, University of
Michigan Medical Center, Ann Arbor,
Michigan
*Principles of Postoperative Care; Management of
Wound Complications*

Patricia Braly, MD
Professor and Director, Gynecologic Oncology,
LSU Medical School, New Orleans, Louisiana
Abscess, Hematoma, and Lymphocyst

Eva Chalas, MD
Associate Professor, Department of Obstetrics
and Gynecology, State University of New
York at Stony Brook, Stony Brook, New York
Vascular Access

Daniel L. Clarke-Pearson, MD
James M. Ingram Professor of Gynecologic
Oncology, Duke University School of
Medicine; Director of Gynecologic Oncology,
Duke Medical Center, Durham, North
Carolina
Venous Thromboembolic Complications

Robert L. Coleman, MD, FACOG, FACS
Assistant Professor, Department of Obstetrics
and Gynecology, Division of Gynecologic
Oncology, University of Texas Southwestern
Medical Center, Dallas, Texas
The Retroperitoneal Mass

Gunter Deppe, MD
Director, Gynecologic Oncology, and
Professor, Department of Obstetrics and
Gynecology, Wayne State University School of
Medicine, Detroit, Michigan
Preoperative Care

Alton V. Hallum III, BSc, MD
Clinical Assistant Professor, University of
Arizona College of Medicine, Department of
Obstetrics and Gynecology, Tucson, Arizona
Gastrointestinal Tract Complications

Allan J. Jacobs, MD
Professor of Obstetrics and Gynecology,
Albert Einstein College of Medicine, Bronx;
and Chairman, Department of Obstetrics and
Gynecology, Beth Israel Medical Center, New
York, New York
Bleeding and Anemia in the Surgical Patient

Edward R. Kost, MD
Instructor of Obstetrics and Gynecology and
Fellow in Gynecologic Oncology, Department
of Obstetrics and Gynecology, Division of
Gynecologic Oncology, Washington University
School of Medicine, St. Louis, Missouri
Hemorrhage

Heather Lafferty, MD
Third-Year Resident, Obstetrics and
Gynecology, University of Miami School of
Medicine, and House Staff Officer, Jackson
Memorial Hospital, Miami, Florida
Postoperative Genitourinary Tract Complications

John M. Malone, Jr., MD
Associate Professor of Obstetrics and
Gynecology, Wayne State University, and
Attending Jr., Hutzel Hospital, Detroit
Medical Center, Detroit, Michigan
Wound Closure

Vinay K. Malviya, MD
Wayne State University School of Medicine,
Detroit, Michigan
Bowel Preparation

S. Gene McNeeley, Jr., MD
Associate Professor, Wayne State University
School of Medicine; Chief, Division of
Gynecology, Department of Obstetrics and
Gynecology; and Chief, Department of
Gynecology, Wayne State University, Hutzel
Hospital, Detroit Receiving Hospital,
University Health Center, Detroit, Michigan
Prophylactic Antibiotics

Adnan R. Munkarah, MD
Assistant Professor, Department of Obstetrics
and Gynecology, Division of Gynecologic
Oncology, Wayne State University School of
Medicine, Detroit, Michigan
Preoperative Care

David G. Mutch, MD
Associate Professor of Obstetrics and
Gynecology and Director, Division of
Gynecologic Oncology, Department of
Obstetrics and Gynecology, Washington
University School of Medicine, St. Louis,
Missouri
Hemorrhage

Peggy A. Norton, MD
Associate Professor, Department of Obstetrics
and Gynecology, University of Utah School of
Medicine, Salt Lake City, Utah
Urologic Complications

George J. Olt, MD
Assistant Professor, Division of Gynecologic
Oncology, Pennsylvania State University, The
Milton S. Hershey Medical Center, Hershey,
Pennsylvania
Postoperative Bowel Complications

Bruce Patsner, MD, FACOB, FACS
Professor, Clinical Obstetrics-Gynecology,
New Jersey Medical School, UMA-NJ,
Newark, New Jersey
Intraoperative Care

Manuel Penalver, MD
Professor and Chief, Division of Gynecologic
Oncology, Jackson Memorial Hospital Medical
Center, Miami, Florida
Postoperative Genitourinary Tract Complications

Edward Podczaski, MD
Associate Professor, Department of Obstetrics
and Gynecology, Pennsylvania State
University, The Milton S. Hershey Medical
Center, Hershey, Pennsylvania
The Role of the Consultant

John R. Potts III, MD
Professor of Surgery, Program Director in
Surgery, and Vice-Chairman for Educational
Programs, University of Texas–Houston
Medical School, Houston, Texas
Upper Abdominal Complications

Scott B. Ransom, DO, FACOG, FACS
Assistant Professor of Gynecology, Wayne
State University School of Medicine, and
Division Head–Medical Director of Obstetrics
and Gynecology, Henry Ford Health System,
Detroit, Michigan
Prophylactic Antibiotics

Laurie S. Swaim, MD
Assistant Professor, Department of Obstetrics
and Gynecology, University of Texas Health
Science Center–Medical School, Houston,
Texas
Postoperative Neuropathy

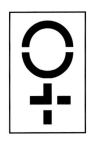

Preface
■ ■ ■ ■ ■ ■ ■

As any experienced surgeon knows, perioperative complications will invariably occur in a finite proportion of cases. Recognizing this fact, an important goal of surgical care is to minimize the occurrence of complications and both to promptly recognize and appropriately manage them when they occur. The goal of this text is to assist students of surgery—whether medical students, residents, fellows, or experienced practitioners—to avoid, recognize, and manage perioperative complications. This text is intended to be a clinically useful, well-referenced text that addresses the more common perioperative complications rather than an exhaustive reference for all potential complications following gynecologic surgery. The authors who contributed to this text were selected for their clinical and academic expertise and interest in teaching.

We would like to acknowledge the assistance of William R. Schmitt of the W.B. Saunders Company in the planning and preparation of this text.

Vicki V. Baker, MD
Gunter Deppe, MD

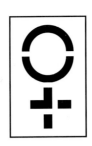

Contents
■ ■ ■ ■ ■ ■ ■

1

Gunter Deppe
Adnan R. Munkarah

CHAPTER

Preoperative Care

The goal of preoperative assessment is to reduce the morbidity of gynecologic surgery. Because most patients are no longer admitted to the hospital the night before surgery, preoperative evaluation and care has to be comprehensive in that every aspect of care is addressed, efficient for the patient and medical care providers, and cost effective. Improvement of preoperative care through better communication between patient and gynecologic surgeon will lead to greater patient satisfaction, lower costs, and better results.

The patient and gynecologic surgeon meet preoperatively to facilitate these goals. The following topics should be discussed:

History with evaluation of physical and mental health status
Nature and extent of disease
Relevant investigations
Extent of actual operation proposed and potential modification process of the operation depending on intraoperative findings
Anticipated benefits, risks, and potential complication of the surgery
Alternative forms of treatment with their risks and results
Preoperative events (anesthesia, blood transfusion, pain therapy)
Psychological preparation and alleviation of anxiety
Informed consent

MEDICAL HISTORY AND HEALTH STATUS EVALUATION

The preoperative care of the patient begins with the careful taking of a complete health history, including the present illness, past illnesses, associated diseases, bleeding tendencies, current medications, and allergies. The gynecologist should attempt to obtain complete data about previous surgical procedures, including the extent of the surgery, the reaction to anesthesia, and the final diagnosis. Any previous gynecologic surgery would be documented in detail with the pathologic diagnosis and subsequent follow-up.

A careful preoperative evaluation may uncover medical conditions that can affect the preoperative course. Studies have shown that a patient's health status before surgery predicts postoperative complications.[1, 2] Good history taking is more effective than laboratory testing alone in screening patients for risk factors and medical problems that predispose to significant

preoperative complications. For example, a patient with a history of unstable angina may have a normal preoperative electrocardiogram but is at significant risk of postoperative myocardial infarction. The gynecologist's task is to explore areas of positive history in depth and determine the need for special testing or different medical consultations. In addition to reviewing the past and present illnesses, a comprehensive review of systems may detect specific symptoms that indicate the existence of a serious undiagnosed illness. This is important especially in the population of elderly patients who have a higher prevalence of medical illnesses such as cardiovascular and respiratory diseases. Exploration of the social history will expose certain habits, such as chronic smoking and alcohol or drug abuse, that increase the patient's physiologic age and consequently influence the recovery after surgery. Thus, it is understandable why good history taking is essential for good surgical results.[3]

A thorough and complete examination is an integral part of the preoperative evaluation. It should include all major systems and search for any factor that may complicate anesthesia or the surgical procedure. The last part should focus on the genitourinary system and try to confirm or reaffirm the working diagnosis. The gynecologist should determine whether the disease process is stable or worsened since the initial evaluation; for example, a patient undergoing surgery for a persistent ovarian cyst needs to be reexamined to confirm that the cyst has not resolved, ruptured, or been confused with a full bladder.

A careful history and physical examination, the patient's age, and the clinical diagnosis will determine the need for specific preoperative testing.

RELEVANT INVESTIGATIONS AND LABORATORY TESTS

Laboratory tests should be ordered selectively to increase efficiency and decrease cost. Preoperative testing may be increased if more invasive operations are planned. A patient's chronologic age is important in determining the risk and benefit of a preoperative test.[4] Abnormal results of preoperative tests occur more frequently in older patients.

A risk-benefit analysis and literature review may help gynecologic surgeons select preoperative tests that will benefit rather than harm patients. The benefit from nonselective laboratory testing is low. For example, the routine ordering of a preoperative chest radiograph is not justified. In fact, Tape and Mushlin[5] reported that of 1000 symptomatic patients younger than 40 years of age, only 0.8% would benefit from a routine preoperative chest radiograph. Similarly, not every patient undergoing a gynecologic surgical procedure needs an electrocardiogram. Nonspecific findings in a low-risk patient may initiate an unnecessary workup that is usually expensive and without proven benefit. The physician should learn to eliminate unwarranted tests to reduce costs and avoid errors.[6] The institution of standard clinical care pathways is definitely helpful in this aspect. These pathways, which usually include standardized orders with limited testing, can be applied to all patients undergoing a specific surgical procedure. Any ordering of additional studies is considered a deviation from the pathway that should be justified based on the patient's risk factors and clinical history. This will push us to practice more economical but also better medicine. An example of standardized orders for vaginal hysterectomy standard care is shown in Table 1–1.

Preoperative testing is mostly performed in an outpatient setting. This requires an additional patient visit to the hospital or clinic for blood drawing and other required testing. The gynecologic surgeon should review the test re-

sults and determine whether the patient is ready for the surgery or needs institution of further corrective action.

The routine referral of all patients with stable medical problems, such as controlled hypertension or diabetes mellitus, to an internist for medical clearance should be avoided. As more emphasis is being placed on primary care in residency training, the young gynecologist should be able to handle these relatively simple problems. However, the gynecologic surgeon should not be reluctant to obtain the opinion of a medical consultant to help in the management of a high-risk patient. When patients are referred by a primary care physician, adequate communication between this physician and the gynecologist speeds up the process of preoperative evaluation and eliminates the duplication of tests. In cases in which abnormal findings necessitate special intraoperative care, the abnormality as well as the planned procedure should be discussed with the anesthesiologist. A preoperative assessment clinic with participation of the primary care physician, the anesthesiologist, and the surgeon might be cost effective and ensure the best possible outcome for surgical patients.[7, 8]

PSYCHOLOGICAL PREPARATION

Gynecologic surgeons must keep in mind the psychological stresses that the patient endures as a result of surgery and hospitalization. For the patient, gynecologic procedures may threaten future childbearing, menstruation, sexual function, and femininity. The patient may experience feelings of vulnerability, insecurity, manipulation, depersonalization, and helplessness, which may lead to anxiety, depression, dependency, and grief; all of this can be associated with loss of sexual function, sexual identity, body image, and self-esteem.[9, 10]

Therefore, the patient's psychological state (history or presence of a psychiatric problem) as well as her physical problems (e.g., discomfort, pain, bleeding) should be addressed during the preoperative consultations.[11] A mental status examination can be part of the preoperative assessment and can explore affective and cognitive functioning. When abnormalities are detected, supportive measures including possible psychotherapeutic consultation can minimize the risk of postoperative complications.

The gynecologic surgeon can influence the patient's emotional response to surgery by addressing anatomy, physiology, sexual response, psychological problems, and fears and expecta-

TABLE 1–1
Vaginal Hysterectomy Standard Orders

Preoperative Tests

Complete blood cell count within 14 days of surgery
Chest radiograph if clinically indicated
Electrocardiogram if older than 50 years of age or clinically indicated

Preoperative Orders

Cefazolin, 2 g, 30 minutes given intravenously piggyback before surgery

Postoperative Orders

Vital signs every 4 hours for 24 hours
Activity: ambulate with assistance on day of surgery
Diet: regular as tolerated
Discontinue Foley catheter 6 hours after surgery
Straight catheterization if unable to void 6 hours after Foley catheter removed
IV: 5% dextrose and 0.45% NaCl with 20 mEq KCl at 100 mL/h
Discontinue IV when tolerating regular diet
Pain medication:
  1. Tylenol 3: 1–2 tablets orally every 4 hours as needed for pain
  2. Demerol: 50–75 mg intramuscularly every 4 hours as needed for severe pain
Routine medications
Anticipate discharge on postoperative day 1

tions in a realistic and positive way. Reassurance is an important part of the preoperative preparation. Alleviation of anxiety by preoperative counseling has been reported by Wilson-Barnett.[12] Rapport and trust should be built between a patient and her gynecologist. The patient needs to be assured of the gynecologic surgeon's technical competence and professional efficiency as well as have his or her complete attention. The patient's confidence is based on genuine understanding and trust.[13] The nursing staff should be involved in reassuring the patient and in trying to relieve her fears and anxiety.

A patient's family is an important part of her support system and needs to be informed, reassured, and supported by the surgeon. The better prepared the patient is psychologically, the smoother will be her postoperative course. The hospital stay will be shorter and the recovery faster, thus benefitting the patient, gynecologist, and hospital in the present managed-care setting.[14, 15]

OPERATIVE INDICATIONS, RATIONALE, AND GOALS

Before taking a patient to the operating room, the gynecologic surgeon must assess the indication, nature, and goals of the planned operation. Thorough knowledge of the basic pathologic lesions and proper preoperative diagnostic workup, laboratory and imaging studies, biopsy results, and slide reviews are essential.

Technical skills of the surgeon are unimportant or harmful if the operation is unindicated, inadequate, or excessive. Occasionally a major operation is performed when a minor one would have been the better choice. Surgical procedures are only justified to correct deformities, to relieve suffering, or to save lives of patients.[16]

The gynecologic surgeon must clearly identify the technical goals (type of operation) and therapeutic goals (benefits for patient) of the planned surgery. The potential advantages of the operation should justify the possible negative consequences. Nature and extent of the disease process and goals of the surgery should be discussed with the patient in detail. Results of appropriate imaging studies and biopsies (Papanicolaou smear, endometrial biopsy) should be reviewed preoperatively and detailed in the medical record.

A competent gynecologic surgeon should be able to select or tailor the specific operation for the individual patient. Gynecologic operations are performed for sterilization, diagnosis (e.g., dilation and curettage), symptoms (e.g., pelvic pain), physical abnormalities (e.g., pelvic mass), and pathophysiologic findings (e.g., endometriosis).

The extent of the operation and its outcome depend on surgical and pathologic findings unknown before surgery. The planned procedure should be discussed with the patient in detail, including the type of incision, the different involved organs, and the expected length of the operation.

The possible complications and risks should be explained in simple, understandable nonmedical language but with compassion and concern so as not to compound the patient's anxiety. In cases in which a malignancy is suspected, the patient should be informed about this possibility as well as the possible need for postoperative adjunctive therapy (e.g., radiation therapy, chemotherapy). The duration of disability and length of recovery should be addressed so that the patient would know what to expect.

Patients need to understand that the type of surgery, the skill of the surgeon and anesthesiologist, the severity of the condition for which the surgery is performed, as well as their own physical health status all contribute to the outcome of surgery.

INFORMED CONSENT

The gynecologic surgeon is required to obtain consent for surgical treatment of every competent patient who is 18 years of age or older. A patient must give permission for any "touching" of her person by another, without which such contact is an "assault" on the person. The gynecologic surgeon must keep in mind that to obtain fully informed consent the patient should be informed about the following:

Diagnosis
Nature and purpose of the proposed operation
Expectations of the recommended procedure and the likelihood of success
Risks and potential complications associated with the surgical procedure
All feasible alternative treatments or procedures, including the option of taking no action, as well as the likelihood of success and the risks associated with each
Relative probability of success for the procedure in understandable terms

Obtaining informed consent should be

viewed as a process, not signing of a consent sheet. Discussion of the risks, benefits, and alternatives to a procedure must take place before surgery and before the patient signs a consent form.[17] Ideally, discussion and obtaining consent for surgery should take place in the gynecologist's office. The patient is given reasonable time to contemplate all the information given and is encouraged to ask questions. A key element in obtaining a valid consent is that the patient fully understands the information provided. The responsibility to obtain informed consent from the patient clearly remains with the gynecologist, and this responsibility cannot be delegated. The presence of a nurse in the room at the time of the discussion with the patient offers additional confirmation. The patient may be reluctant to ask the gynecologist questions about the operation but usually will readily discuss her lack of understanding with the nurse, who in turn can convey to the gynecologist the patient's concerns. It may be relevant to involve the patient's family in counseling.

Special Informed Consent Rules

Failure to obtain a patient's informed consent for a surgical procedure is excused in a medical emergency when the patient is unable to give consent and no one who is authorized to consent on behalf of the patient is readily available. In such an event the gynecologic surgeon should document that the patient is unconscious or incapacitated and suffering from a life-threatening or serious health-threatening situation requiring immediate surgical intervention and that efforts were made to locate and obtain the consent from the patient's next of kin.

Special informed consent rules apply to minors (age defined by the particular jurisdiction where they reside). Basically, minors are unable to consent to gynecologic surgery and the gynecologist must obtain consent from the minor's parent or legal guardian when performing all but emergency surgery. As with all patients, a minor should be fully informed before surgery is done.

Some patients do not want to be informed about the risks or complications of a gynecologic surgical procedure or about its prognosis. It is mandatory for the gynecologist to obtain the patient's signature on a written statement of that fact.

The informed consent loses its power when the surgical procedure far exceeds what has been discussed with the patient. When a patient does not receive enough material information to make an informed decision and an injury occurs, the patient could successfully sue the gynecologist; the presence of a signed consent form is not protective in this situation. The jury decides whether the patient or a reasonably prudent person in the patient's position would have refused surgery if sufficiently informed. Asking the patient to state in her own words the procedure, its goals, and the expected results may help the surgeon detect and clarify any misconceptions.

A patient who is informed of the risks and benefits of a surgical procedure may refuse to undergo that particular treatment. In these circumstances, the gynecologic surgeon should document the informed refusal in the patient's medical record.[18]

The documented counseling session can at times replace a signed consent form. The documentation need not be in great detail but should be a convincing statement that the surgery, with its risks and benefits, has been discussed with the patient.

Informed Consent Forms

A consent form can be very detailed, mentioning all pertinent information regarding risks, benefits, and reasonable alternatives relating to the particular gynecologic operation. The more elective the procedure and the greater the choices of alternative treatments, the more detailed the information should be.

Consent forms for teaching hospitals should mention that residents may either perform the gynecologic procedure or assist in the surgery. Additionally, the gynecologist should explain this to the patient. Residents should explain their role to the patient, stating the care they provide is constantly supervised by the attending physician. If the patient objects, it is necessary to document this objection in the record and prevent violation of the objection.

In preparing a consent form, these general principles should be kept in mind[17, 19, 20]:

1. All commonly occurring risks of the gynecologic procedure should be mentioned, including those with anesthesia (death, brain damage, and paralysis).

2. Medical terms should be explained in a language a lay person can understand.

3. The words "simple," "minor," or "uncomplicated" should be avoided to describe gynecologic surgery.

4. Every consent form should state that no

result has been guaranteed. The use of statistics should be avoided.

5. The patient should be asked to acknowledge in writing that the procedure has been fully explained to her, that she understands the information disclosed, that she had an opportunity to ask questions, and that all questions have been answered to her satisfaction.

6. Ideally, the signatures of both the patient and gynecologic surgeon and the time and date on which the discussion took place should be on the consent form.

7. Each consent form should conclude with the following statement:

I am aware that during my gynecologic operation, other risks or complications not discussed may occur. I also understand that during the proposed operation unforeseen conditions may necessitate additional procedures and I give my permission for their performance. I further realize that no guarantees or promises have been made to me concerning the results of the gynecologic operation.

REFERENCES

1. Duncan PG, Cohen MM, Tweed WA, et al. The Canadian four-centre study of anaesthetic outcomes: III. Are anaesthetic complications predictable in day surgical practice? Can J Anaesth 1992;39:440–448.
2. Pedersen T, Eliasen K, Henriksen E. A prospective study of mortality associated with anesthesia and surgery: risk indicators of mortality in hospital. Acta Anaesth Scand 1990;34:176–182.
3. Charlson ME, MacKenzie CR, Gold JP. Preoperative autonomic function abnormalities in patients with diabetes mellitus and patients with hypertension. J Am Coll Surg 1994;179:1–10.
4. Velanovich V. Preoperative laboratory screening based on age, gender, and concomitant medical diseases. Surgery 1994;115:56–61.
5. Tape TG, Mushlin AI. How useful are routine chest x-rays of preoperative patients at risk for postoperative chest disease? J Gen Intern Med 1988;3:15–20.
6. Macario A, Roizen MF, Thisted RA, et al. Reassessment of preoperative laboratory testing has changed the test-ordering patterns of physicians. Surg Gynecol Obstet 1992;175:539–547.
7. Gibby CL, Gravenstein JS, Layon AJ, Jackson KI. How often does the preoperative interview change anesthetic management? Anesthesiology 1992;77:A1134.
8. MacPherson DS. Preoperative laboratory testing: should any tests be "routine" before surgery? Med Clin North Am 1993;77:289–308.
9. Bauchmann GA. Psychosexual aspects of hysterectomy. Womens Health Issues 1990;1:41–49.
10. American College of Obstetricians and Gynecologists. Sexual Dysfunction: Technical bulletin No. 211. Washington, DC, American College of Obstetricians and Gynecologists, September 1995.
11. Wolfer JA, Davis CE. Assessment of surgical patients' preoperative emotional condition and postoperative welfare. Nurs Res 1970;19:402–414.
12. Wilson-Barnett J. Interventions to alleviate patients' stress: a review. J Psychosom Res 1984;28:63–72.
13. Buckner F. The physician–patient relationship. J Med Pract Manage 1994;10:59–62.
14. Egbert LD, Baht GE, Welch CE, Bartlett MK. Reduction of postoperative pain by encouragement and instruction of patients: a study of doctor–patient rapport. N Engl J Med 1964;270:825–827.
15. Munday IT, Desai PM, Marshall CA, et al. The effectiveness of preoperative advice to stop smoking: a prospective controlled trial. Anaesthesia 1993;48:816–818.
16. TeLinde RW, Mattingly RF. Operative Gynecology, 4th ed. Philadelphia, JB Lippincott, 1970.
17. American College of Obstetricians and Gynecologists. Ethical Dimensions of Informed Consent: ACOG Committee Opinion 108. Washington, DC, American College of Obstetricians and Gynecologists, May 1992.
18. American College of Obstetricians and Gynecologists. Department of Professional Liability: Informed Consent. Technical bulletin No. 166. Washington, DC, American College of Obstetricians and Gynecologists, December 1995.
19. Nora PF. Professional Liability Risk Management: A Manual for Surgeons. Developed by the Professional Liability Committee. Chicago, American College of Surgeons, 1991, pp 105–128.
20. American College of Obstetricians and Gynecologists. Department of Professional Liability: Informed Consent: The Assistant. Washington, DC, American College of Obstetricians and Gynecologists, 1988.

2

CHAPTER

S. Gene McNeeley, Jr.
Scott B. Ransom

Prophylactic Antibiotics

Hysterectomy and abortion are the most frequently performed elective surgical procedures in women of reproductive age. Since legalization of abortion, suction curettage is recognized as a very safe method of pregnancy termination and serious complications are rare. Hysterectomy is the treatment of choice for most gynecologic malignancies; and because of the low rate of morbidity and mortality, hysterectomy is important for the treatment of benign conditions of the female pelvis. Improved surgical techniques (gentle handling of tissues, minimizing of pedicle size, and obtaining excellent hemostasis) and improved surgical instruments and suture materials decrease post-hysterectomy morbidity. This is due to decreased bacterial contamination, to minimizing the presence of foreign bodies, and to minimizing the amount of devascularized or necrotic tissue.

As early as 1946, antibiotics were administered in hopes of further preventing postoperative infection. Although early retrospective reports suggested that even single-dose preoperative prophylactic antibiotics significantly reduced hysterectomy-associated infection, the benefit of prophylactic antibiotics was not clearly demonstrated until the 1980s for vaginal hysterectomy and until the 1990s for abdominal hysterectomy. In this chapter the microbiology, pathogenesis, and prevention of common soft tissue infections of the pelvis (post-hysterectomy pelvic cellulitis and post-abortion endometritis) and infections of the abdominal incision are reviewed.

BACTERIAL FLORA OF THE VAGINA AND BACTERIAL CONTAMINATION OF SOFT TISSUES

The bacteria responsible for post-hysterectomy soft tissue infections arise from what is considered the normal flora of the vagina and cervix. In the case of abdominal hysterectomy, the skin is also a common source of bacterial contamination. Throughout the 1970s and 1980s, qualitative and quantitative studies defined the cervical and vaginal flora and, more importantly, those environmental and host influences that modified the flora. By using contemporary techniques, five to seven species of bacteria are commonly recovered from the vagina of healthy women, with more anaerobes being recovered than aerobes.[1, 2] Likewise, the mean bacterial count for anaerobes is approximately

10^9 colony-forming units per gram of vaginal material compared with 10^8 colony-forming units per gram of vaginal material for the aerobic isolates. The most common isolates are *Lactobacillus* species and *Corynebacterium* species, both recognized as nonpathogenic and important for maintaining a normal flora in healthy women. Potential aerobic pathogens frequently recovered from the vagina include *Staphylococcus aureus; Staphylococcus epidermidis; Escherichia coli*; groups A, B, and C *Streptococcus*, and *Enterococcus faecalis*. Commonly recovered anaerobes include *Peptostreptococcus* species, *Bacteroides fragilis, Prevotella* species, and *Clostridum* species. A more thorough list of potential pathogens is seen in Table 2–1. Infections are usually mixed polymicrobial infections involving two or more aerobic and anaerobic pathogens. Postabortion infections are frequently associated with *Neisseria gonorrhoeae* and *C. trachomatis*.

Numerous environmental influences on the cervical and vaginal flora have been reported. Hormonal influences are significant. When compared to cultures in woman of reproductive age, cervical and vaginal cultures of prepubertal girls tend to yield a higher prevalence of anaerobic gram-negative rods (i.e., *Bacteroides fragilis*) and *Clostridium* species. The prevalence of diphtheroids and *Staphylococcus epidermidis* is comparable to that in menstruating women.[3, 4] These findings are similar to those seen in postmenopausal women not on hormone replacement. In addition, the vagina of postmenopausal women is less frequently colonized with *Lactobacillus* species and more fre-

TABLE 2–1
Pathogens Recovered From Gynecologic Infections

Aerobic Bacteria	Anaerobic Bacteria
Gram-positive cocci	Gram-positive cocci
Enterococcus faecalis	*Peptostreptococcus* species
Streptococcus agalactiae	*Peptostreptococcus tetradius*
Streptococcus species	Gram-positive bacilli
Staphylococcus aureus	*Clostridium* species
Staphylococcus epidermidis	*Bifidobacterium* species
Gram-negative bacilli	Gram-negative cocci
Escherichia coli	*Veillonella parvula*
Enterobacter species	Gram-negative bacilli
Klebsiella species	*Bacteroides* species
Proteus species	*Bacteroides fragilis*
Acinetobacter species	*Prevotella bivia*
Citrobacter species	*Prevotella melaninogenica*
Pseudomonas species	*Fusobacterium* species
Haemophilus influenzae	
Gram-positive bacilli	
Diphtheroids	

quently colonized with facultative gram-negative rods. Fewer species are recovered from postmenopausal women not taking hormone replacement when compared with women on hormone replacement and menstruating women.[5-7] The microflora of women on hormone replacement is strikingly similar to that of women of reproductive age.

Studies of the vagina of pregnant women failed to reveal clinically significant changes of the cervical and vaginal flora during pregnancy. However, during the early postpartum period there is a significant reduction in *Lactobacillus* species and significant increases in gram-negative anaerobes, gram-positive anaerobes, and facultative gram-negative rods. Likely causes for the changes include trauma, lochia, and rectal contamination during delivery. These changes are transient, and the vaginal flora returns to normal.[8]

Both vaginal and abdominal hysterectomy result in significant changes in the vaginal flora. When compared with preoperative cultures, post-hysterectomy cultures reveal a 50% reduction of *Lactobacillus* species, a twofold to threefold increase in *Escherichia coli* and other facultative gram-negative rods, and a twofold to fourfold increase in the prevalence of *Bacteroides fragilis*. This is of practical clinical importance because the shift toward a more virulent flora is compounded by disruption of the mucosal barrier, allowing immediate access to pelvic soft tissues.[9, 10] Before opening the vagina during abdominal hysterectomy, the peritoneal fluid contains 10^4 colony-forming units of skin flora per milliliter of fluid. After opening the vaginal vault, colony counts exceed 10^5 colony-forming units per milliliter. The magnitude of contamination is dependent on the duration of surgery, the use of a vaginal preparation, and the administration of prophylactic antibiotics.[11] In a prospective study, the incidence of infectious morbidity directly correlated with the peritoneal fluid bacterial count. Forty-two percent of women with total bacterial counts exceeding 10^4 colony-forming units per milliliter experienced postoperative infectious morbidity. The relative risk of developing postoperative morbidity in women who did not receive prophylaxis was 7.69 when compared with women who received prophylactic antibiotics. Total bacterial counts and counts of the microaerophilic species were significantly associated with increasing risk of infection.[12]

There is no consensus on the effect of short-term antibiotic therapy or prophylaxis on the cervical and vaginal flora. Grossman and Adams did not detect significant differences between pretreatment and post-treatment cultures in women receiving penicillin and cefazolin.[13] Ohm and Galask reported an increased prevalence of cephalosporin-resistant species (*Pseudomonas aeruginosa, Enterobacter* species, and *Streptococcus faecalis*) in women who received cephalosporins.[9]

Modest information is available regarding the effect of immune suppression and genital cancer on the vaginal flora. As a general statement, immune suppression is not associated with significant changes in the vaginal flora.[14] On the other hand, there are significant changes in women with genital cancer. There appears to be a significant reduction in the prevalence of colonization with *Staphylococcus epidermidis* and *Lactobacillus* species and increased colonization with virulent pathogens, including *E. coli, B. fragilis, Clostridium perfringens*, and *Fusobacterium nucleatum*.[15, 16]

Widely recognized risk factors for postoperative infections are noted in Table 2–2.

ANTIBIOTIC PROPHYLAXIS IN HYSTERECTOMY

Vaginal Hysterectomy

The use of prophylactic antibiotics was first reported in vaginal hysterectomy by Allen in 1949. He used penicillin vaginal suppositories to reduce febrile morbidity from 17% in a control group to 8% in the treatment group.[17] The early studies evaluating the use of prophylactic antibiotics in vaginal hysterectomy concluded that multiple-day regimens dramatically reduced the infectious morbidity. Goosenberg compared a 5-day trial of either chloramphenicol or penicillin with streptomycin. The infectious morbidity was 77.5% in the control group, 52.5% in the chloramphenicol group,

TABLE 2–2
Risk Factors for Postoperative Infections

Chronic obstructive pulmonary disease
Acute viral upper respiratory tract infection
Bowel obstruction
Urinary tract obstruction
Diabetes mellitus
Chronic renal failure
Malnutrition
Asplenia
Sickle cell disease
General anesthesia
Immunosuppressants (i.e., cyclosporine)
Radiation therapy

and 7.5% in the penicillin and streptomycin group.[18] Similarly, Allen and colleagues showed that a 3-day regimen of cephalothin reduced the morbidity from 50% in the control group to 4% in the study group.[19] A number of studies conducted in the early 1970s proved that long-term antibiotic therapy significantly reduced the febrile morbidity, length of hospital stay, and serious pelvic infections associated with vaginal hysterectomy.[9, 20–26] In addition, the overall success of long-term antibiotics in preventing morbidity generally replaced concerns of resistant organisms, antibiotic toxicity, and costs until reports revealed an increased colonization of the treated patients by aerobic and anaerobic organisms.[27, 28] Ledger and co-workers and Glover and associates compared the efficacy of long- and short-term regimens of antibiotic prophylaxis and found similar effectiveness in the reduction of morbidity associated with vaginal hysterectomy.[29–31]

Burke and colleagues suggested that bacterial contamination occurs at the time of tissue damage and that "supplements to host resistance serve no purpose if they are delivered for periods longer than four hours after the end of the period of active bacterial contamination of tissue or bloodstream."[32, 33] Subsequently, multiple studies have indicated no differences in the efficacy of single-dose versus short-term antibiotic prophylaxis in vaginal hysterectomy.[34–36] That is, the single-dose prophylaxis appears to be as effective in reducing febrile morbidity, hospital stay, and serious pelvic infections when compared with the prolonged use of antibiotics for prophylaxis.[37–39]

The antibiotic of choice for prophylaxis in vaginal hysterectomy has not been established. In vaginal hysterectomy, the choice of antibiotic should be concerned with the wound or interstitial fluid concentrations of antibiotic. Specifically, the antibiotic of choice should be present at the surgical site for prevention of morbidity.[40] Similarly, the antibiotic chosen should be effective against commonly found infectious organisms at the surgical site. The vaginal infections tend to be polymicrobial and include a wide variety of aerobic and anaerobic pathogens. Although the choice of antibiotic should be adequate against the common organisms invading the vagina, many studied antibiotics have limited in vitro effectiveness on the common organisms. Ampicillin is not effective against most *Pseudomonas*, *Klebsiella*, *Enterobacter*, and *Proteus* species. Cephalosporins have limited activity against many anaerobic species. Metronidazole is only effective in vitro against anaerobic species. Although these antibiotics have proven poor effectiveness in vitro against many common organisms that harbor in the vagina, it appears that aerobic and anaerobic organisms are dependent on the presence of each other; the reduction of one type of bacteria may preclude infection by others. Thus, the choice of a prophylactic antibiotic is relatively simple because any antibiotic that is effective against aerobic or anaerobic flora would probably be effective in reducing postoperative infections.[41]

The recommended prophylactic antibiotic regimen in vaginal hysterectomy is 1 or 2 g of cefazolin administered intravenously in the operating room after intravenous line placement and before anesthesia. If a woman is allergic to cephalosporins, 100 mg of doxycycline is given orally at bedtime with another, identical oral dose 3 to 4 hours before the scheduled procedure. A 200-mg dose of doxycycline given intravenously preoperatively was not found to be effective.[42] The third drug of choice would include 900 mg of clindamycin intravenously preoperatively.[43] The cost-effectiveness of prophylactic antibiotics has been shown to be significant.[44] The final choice of the antibiotic should consider the relative cost of the antibiotic with its marginal effectiveness. That is, given two identically equivalent antibiotics for effective prophylactic use, the less expensive antibiotic should be the drug of choice. Personnel at the hospital where the surgical procedure occurs should provide information regarding the relative cost of commonly used antibiotics at that institution for appropriate selection.

Abdominal Hysterectomy

The use of prophylactic antibiotics in abdominal hysterectomy has been controversial owing to a variety of outcomes in randomized trials. When compared with vaginal hysterectomy, the benefits of prophylactic antibiotics remain relatively controversial. The potential for bacterial contamination for abdominal hysterectomy is different from that for vaginal hysterectomy. The apparent effectiveness of prophylactic antibiotics in abdominal hysterectomy seems to be associated with the overall infection rate in the patient population being investigated.[45] A population with a high risk for postoperative infection tends to show a significant reduction of infectious morbidity with antibiotics; conversely, a population with a low incidence of infection would require a large number of patients to demonstrate a significant reduction.[46–50] That is, when considering the option of the use of antibiotics for abdominal hysterectomy, the population risk should be considered when evaluating the option.

Mittendorf and coworkers[51] performed a meta-analysis of the use of prophylactic antibiotics for abdominal hysterectomy and found significant benefit. Overall, 21.1% (373 of 1768) of the patients evaluated who did not receive antibiotic prophylaxis had serious infections, whereas 9.0% (166 of 1836) of patients who received an antibiotic had a serious infection. The differences in the prevalence of infection between women who received prophylaxis and women who did not receive prophylaxis were found to be statistically significant. Therefore, the use of prophylactic antibiotics should be strongly considered, particularly for high-risk populations.

The specific choice of antibiotic for prophylaxis is controversial. Mittendorf and coworkers evaluated the use of cefazolin, metronidazole, and tinidazole and found 11.4% (70 of 615), 6.3% (17 of 269), and 5.0% (5 of 101) infectious morbidity rates, respectively.[51] Chemoprophylaxis with cephalosporins was found to be effective in preventing post-hysterectomy infectious complications. A single preoperative injection of a first- (cefazolin) or second-generation (cefoxitin) cephalosporin, when administrated intravenously, was shown to be effective at reducing postoperative febrile and serious infectious morbidity.[52] Similarly, Tanos and associates concluded that single-dose intravenous cefonicid, when given preoperatively, is as safe and effective as a multiple-dose regimen of cefazolin in patients undergoing elective abdominal hysterectomy.[53]

In conclusion, the antibiotic of choice for abdominal hysterectomy is controversial. The use of prophylaxis is particularly helpful for the high-risk population; however, the relatively low risks associated with the use of antibiotics correlated with the potential infectious morbidity prevention should indicate a strong argument for the usefulness of prophylaxis even in the low-risk population. The current recommendation for the use of prophylactic antibiotics in abdominal hysterectomy parallels that for vaginal hysterectomy.

Radical Abdominal Hysterectomy

Patients undergoing radical pelvic surgery, including radical hysterectomy, are at significant risk for infectious morbidity. Poor nutritional status, immune suppression, prolonged opera-

tive time, and the potential for bacterial contamination from multiple sites (skin, vagina, and bowel) are important reasons for the increased postoperative morbidity. Infections occur in 43% to 81% of women undergoing surgery for gynecologic cancer.[54, 55] In a placebo-controlled study, Hemsell and associates[37] reported the incidence of infection in the placebo group to be 27% and the incidence of infection was significantly reduced with single-dose prophylaxis. Additional retrospective and prospective studies indicate that antibiotic prophylaxis significantly reduces the incidence of incisional and pelvic soft tissue infections.[56–58] We recommend a single intravenous dose of cefazolin administered before the incision is made.

ANTIBIOTIC PROPHYLAXIS FOR ABORTION

Infection is the most common serious complication of abortion, occurring in 1% to 30% of women undergoing induced abortion. Risk factors for developing endometritis include nulliparity, advanced gestation, a history of pelvic inflammatory disease, bacterial vaginosis, and genital colonization with *N. gonorrhoeae, C. trachomatis, Mycoplasma hominis,* and group B *Streptococcus.* In a placebo-controlled study, Sonne-Holm noted that women with a history of pelvic inflammatory disease were more likely to develop postabortion endometritis if antibiotic prophylaxis was not administered.[56] Gonococcal and chlamydial infections of the cervix are significant risk factors for postabortion endometritis. Genital colonization occurs more frequently with *C. trachomatis* and is likely the most important risk factor for developing endometritis, which occurs in up to 20% of *Chlamydium*-infected women.[57–59] In a study of *Chlamydium*-negative women, Hamark[60] found that bacterial vaginosis was the most important risk factor for developing postabortion endometritis. Preabortion treatment with metronidazole significantly reduced the risk of postabortion infection.[61]

As reviewed by Grimes and coworkers,[62] early data did not convincingly demonstrate that prophylactic antibiotics significantly prevented postabortion infections. Subsequently, single-dose doxycycline and multiple-dose doxycycline and metronidazole were shown to significantly reduce the incidence of infection after first-trimester abortion.[63–65] We recommend preoperative testing and treatment for *N. gonorrhoeae* and *C. trachomatis* in women at risk for sexually transmitted diseases and preoperative treatment of women with bacterial vaginosis. Women undergoing abortion should receive perioperative prophylaxis with doxycycline, 200 mg before surgery and 100 mg 12 hours later.

REFERENCES

1. Larsen B, Galask RP. Vaginal microbial flora: practical and theoretic relevance. Obstet Gynecol 1980;55:100S–113S.
2. Bartlet JG, Onderdonk AB, Drude E, et al. Quantitative bacteriology of the vaginal flora. J Infect Dis 1977;136:271.
3. Hammerschlag MR, Alpert S, Onderdonk AB, et al. Anaerobic microflora of the vagina in children. Am J Obstet Gynecol 1978;126:853.
4. Hammerschlag MR, Alpert S, Rosner I, et al. Microbiology of the vagina in children: normal and potentially pathogenic organisms. Pediatrics 1978;62:57.
5. Osborne NG, Wright RC, Grulin L. Genital microbiology: a comparative study of premenopausal women with postmenopausal women. Am J Obstet Gynecol 1979;1:597.
6. Larsen B, Gopelrud CP, Petzold CR, et al. Effect of estrogen treatment on the genital flora of postmenopausal women. Obstet Gynecol 1982;60:20.
7. Molander U, Milson I, Mellstrom D, et al. Effect of oral estrogen on vaginal flora and cytology and urogenital symptoms in the post-menopause. Maturitas 1990;12:113.
8. Gopelrud CP, Ohm MJ, Galask RP. Aerobic and anaerobic flora of the cervix during pregnancy and the puerperium. Am J Obstet Gynecol 1978;126:858.
9. Ohm MJ, Galask RP. The effects of antibiotic prophylaxis on patients undergoing vaginal operations: II. Alterations of the microbial flora. Am J Obstet Gynecol 1975;123:597.
10. Ohm MJ, Galask RP. The effect of antibiotic prophylaxis on patients undergoing total abdominal hysterectomy: II. Alterations of microbial flora. Am J Obstet Gynecol 1976;125:448.
11. Helm CW, McDonald C, Houang ET. Bacterial contamination during abdominal hysterectomy. J Obstet Gynecol 1986;6:S64.
12. Houang ET, Ahmet Z. Intraoperative wound contamination during abdominal hysterectomy. J Hosp Infect 1991;19:181.
13. Grossman JH III, Adams RL. Vaginal flora of women undergoing hysterectomy with antibiotic prophylaxis. Obstet Gynecol 1979;53:23.
14. Ohm MJ, Scott JR, Galask RP. Cervical-vaginal flora of immunosuppressed renal transplant patients. Am J Obstet Gynecol 1978;130:49.
15. Blythe JG. Cervical bacterial flora of patients with gynecologic malignancies. Am J Obstet Gynecol 1978;131:438.
16. Mead PB. Cervical-vaginal flora of women with invasive cervical cancer. Obstet Gynecol 1978;52:601.
17. Houang ET. Antibiotic prophylaxis in hysterectomy and induced abortion: a review of the evidence. Drugs 1991;41:19.
18. Goosenberg J. Prophylactic antibiotics in vaginal hysterectomy. Am J Obstet Gynecol 1969;105:503.
19. Allen J, Rampone JF, Wheeless C. Use of a prophylactic antibiotic in elective major gynecologic operations. Obstet Gynecol 1972;39:218.
20. Bolling DR, Plunkett GD. Prophylactic antibiotics for vaginal hysterectomies. Obstet Gynecol 1973;41:689.
21. Harralson JD, Van Nagell JR, Roddick JW, Sprague AD. The effect of prophylactic antibiotics on pelvic infection following vaginal hysterectomy. Am J Obstet Gynecol 1974;120:1046.
22. Ledger WJ, Sweet RL, Headington JT. Prophylactic cephaloridine in the prevention of postoperative pelvic infections in premenopausal women undergoing vaginal hysterectomy. Am J Obstet Gynecol 1973;115:766.
23. Thomsen RJ. Prophylactic antibiotics for vaginal surgery: a historical addendum. Am J Obstet Gynecol 1973;117:1034.
24. Forney JP, Morrow CP, Townsend DC, Disaia PJ. Impact of cephalosporin prophylaxis on conization—vaginal hysterectomy morbidity. Am J Obstet Gynecol 1976;125:100.
25. Boyd ME, Garceau R. The value of prophylactic antibiotics for vaginal hysterectomies. Am J Obstet Gynecol 1976;125:581.
26. Kamal A, Spence MR, King TM. Prophylactic antibiotics in vaginal hysterectomy: a review. Obstet Gynecol Survey 1982;37:207.
27. Breeden JT, May JE. Low dose prophylactic antibiotics in vaginal hysterectomy. Obstet Gynecol 1974;43:379.
28. Grossman JH III, Adams RL. Vaginal flora in women undergoing hysterectomy with antibiotic prophylaxis. Obstet Gynecol 1979;53:23.
29. Ledger WJ, Gee C, Lewis WP. Guidelines for antibiotic prophylaxis in gynecology. Am J Obstet Gynecol 1975;121:1038.
30. Ledger WJ, Boice C, Yonekura L, Dizerega G. Vaginal hysterectomy. South Med J 1977;70:40.
31. Glover MW, Nagell JR Jr. The effect of prophylactic ampicillin on pelvic infection following vaginal hysterectomy. Am J Obstet Gynecol 1976;126:385.
32. Burke JF. Preventing bacterial infection by coordinating antibiotic and host activity: a time-dependent relationship. South Med J 1977;70:24.
33. Burke JF. The effective period of preventive antibiotic action in experimental incisions and dermal lesions. Surgery 1961;50:161.
34. Lett WJ, Ansbacher R, Davison BL, Otterson WN. Prophylactic antibiotics for women undergoing vaginal hysterectomy. J Reprod Med 1977;19:51.
35. Mendelson J, Portnoy J, De Saint Victor JR, Gelfand MM. Effect of single and multidose cephradine prophylaxis on infectious morbidity of vaginal hysterectomy. Obstet Gynecol 1979;53:31.
36. Hamod KA, Spence MR, Rosenshein NB, Dillon MB. Single and multidose prophylaxis in vaginal hysterectomy: a comparison of sodium cephalothin and metronidazole. Am J Obstet Gynecol 1980;136:976.
37. Hemsell DL, Heard ML, Nobles BJ, Hemsell PG. Single-dose cefoxitin prophylaxis for premenopausal women undergoing vaginal hysterectomy. Obstet Gynecol 1984;63:285.
38. Berkeley AS, Freedman KS, Ledger WJ. Comparison of cefotetan and cefoxitin prophylaxis for abdominal and vaginal hysterectomy. Am J Obstet Gynecol 1988;158:706.
39. Regallo M, Scalambrino S, Negri I, et al. Cefotetan versus piperacillin in the prophylaxis of abdominal and vaginal hysterectomy: a prospective randomized study. Drugs Exp Clin Res 1989;15:315.
40. Neu HC. Clinical pharmacokinetics in preventive antimicrobial therapy. South Med J 1977;70:14.
41. Hamod KA, Spence MR, King TM. Prophylactic antibiotics in vaginal hysterectomy: a review. Obstet Gynecol Survey 1982;37:207.
42. Hemsell DL, Hemsell PG, Nobles BJ. Doxycycline and

cefamandole prophylaxis for premenopausal women undergoing vaginal hysterectomy. Surg Gynecol Obstet 1985;161:462.

43. Hemsell DL. Prophylactic antibiotics in gynecology and obstetric surgery. Rev Infect Dis 1991;13(suppl 10):S821.

44. Shapiro M, Schoenbaum SC, Tager IB, et al. Benefit-cost analysis of antimicrobial prophylaxis in abdominal and vaginal hysterectomy. JAMA 1983;249:1290.

45. Duff P. Antibiotic prophylaxis for abdominal hysterectomy. Obstet Gynecol 1982;60:25.

46. Polk BF, Tager I, Shapiro M, et al. Randomized clinical trial of perioperative cefazolin in preventing infection after hysterectomy. Lancet 1980;1:327.

47. Grossman J III. Prophylactic antibiotics in gynecologic surgery. Obstet Gynecol 1979;53:537.

48. Tanos V, Rojansky N, Anteby SO. Comparison of cefonicid and cefazolin prophylaxis in abdominal hysterectomy. Gynecol Obstet Invest 1994;37:115.

49. Senior CC, Steigrad SJ. Are preoperative antibiotics helpful in abdominal hysterectomy? Am J Obstet Gynecol 1992;154:1004.

50. Mamsen A, Hansen V, Moller BR. A prospective randomized double blind trial of ceftriaxone versus no treatment for abdominal hysterectomy. Eur J Obstet Gynecol Reprod Biol 1992;47:235.

51. Mittendorf R, Aronson MP, Berry RE, et al. Avoiding serious infections associated with abdominal hysterectomy: a meta-analysis of antibiotic prophylaxis. Am J Obstet Gynecol 1993;169:1119.

52. Tanos V, Rojansky N. Prophylactic antibiotics in abdominal hysterectomy. J Am Coll Surg 1994;179:593.

53. Tanos V, Rojansky N, Anteby SO. Comparison of cefonicid and cefazolin prophylaxis in abdominal hysterectomy. Gynecol Obstet Invest 1994;37:115.

54. Ledger WJ, Reite A, Headington JT. Infection on an inpatient gynecology service. Am J Obstet Gynecol 1972;113:662.

55. McNeeley SG, Hopkins MP, Ehlerova B, et al. Infection on a gynecologic oncology service. Gynecol Oncol 1990;37:183.

56. Sonne-Holm S, Heisterberg L, Hebjorn S, et al. Prophylactic antibiotics in first trimester abortions: a controlled clinical trial. Am J Obstet Gynecol 1981;139:693.

57. Burkman R, Atienza MF, King TM. Culture and treatment results in endometritis following elective abortion. Am J Obstet Gynecol 1977;128:556.

58. Qvistgad E, Skaug K, Jerve E, et al. Pelvic inflammatory disease associated with *Chlamydia trachomatis* infection after therapeutic abortion. Br J Vener Dis 1983;59:189.

59. Houang ET. Antibiotic prophylaxis in hysterectomy and induced abortion. Drugs 1991;41:19.

60. Hamark B. Postabortal endometritis in chlamydia-negative women: association with preoperative signs of infection. Gynecol Obstet Invest 1991;31:102.

61. Larson PG, Platz-Christensen JJ, Thejls H, et al. Incidence of pelvic inflammatory disease after first-trimester legal abortion in women with bacterial vaginosis after treatment with metronidazole: a double-blind randomized study. Am J Obstet Gynecol 1992;166:100.

62. Grimes DA, Schulz KF, Cates W Jr. Prophylactic antibiotics for curettage abortion. Am J Obstet Gynecol 1984;150:689.

63. Heisterberg L, Peterson K. Metronidazole prophylaxis in elective first trimester abortion. Obstet Gynecol 1985;65:371.

64. Darj E, Stralin E-B, Nilsson S. The prophylactic effect of doxycycline on postoperative infection rate after first trimester abortion. Obstet Gynecol 1987;70:755.

65. Levallois P, Rioux J-E. Prophylactic antibiotics for suction curettage abortion: results of a clinical controlled trial. Am J Obstet Gynecol 1988;158:100.

3

Vinay K. Malviya

CHAPTER

Bowel Preparation

Preparation of the colon for elective surgery is a topic of interest to the gynecologist as well as the gynecologic oncologist and the general surgeon. Emphasis on its importance is based on the observation that poor bowel preparation is the single most important factor in the pathogenesis of anastomotic dehiscence after large bowel resections[1] and that patients with a clean large bowel have a lower incidence of postoperative sepsis[2] and need for defunctional colostomy.

Entry into the colon with gross fecal contamination and the resection and reanastomosis of an unprepped colon are associated with significant postoperative complications. Primary repairs and reanastomosis of an unprepped colon are often followed by leakage, abscess, or fistulization. Anastomotic leakage after resection and reanastomosis of an unprepped colon is reported to range from 15% to 40%. It is generally accepted that infectious complications after colorectal surgery are reduced when satisfactory bowel preparation has been achieved. A variety of regimens to achieve satisfactory bowel preparation have been reported in the literature that are designed to purge solid fecal matter, reduce the quantity of bacteria, and reduce the concentration of bacteria.

In this age of limited Medicare and Medicaid reimbursements and frequent denial of payments for preoperative hospital days by third-party payers, surgeons have been prompted to seek efficient methods of reliable, easy-to-follow bowel preparation regimens that can be performed on an outpatient basis. Preoperative bowel preparation can be transferred effectively from the inpatient to the ambulatory setting without significantly increasing morbidity from either the preparation or the subsequent surgery in most patients with nonobstructing gastrointestinal tract lesions.

INDICATIONS FOR PREOPERATIVE BOWEL PREPARATION

A number of situations are encountered by the gynecologic surgeon in which bowel preparation should be considered (Table 3–1). The specific regimen that is prescribed is based on patient tolerance, cost-effectiveness, and efficacy.

Although most patients tolerate mechanical bowel preparation without difficulty, there are situations in which it is not safe nor feasible. Saline lavage and osmotic cathartics are contraindicated in gastric outlet obstruction, com-

TABLE 3–1
Indications for Bowel Preparation

Endometriosis
Known or suspected pelvic inflammatory disease
Planned bowel resection, bypass, or reanastomosis
Anticipated adhesions
Exenteration
Enteric radiation injury
Surgery for repair of a fistula

plete large bowel obstruction, emergent situations with bowel perforations, toxic colitis or megacolon, and hepatic cirrhosis. Patients with impaired swallowing and those who are unable to understand or follow instructions are poor candidates for osmotic cathartic preparations. Patients with chronic hepatic or renal failure require close supervision because of their susceptibility to fluid and electrolyte alterations.

METHODS OF BOWEL PREPARATION

The ideal method of mechanical bowel preparation should be safe and inexpensive, provide good cleansing, cause little or no patient discomfort, cause minimal electrolyte imbalance, and be simple to follow.

Cathartics and Enemas

The traditional method of bowel preparation consists of a low-residue diet, cathartics, and enemas beginning 2 to 5 days preoperatively (Table 3–2). Prospective studies have demonstrated that cathartics and enemas to provide mechanical cleansing provide good to excellent cleaning in only 70% of patients, may result in significant patient discomfort or metabolic alterations, and require 2 to 3 days.

Saline Lavage Methods

Saline lavage was described in 1970, and it provides good-to-excellent results in approximately 90% of patients.[3] This method of bowel preparation requires the placement of a nasogastric tube followed by the administration of large volumes of normal saline. Apart from the nursing care that is required, this regimen may cause rapid intravascular volume expansion, which is relatively contraindicated in patients

TABLE 3–2
Cathartic and Enema Regimen

Preoperative day 1	Full liquid diet 30 mL of castor oil or magnesium sulfate or one Bisacodyl tablet orally at 3 PM*
Preoperative day 2	Clear liquid diet Repeat oral cathartic* Saline enemas (1.5 L) at bedtime and repeat until clear return
Preoperative day 3	Clear liquid diet Repeat purgative* and enema NPO after midnight Evacuate bowel 1 h before operation

Patients may be given preoperative oral antibiotics: 1 g of neomycin, 1 g of erythromycin base at 9 hours, 18 hours, and 19 hours *before the planned operation*

*Magnesium citrate (300 mL) or Fleet Phospho-Soda (15 mL) may be substituted.

with compromised cardiovascular or renal status.[4–7]

Osmotic Cathartics

Several investigators have reported the use of mannitol as a nonabsorbent osmotic agent. An isotonic solution of 5% mannitol, which is pleasant tasting, cleans the bowel adequately, although 4 L of this solution is required to achieve satisfactory results.[8] Only 1 L of mannitol is required when hypertonic mannitol solution (10%) is used, but fluid and electrolyte alterations are common problems in this group of patients. In addition, mannitol is associated with an increased incidence of infectious complications, with an increased wound infection rate with *Escherichia coli*, and leads to production of combustible colonic gas.[8, 9] The production of this gas can be reduced with oral antibiotics, but its reduction with the use of parenteral antibiotics alone, before surgery, is inadequate.

Two polyethylene glycol electrolyte lavage solutions, originally described by Davis and colleagues in 1980 and marketed as GoLYTELY and Colyte, have gained wide acceptance.[10] The ingestion of 4 L of this solution provides good-to-excellent cleansing in 95% of patients and causes minimal fluid or electrolyte changes. This solution is well tolerated by patients and is not associated with combustible gas formation (see Table 3–2).[3] A sulfate-free electrolyte lavage solution, NuLytely, has also become available. It is formulated for improved taste and has further reduced water and electrolyte changes (Table 3–3).

TABLE 3–3
Composition of Isotonic Lavage Solutions

Composition	GoLYTELY	Colyte	NuLytely
Volume	4L	4L	4L
Polyethylene glycol 3350	236 g	60 g	420 g
Sodium sulfate	22.7 g	5.68 g	
Sodium bicarbonate	6.74 g	1.68 g	5.72 g
Sodium chloride	5.86 g	1.46 g	11.2 g
Potassium chloride	2.96 g	0.745 g	1.48 g
Taste	Mildly salty	Flavored	Mineral water

Total gut perfusion with isotonic solutions causes minimal changes in plasma electrolytes and has been used as a preparation for colonic surgery with excellent results. This regimen of bowel preparation is simple and straightforward (Table 3–4). It is recommended that, for best results, patients be placed on a clear fluid diet (e.g., gelatin, clear soup, apple juice) and the solution be chilled before use. The rate of administration of polyethylene glycol solution is 240 mL (8 fl oz) every 10 minutes. Rapid drinking of each portion is preferred rather than sipping it continuously. The first bowel movement usually occurs 1 hour after start of administration, and bowel cleansing is completed within 6 to 8 hours. Administration of the solution is continued until the watery stool is clear and free of solid matter. This normally requires the consumption of approximately 4 L of polyethylene glycol solution, although more or less may be required in a few patients.

TABLE 3–4
Bowel Preparation Regimen Using an Osmotic Cathartic

2 Days Before Surgery:
Low-residue diet

1 Day Before Surgery:
Liquid diet
Prochlorperazine (Compazine), 10 mg orally, before beginning preparation
Metoclopramide (Reglan), 10 mg orally, before beginning preparation. Repeat every 6 h, as needed, for nausea.
Begin GoLYTELY/NuLytely/Colyte in the morning and complete by noon. Drink 4 L or until the rectal effluent is clear. The preparation tastes better when chilled or served on ice. The addition of Kool-Aid or lemonade may further improve the taste.
Take nothing by mouth after midnight.
Antibiotics should be administered *after* completion of the preparation regimen so that the rapid transit time associated with the evacuation of solid fecal material does not interfere with the action of the antibiotic.

The polyethylene glycol solution is almost inert with respect to water retention, sodium absorption, and intestinal secretion. Patients on clear fluids before the preparation required 0.4 L less lavage solution and finished the preparation 9 hours sooner than those who were on clear liquids for a shorter time. These patients, however, required an average of 18.6 mEq more potassium replacement before surgery because a clear liquid diet supplies little potassium. The use of metoclopramide (Reglan), 15 mg given orally, intravenously, or intramuscularly, reduced abdominal distention, fullness, and nausea. It can be repeated every 6 hours for persistent nausea and fullness.[11]

The use of 5 mg bisacodyl (Dulcolax) has been shown in one study to reduce the volume of polyethylene glycol solution required to mechanically cleanse the bowel to 2 L, thereby improving patient compliance.[12] The patients using polyethylene glycol required a minimum of nursing care and were able to care for themselves because they were not restricted from activity.

No modification of the above preparation is necessary in patients with stomas. Care is taken to prevent leakage of stool through the stoma. For patients undergoing removal of the stoma the physician should order enemas through the stoma and the rectal stump after the lavage to clear any remaining mucus or sediment.

USE OF ANTIBIOTICS IN BOWEL PREPARATION

A survey of colorectal surgeons revealed that 88% recommended oral antibiotics combined with systemic antibiotics in addition to mechanical bowel cleansing before colonic surgery.[13] The ideal antibiotic regimen for use with mechanical bowel preparations has not been defined (Table 3–5). This notwithstanding, many surgeons express the opinion that use of a mechanical bowel preparation and antibiotics is associated with a lower incidence of infection versus use of the same preparation without antibiotics. Studies of antibiotics with an appropriate spectrum have shown higher infection rates in groups of patients with less effective cleansing, but the difference frequently failed to reach statistical significance owing to the small number of patients participating and the low modern rates of infection of 5% to 10%.[3, 14] It has been difficult to demonstrate that a combination of oral and systemic

TABLE 3–5
Recommendations for Antimicrobial Prophylaxis for Colonic Surgical Procedures

Oral:
Erythromycin 1 g, and neomycin, 1 g, 1 day before operation
Metronidazole, 1 g, and neomycin, 1 g, 1 day before operation
The antibiotics are administered 9, 18, and 19 hours before the time of surgery.
Parenteral:
A single parenteral dose of an aerobic agent + an anaerobic agent is given, followed by a second dose if procedure lasts 6 h beyond first dose.
Aerobic Agent
Gentamicin, 2 mg/kg
Aztreonam, 1 g
Cefotaxime, 1 g
Ceftizoxime, 1 g
Ceftriaxone, 1 g
Anaerobic Agent
Clindamycin, 900 mg
Metronidazole, 500 mg
Alternatively:
A single parenteral dose of an agent with aerobic and anaerobic coverage is given, followed by second dose if procedure lasts 6 h beyond first dose.
Ampicillin-sulbactam, 2 g/1 g
Imipenem-cilastin, 1 g
Ticarcillin-clavulanate, 3 g/100 mg

antibiotics is better than either one or the other. Three prospective randomized studies[15–17] have shown statistically significant reduction in the risk of infection, with the addition of a systemic cephalosporin to oral neomycin-erythromycin base. Other studies[18–20] have also confirmed this observation.

Condon and colleagues,[21, 22] in a 5-year multicenter trial, found no statistical difference between the group receiving systemic antibiotics if the appropriate mechanical cleansing and oral antibiotic therapy were employed. They, however, since then have changed their approach and add a second-generation cephalosporin to oral neomycin-erythromycin base regimen for low anterior resection, because the incidence of serious complications of short-term systemic second-generation cephalosporin therapy is low.[23] In Solla and Rothenberger's survey,[13] only 3% of surgeons used oral antibiotic prophylaxis alone, 8% of surgeons used systemic antibiotics alone, whereas 89% of surgeons used both types. Although many seek improved methods of mechanical bowel preparation to obtain a clean bowel, there are nonconformists who question its use, especially in light of present-day systemic antibiotics.[24]

CONCLUSION

Complications relating to bowel preparation are reported with a low incidence. The most common problem in most series was the inability to drink the cleansing preparation, and this varied from 0% to 25%. Difficulties with fluid and electrolyte balance occurred in 10% of patients receiving cathartics and enemas and in 5% of patients with polyethylene glycol lavage.[3]

The achievement of excellent clinical results in colorectal surgery is from an approach that includes mechanical bowel preparation, use of antibiotics, peritoneal lavage, the technique of anastomosis, the use or nonuse of drains, and the judicious use of a defunctional stoma.

REFERENCES

1. Hawley PR, Hunt TK, Dunphy JE. Etiology of colonic anastomotic leaks. Proc R Soc Med 1970;63(suppl):28–30.
2. Burton RC. Postoperative wound infection in colonic and rectal surgery. Br J Surg 1973;60:363–365.
3. Beck DE, Fazio VW. Current preoperative bowel cleansing methods: results of a survey. Dis Colon Rectum 1990;33:12–15.
4. Chung RS, Gurill NJ, Berglund EM. A controlled clinical trial of whole gut lavage as a method of bowel preparation for colonic operations. Am J Surg 1979;137:75–81.
5. Crapp AR, Tillotson P, Powis SJ, et al. Preparation of the bowel by whole-gut irrigation. Lancet 1975;2:1239–1240.
6. Keighley MR. A clinical and physiological evaluation of bowel preparation for elective colorectal surgery. World J Surg 1982;6:464–470.
7. Keighley MR, Taylor EW, Hares MM, et al. Influence of oral mannitol bowel preparation on colonic microflora and the risk of explosion during endoscopic diathermy. Br J Surg 1981;68:554–556.
8. Hares M, Alexander-Williams J. The effect of bowel preparation on colonic surgery. World J Surg 1982;6:175–181.
9. Wolfe BG, Beart RW Jr, Dozois RR, et al. A new bowel preparation for elective colon and rectal surgery: a prospective randomized clinical trial. Arch Surg 1988;123:895–900.
10. Davis GR, Santa Ann CA, Morawski SG, et al. Development of a lavage solution associated with minimal water and electrolyte absorption or secretion. Gastroenterology 1980;78:991–995.
11. Murray S, Preuss M, Schultz F. How do you prep the bowel without enemas? Am J Nurs 1992;92:66–67.
12. Adams WJ, Meagher AP, Lubowski DZ, King DW. Bisacodyl reduces the volume of polyethylene glycol solution required for bowel preparation. Dis Colon Rectum 1994;78:229–234.
13. Solla JA, Rothenberger DA. Preoperative bowel preparation: a survey of colon and rectal surgeons. Dis Colon Rectum 1990;33:154–159.
14. Fleites RL, Marshal JB, Eckhauser ML, et al. The efficacy of polyethylene glycol–electrolyte lavage solution versus traditional mechanical bowel preparation for elective colonic surgery: a randomized, prospective, blinded trial. Surgery 1985;98:708–717.
15. Coppa GE, Eng K, Gouge TH, et al. Parenteral and oral antibiotics in elective colon and rectal surgery. Am J Surg 1983;145:62–65.
16. Washington JA II, Dearing WH, Judd ES, et al. Effect of preoperative antibiotic regimen on development of infection after intestinal surgery: prospective, randomized, double-blind study. Ann Surg 1974;180:567–571.
17. Stone HH, Hooper CA, Kolb LD, et al. Antibiotic prophylaxis in gastric, biliary and colonic surgery. Ann Surg 1976;184:443–440.
18. Peck JJ, Fuchs PC, Gustafson ME. Antimicrobial prophylaxis in elective colon surgery: experience of 135 operations in a community hospital. Am J Surg 1984;147:633–637.
19. Pello JM, Beauregard W, Shaika K, Camishion RC. Colon operations without wound infections: principles and techniques of 101 cases. Am Surg 1984;50:362–365.
20. Portnoy J, Kagan E, Gordon PH, Mendelson J. Prophylactic antibiotics in elective colorectal surgery. Dis Colon Rectum 1983;26:310–313.
21. Condon RE, Bartlett JG, Nichols RL, et al. Preoperative prophylactic cephalothin fails to control septic complications of colorectal operations: results of controlled clinical trial. A Veterans Administrative cooperative study. Am J Surg 1979;137:58–74.
22. Condon RE, Bartlett JG, Greenlee H, et al. Efficacy of oral and systemic antibiotic prophylaxis in colorectal operations. Arch Surg 1983;118:496–502.
23. Condon RE. Antibiotic bowel preparation for surgery. In: Confronting Infection, Cases and Commentary, Wilmington, DE, Stuart Pharmaceuticals, 1987, vol 5., pp 1–12.
24. Irving AD, Scirmgeour D. Mechanical bowel preparation for colonic resection and anastomoses. Br J Surg 1987;74:580–581.

4

Edward Podczaski

CHAPTER

The Role of the Consultant

In addition to an active role in the primary care of women, the obstetrician-gynecologist is often called on to provide advice to colleagues. The American Board of Obstetrics and Gynecology has emphasized that its physicians have the capability to perform major gynecologic procedures, manage obstetric complications, and perform the essential diagnostic procedures required of a consultant in obstetrics and gynecology. Candidates are expected to demonstrate a level of competence that allows them to serve as consultants to other physicians in their community.[1]

The increasing scrutiny of medicine has directed attention at consultation as a component of the health care process. The skills and process of consultation are learned through experience and observation of senior clinicians. We interact with other physicians by performing and obtaining consultations. The effectiveness of our consultations determines how other physicians perceive our competence, influences future referrals, and ultimately affects compliance with our recommendations.

A *consultation* should be distinguished from a *referral*, although these terms have often been used interchangeably. A consultation is a request by an attending physician to obtain the opinion of a specialist on diagnosis or patient management. The attending physician is expected to continue the medical supervision of the patient. A referral is a request for another physician to assume direct responsibility for all or a portion of the patient's care. A referral may be directed at a specific problem or at complete care for the patient.[2]

The opinions and reports of the Judicial Council of the American Medical Association contain the most comprehensive listing of responsibilities for the consultant and respective attending physician.[3] This document lists the following ethical principles of consultation:

1. Consultations should be encouraged in case of serious illness or difficult conditions.
2. In every consultation, the benefit to the patient is of primary importance.
3. The consultant should not assume primary care of the patient without the consent of the referring physician.
4. The consultation should be done punctually.
5. Discussions in consultation should be with the attending physician and with the patient only with the prior consent of the attending physician.
6. Conflicts of opinion between the attending physician and the consultant should

be resolved by a second consultation or withdrawal of the consultant; however, the consultant has the right to present his or her opinion to the patient in the presence of the attending physician.

Consultation is a formal process that should be requested and provided according to accepted guidelines. The attending physician should submit a written request to the consultant that specifies the reason for the consultation and provides any other pertinent information. The patient should also be notified that a consultation has been requested.[2, 4] Consultations are obtained on request of the patient, in doubtful or difficult cases, or when they enhance the quality of medical care. Ordinarily a legal duty to obtain a consultation arises when, after a reasonable length of time and effort on the part of the attending physician, the diagnosis is unusually difficult and uncertain, the therapy is ineffective, or the patient requests a consultation.[5] Consultations are primarily for the benefit of the patient and are requested by the attending physician.

The process of consultation can be viewed in terms of the initial contact, completion of the consultation report, and follow-up.[2] The initial contact begins with the question(s) to be answered by the consultant. A precise understanding of the reason for the consultation is of major importance to provide optimal service to the patient and the referring physician. In a series of medical and subspecialty consultations at the Brigham and Women's Hospital in Boston, the consultant and referring physician had totally different impressions as to the reason for the consultation or the principal clinical issue in 14% of the cases.[6]

Regardless of how the request for consultation is communicated, the urgency of the consultation must be determined. Emergent or urgent consultations should be directly discussed between physicians. Such a determination can prevent subsequent problems in communication and delays in appropriate care.

At the time of initial patient contact, the consultant should identify himself or herself as a consultant and indicate the service represented and the reason for the consultation. The consultant should review the medical record, obtain any additional history necessary, examine the patient, and review the pertinent radiologic and laboratory studies. The actual consultation should include a brief summary of the history, hospital course, and physical examination. Most of the emphasis should be placed on the impressions, specific recommendations, and a discussion of how the conclusions were reached and their rationale.

Requesting physicians value clarity and brevity but also appreciate consultants who share their insights without condescension. It is counterproductive for the consultant to criticize the attending physician because of perceived differences in knowledge or philosophy of care. The "malignant" consultant has a limited clinical "life span" and faces extinction by disuse. Open communication between the consultant and the attending physician has always been of great importance. There is no substitute for direct contact, especially in cases in which the consultant's recommendations are controversial or crucial.

The frequency of follow-up visits and of future care is based on the nature of the problem prompting the consultation. The type and frequency of follow-up should be specifically addressed in the initial consultation. Compliance with the consultant's recommendations is more likely with more frequent follow-up documented with progress notes. A written note should document when the consultant will no longer follow the patient or that the consultation is complete.[2]

In an effort to improve the effectiveness of medical consultation, Goldman and colleagues have provided the following "Ten Commandments" of consultation[7]:

1. Determine the question
2. Establish urgency
3. Look for yourself
4. Be as brief as appropriate
5. Be specific
6. Provide contingency plans
7. Thou shalt not covet thy neighbor's patient
8. Teach with tact
9. Talk is cheap and effective
10. Follow-up

An increasing literature has evaluated the effectiveness of the consultation process. The outcome event analyzed by this literature has usually been compliance with the consultant's recommendations. Compliance with medical consultations ranged from 54% to 77% in academic hospitals.[2] Major determinants of compliance included answering the central question of the consult, promptness, a limited number of recommendations, the severity of the patient's illness, contact with the referring physician, and frequent follow-up.[2, 8] Most of these variables are determined by the attitude and skills of the consultant. The manner in which the consultation is performed directly affects its outcome.

An intraoperative consultation can result from unanticipated findings at surgery (e.g., ovarian cancer) or from a surgical complication (e.g., intractable bleeding during cesarean section). Intraoperative findings are appreciated by the eyes and hands of the operating surgeon. Occasionally, frozen section diagnosis contributes a more complete appreciation of any unanticipated pathologic process. This situation requires significant clinical acumen and must consider the patient's overall condition, the pathologic process, its treatment under the prevailing circumstances, and the necessary surgical procedure. The central problem prompting the consultation needs to be urgently and appropriately evaluated in terms of the individual patient. The consultant needs to make sure that the problem is within the scope of his or her practice and intervene surgically, if indicated. In an emergent situation, obviously, a verbal consultation is expected. However, this should be followed by a formal, written note. If the consultant performs surgery, the physician should be available to discuss the situation with the family. The consultant should also provide necessary follow-up in the postoperative interval, in addition to any further care required after discharge from the hospital.

The consultant and the attending physician share legal responsibility for the care of the patient based on the proportion of knowledge, control, and the foreseeability of potential harm.[9] Failure to choose an appropriate consultant can potentially create liability for the referring physician, especially if the choice of consultants was based on considerations other than competence. The attending physician should also be notified when the consultation is completed or when follow-up will no longer be provided. Lack of adequate notification may be misconstrued as abandonment.

The attending physician retains responsibility for the overall management of the patient. As such, the therapeutic recommendations of the consultant should not be discussed with the patient without the specific approval of the attending physician. The consultant needs to resolve any differences of opinion with the referring physician before discussing the recommendations with the patient. If irreconcilable differences of opinion exist, they should be specifically cited in the chart with a request for another opinion to resolve the situation. If the difference of opinion is not resolved, the consultant should indicate his or her intention to withdraw from the case because of a disagreement in diagnosis or management and indicate that it is the patient's prerogative to seek another opinion. However, the consultant does have a right to give an opinion to the patient in the presence of the attending physician.

Such guidelines appear to pertain to the care of hospitalized patients.[10] In such circumstances, a consultant may examine a patient, review the chart, and leave without explaining the findings and recommendations to the patient. Communication with the attending physician is rapid, and the consultant's findings can be promptly discussed with the patient. However, outpatient visits to a consultant's office may require some change in this format. Fortunately, contact with the referring physician at the time of consultation can clarify the situation. It would be unreasonable to expect a patient to keep an appointment with a specialist, pay for the visit, and leave the office without some discussion of the consultant's findings and recommendations.

REFERENCES

1. American Board of Obstetrics and Gynecology. Bulletin for 1994. Dallas, American Board of Obstetrics and Gynecology, 1994, p 7.
2. Gross R, Kammerer WS. General medical consultation service: the role of the internist. In: Kammerer WS, Gross R, eds. Medical Consultation: The Internist on Surgical, Obstetric, and Psychiatric services, 2nd ed. Baltimore, Williams & Wilkins, 1990, pp 1–8.
3. American Medical Association. Opinions and Reports of the Judicial Council. Chicago, American Medical Association, 1972, pp 51–52.
4. American College of Obstetricians and Gynecologists. Standards for Obstetric-Gynecologic Services, 7th ed. American College of Obstetricians and Gynecologists, Washington, DC, 1989, pp 90–91.
5. Abrams FR, Barclay ML, Cain JM, et al. Exploring Medical-Legal Issues in Obstetrics and Gynecology. Washington, DC, APGO Medical Education Foundation, 1994, p 212.
6. Lee T, Pappius EM, Goldman L. Impact of inter-physician communication on the effectiveness of medical consultations. Am J Med 1983;74:106.
7. Goldman L, Lee T, Rudd P. Ten commandments for effective consultations. Arch Intern Med 1983;143:1753.
8. Sears CL, Charlson ME. The effectiveness of a consultation: compliance with initial recommendations. Am J Med 1983;74:870.
9. Dunn JD. Practice with co-providers. In: American College of Legal Medicine. Legal Medicine: Legal Dynamics of Medical Encounters, 2nd ed. St. Louis, Mosby–Year Book, 1991, pp 434–439.
10. Graber GC, Beasley AD, Eaddy JA. The scope of professional responsibility. In: Ethical Analysis of Clinical Medicine: A Guide to Self-evaluation. Baltimore, Urban & Schwarzenberg, 1985, pp 113–158.

5

Bruce Patsner

CHAPTER

Intraoperative Care

The goal of any surgical procedure, gynecologic or otherwise, is to perform the appropriate operation after obtaining informed consent and evaluating the patient preoperatively in the proper manner. Because surgery is controlled trauma, the best interests of both physician and patient are served when surgery is performed as anatomically, hemostatically, and expeditiously as possible. In a perfect world, all surgery would go smoothly without perioperative complications and everyone would be satisfied with the outcome. Moreover, patient and physician expectations about what surgery will or might accomplish would always be reasonable.

Unfortunately, gynecologic surgery is not performed in the best of all possible worlds. Intraoperative problems are lessened to some degree by thoughtful preoperative patient selection and preparation. However, even under ideal circumstances with the best planning, problems are encountered intraoperatively. Expecting that the unexpected might happen and being prepared helps ensure a satisfactory outcome, as does attention to surgical anatomy and technique.

The most meticulous preoperative preparation and postoperative care of the gynecologic surgery patient will go to waste if the intraoperative care is poor. From the moment the patient is brought into the operating room, the surgeon must assume ultimate responsibility for what happens until the patient arrives in the postanesthesia unit. The gynecologic surgeon must be sure that the scrub nurse and circulating nurses are familiar with his or her operative routine and equipment. Special equipment should be requested in advance. Communication is essential among all members of the operative team.

The type of anesthesia should be agreed on ahead of time for each case. Debating the relative merits of regional versus general anesthesia or if the patient does or does not require intubation for a short procedure such as conization should not occur in the operating room. These issues should be discussed and decided in advance.

Once in the operating suite, appropriately medicated, and under suitable anesthesia, the patient should be properly positioned. The critical determining factor for positioning the patient is the operation to be performed and the length of time needed to complete the surgery. The dorsal lithotomy position may be used with traditional "candy cane" stirrups or with Allen-type exenteration stirrups. This position is ideal for patients who are undergoing vulvo-vaginal or laparoscopic procedures. Patients undergoing lengthy operative procedures, very obese patients, and patients with spine or orthopedic conditions that may be aggravated by having the hips flexed are better served by Allen stirrups. Proper use of exenteration-type stirrups requires that the calf not rest against the back of the stirrups or the patient may develop footdrop or even muscle necrosis. The leg should "float" in the stirrup, with all pressure ideally on the ball of the foot (or heel, if not possible). The legs should be raised above the level of the trunk so that venous pooling in the legs and thighs is minimized.

Much ado is made about "proper" vaginal and skin preparation for gynecologic surgery. However, there are few randomized, prospective data to support any particular practice. Ostensibly, all preoperative preparations of the vagina and abdominal wall are done to lessen the risk of infections. The use of prophylactic cephalosporin antibiotics before hysterectomy or extended pelvic operations has demonstrably lessened the infection rate after vaginal and, to a lesser extent, abdominal hysterectomy.[1, 2] Comparison of study results regarding the efficacy of various vaginal and abdominal preparations is difficult because of the inconsistent use of prophylactic antibiotics and less reactive suture materials (e.g., Vicryl or Dexon as opposed to plain or chromic catgut suture). Still, some general conclusions may be drawn from the existing data, keeping in mind that operative site (pelvis, abdominal wall) infection is as much a function of what is done *under* the skin (e.g., use of cautery, drains, dead space, operative time, tissue trauma) and what is present in the wound or pelvis as it is a function of what is on the skin of the surgeon and patient. A shower the night before surgery using an antiseptic soap has been shown to decrease the incidence of wound infection in patients undergoing chest surgery and may be of benefit in patients undergoing pelvic surgery.[3] Douching may be useful before vulvovaginal procedures, although there are no prospective, randomized data on its usefulness before abdominal procedures. Shaving causes microtrauma to the skin and may increase the likelihood of wound infection unless it is done immediately before incision and restricted only to hair that might be incorporated into the wound. The difference in wound infection rate between hair clipping (2%) and shaving (1%) performed immediately before surgery is not statistically or clinically significant.[4] A 2-minute hand scrub with chlorhexidine solution (Hibiclens) is as effective as a longer 5- to 10-

minute scrub in reducing the bacterial count of microorganisms. Regardless of the duration of the scrub, the surgeons' nails should be kept short and hands in good condition. Surgeons with an active hand dermatitis, cellulitis, or abscess should not operate until such conditions have resolved. No data exist to support the concept that paper drapes have a lower infection rate than cloth drapes even though the former are less "absorbent." There are also no data to support a lower wound infection rate with the general use of plastic barrier drapes, although they are useful in isolating specific areas (e.g., colostomy stoma) from the operative field. Prepping the abdominal wall the night before surgery adds nothing to an abdominal wall preparation in the operating room. Given the fact that virtually all patients are day-of-surgery admissions, the era of such extensive skin preparation (other than a shower) is probably gone forever. The critical goal of abdominal wall preparation is reduction of bacterial counts at the planned operative site.[5] A variety of agents are available for abdominal wall preparation, and each agent has unique advantages and disadvantages. However, no single agent has been demonstrated clinically superior (Table 5–1). In general, painting with an antiseptic agent is as good as scrubbing.

The importance of protection of the surgeon from acquiring a viral or bacterial infection from the patient needs no emphasis. Glove puncture may occur in up to 60% of all surgical procedures, and the likelihood increases in direct proportion to the length of operative time and amount of needle handling. No glove can prevent penetrating injury from scalpel or needles, but heavier gloves such as orthopedic ones may minimize contamination of the surgeons' hands from body fluids from the patient. Double gloving is an alternative, though there are little prospective data to as-

sess the efficacy of this practice. Protective eyewear, if the surgeon does not wear glasses, is also an excellent practice. The surgeon should *always* follow universal precautions.

CHOICE OF INCISION

Once the patient has been properly positioned and the abdomen or perineum or both prepped and draped, the next step is to make the incision. Before doing so, the surgeon must ensure that the Mayo stand is properly positioned and the necessary instruments ready. In addition, Bovie cautery and suction apparatus must be positioned so that the surgeon may reach for either without constantly interfering with the visibility of the surgical field and of that of the assistants and without reaching across the wound. For a right-handed surgeon who operates on the patient's left side, the Bovie cautery and suction should be handed off the top of the field and positioned near his or her right (operating) hand.

Surgical incisions for gynecologic abdominal operations may be divided into either vertical or transverse incisions. For all intents and purposes, pararectus, paramedian, and rectus-splitting incisions are seldom indicated and rarely used unless a prior scar in that area exists or there is a hernia in a prior scar. The decision to use a vertical or transverse abdominal incision is generally based on three factors: (1) the presence of a prior surgical incision, (2) the need or anticipated need to operate above the umbilicus or in the upper abdomen, and (3) whether a transverse incision will provide adequate exposure to allow the safe resection of any pelvic pathologic process if the pelvis is the only planned area of surgery. The decision to use a vertical incision is not mandated by a known or suspected gynecologic malignancy but by consideration of several factors (Table

TABLE 5–1
Abdominal Skin Preparations

Agent	% Immediate Reduction in Skin Bacteria	% Reduction in Skin Bacteria After 3 Hours
Liquid soap	40	0
Povidone liquid soap	90	20
Chlorhexidene detergent	75	70
Povidone aqueous solution	97	75
Hexachlorophene detergent	40	91
Isopropyl alcohol 60%	96	90
Isopropyl alcohol 70%	99.3	99.1
Isopropyl alcohol (70%) + chlorhexidene (0.5%)	99.4	99.7

TABLE 5–2
General Guidelines for the Selection of Transverse or Vertical Abdominal Incisions

Vertical

Applicable for *any* pelvic procedure

Permits rapid abdominal entry, which may be important in cases of abdominal pain or bleeding or uncertain etiology

Indicated in cases of known or suspected ovarian cancer, intestinal obstruction, or abdominal mass of uncertain etiology

Transverse

Appropriate for benign adnexal surgery if the mass is not too large

Provides acceptable exposure for radical hysterectomy, extrafascial hysterectomy with pelvic lymph node sampling, and surgery for endometriosis or pelvic infection

5–2). Patients undergoing radical hysterectomy and many patients with uterine malignancy do not invariably require para-aortic node sampling so that the primary operation can be safely performed using a transverse incision.

The advantages of a vertical midline incision are clear: it is often the simplest, fastest, and least hemorrhagic abdominal incision. A vertical incision provides excellent pelvic exposure, although less lateral pelvic exposure than a Maylard incision. Because it may be easily extended, it is the incision of choice for patients with known or suspected gynecologic cancers that may require access to the supraumbilical areas, particularly the bowel and hemidiaphragms. Disadvantages of the vertical midline incision include a poorer cosmetic appearance compared with a low transverse incision (particularly one below the pubic hair line) and the higher wound hernia rate. The vertical incision hernia rate of 7% is roughly equivalent for interrupted and continuous suturing, with the latter technique now favored because of increased speed of closure.[6]

Several technical points about vertical midline incisions for gynecologic surgery must be emphasized. The abdominal cavity should be entered at the apex of the incision to avoid injury to either the bladder or pelvic organs, followed by extension of the incision toward the pubic symphysis to maximize pelvic exposure. In patients with a large panniculus who are not undergoing panniculectomy,[7] it is important to pull the panniculus *down* past the pubis. In this situation, the skin incision should be made above the portion of the abdominal wall pulled below the pubis to avoid a "buttonhole" or through-and-through incision.

When the abdomen is entered by means of a laparotomy, the skin incision should be made with a single bold stroke to the fascial layer. This technique minimizes surgical dead space and lessens the risk of postoperative infection.[8] The tradition of using two knives (e.g., one for the skin and one for the subcutaneous tissue and fascia) does not provide a significant lessening of the risk of wound infection compared with use of a single knife.

After incision of the rectus fascia, the rectus muscles should be gently separated, taking care to avoid lacerating the vessels that penetrate the undersurface of the muscle. The peritoneum should not be entered bluntly but rather by careful scalpel dissection. It is preferable to enter the abdominal cavity at the apex of the incision, followed by extension of the peritoneal incision toward the pubic symphysis.

There are several transverse lower abdominal incisions from which the gynecologic surgeon may choose. As a rule, transverse incisions offer several advantages compared with vertical incisions: (1) cosmetic results are superior because they more closely follow Langer's lines; (2) wound strength is high and hernia and dehiscence rates are negligible because the tension on the wound by abdominal muscles is parallel and not at right angles to the incision; and (3) pulmonary complications are lower because there is less interference with respiration.

The most commonly used transverse abdominal incisions in gynecology are the Pfannenstiel, Maylard, and Cherney.[9] Pictures of these incisions in various textbooks notwithstanding, they may all be made at the *same* level on the abdominal wall. The differences among these incisions relate to how the rectus abdominis musculature and the incision of the peritoneum are handled. The exact level of the skin incision and its length are individualized to allow varying degrees of lateral exposure and access to the mid and upper abdomen.

The Pfannenstiel incision involves transverse incisions in the skin, subcutaneous tissue, and anterior rectus sheath; separation of the rectus muscles in the midline; and a vertical peritoneal incision. The Maylard incision differs in that rectus muscles are divided transversely with cautery (the inferior epigastric vessels may be preserved) and the peritoneum is divided transversely; this allows maximal lateral pelvic exposure and is ideally suited for radical hysterectomy or benign cases that may require extensive retroperitoneal dissection. The Cherney incision involves separation of the rectus

TABLE 5–3
Routine Evaluations Performed at the
Time of Laparotomy

Palpation of pelvic organs
Palpation of pelvic sidewalls and aortocaval areas for
  enlarged lymph nodes
Palpation of the surfaces of the stomach, liver,
  diaphragm, pancreas
Assessment of the gallbladder and gentle ballottement to
  detect stones
Inspection of the small bowel from the ileocecal junction
  proximally to the ligament of Treitz
Inspection of the colon, appendix, and omentum

TABLE 5–4
Factors to Consider in Choice of Retractor

Type of incision (vertical versus transverse)
Anticipated length of incision
Benign versus cancer case
Anticipated procedures (e.g., need for access to mid and
  upper abdomen)
Body habitus of patient

muscles from their attachment to the pubic bone and a transverse peritoneal incision.

EXPLORING THE ABDOMEN

The opportunity to inspect the abdomen and pelvis at the time of laparotomy provides the gynecologist an opportunity to evaluate the patient for occult disease. A thorough exploration of the abdomen and pelvis should become a habit that is standard practice.

Approaches to exploring the pelvis and upper abdomen vary from surgeon to surgeon but must include a number of organs and surfaces (Table 5–3). These findings should be specifically noted in the operative note dictation.

Cytologic washings with heparinized saline should be obtained from the cul de sac and paracolic gutters whenever cancer is present or suspected. Suspicious areas on any peritoneal or visceral surface should be sampled.

RETRACTORS

The decision as to which retractor to use for gynecologic abdominal and pelvic operation is dictated by several factors (Table 5–4). For thin or average-sized patients undergoing surgery for benign disease or limited pelvic malignancy through a transverse incision, many surgeons will use self-retaining retractors such as the Balfour, Harrington, or O'Connor-O'Sullivan. All of these retractors provide pelvic exposure and come with an upper arm extension to allow the intestines to be "self retained." For a deeper pelvis, the deep blades should be selected but care must be taken to avoid undue pressure on the psoas muscle or pelvic sidewall to avoid nerve injury (see Chapter 22).

When operating on a morbidly obese patient or a patient in whom a long vertical incision is required or when performing a complicated pelvic operation in which minimizing the amount of retraction by the surgical assistants is desirable, use of the Bookwalter retractor is recommended. This is a self-retaining retractor that attaches to the rail on the surgical table and has a variety of "rings" of different sizes and shapes that are secured to the side rails by either a flex bar or a straight metal rod. Six or more fixed or flexible blades may then be attached to the ring and superb pelvic and abdominal exposure obtained (Figs. 5–1 and 5–2).

The Bookwalter retractor may be adjusted at any time during surgery by the surgeon, because virtually the entire retractor is on the field and is sterile. Care should be taken to avoid packing off too vigorously to avoid psoas muscle compression.

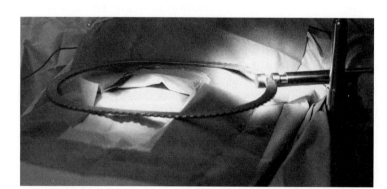

FIGURE 5–1
The Bookwalter retractor consists of a ring that is attached to a sidearm on the operating table.

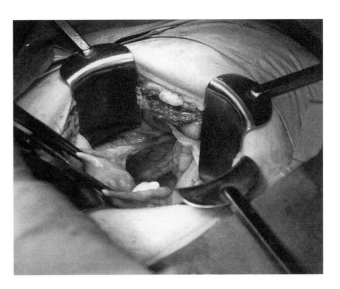

FIGURE 5-2
The Bookwalter retractor permits considerable flexibility in the placement of body wall retractors to provide optimal surgical exposure.

After placement of the abdominal wall retractor, the bowel is usually packed into the upper abdomen using moist laparotomy pads. Although many techniques may be used, it is helpful to employ a method that keeps the bowel out of the operative field with the minimum number of lap pads. One technique is to pack the cecum into the right gutter with the first lap pad followed by packing of the sigmoid and descending colon into the left gutter with the second lap pad. The third laparotomy pad is used to pack the small bowel into the upper abdomen. "Tight" packing of the intestine should be avoided because this may impair venous return and make ventilation of the patient more difficult.

CHOICE OF INSTRUMENTS

An amazing variety of clamps are available for open pelvic and abdominal surgery, including the Heaney-Ballantine, Wertheim, Masterson, Kocher, Rochester, Kelly, Moynihan, and Coppleson, among others. Clamps differ in length, shape, degree of tissue trauma, the presence of toothed end, serrations, and cost. Interpretation of supposed advantages of one clamp as compared with another is difficult, given that surgical speed, technique, and prophylactic antibiotics and the use of less-reactive suture materials are potential confounding variables that are rarely taken into account. Regardless of the clamp used, the pedicle must be cut and tied or suture ligated, and ultimately undergoes necrosis.

In general, surgeons use the clamps they were trained to use and with which they are comfortable. There is no obvious advantage in using a clamp that is larger than necessary or in having surgical pedicles larger than needed. In the only study which prospectively compared post-hysterectomy infection rates with respect to the use of Masterson, Heaney and Wertheim clamps (all of which yield different sized pedicles), no difference could be documented.[10] There is no surgical advantage to be gained from doubly or triply clamping vascular pedicles as is routinely illustrated in many current textbooks of gynecologic surgery. The application of multiple clamps to control "back-bleeding" or to secure the suture simply results in larger tissue pedicles with larger areas of necrosis.

Finally, regardless of the surgical clamp used, the wound healing process in the pelvis or anywhere else in the abdominal cavity can only be expedited by minimizing the amount of Bovie cautery (electrosurgical scalpel) for cutting and using the standard steel scalpel whenever possible.[11]

SUTURE SELECTION

Significant advances in suture materials have occurred in the past decade that have impacted on surgical practice. Prior to 1970, other than stainless steel, the only suture materials that were available were natural materials such as cotton, silk, and catgut. The first synthetic absorbable suture available in the United States was Dexon (1970) followed by Vicryl (1974) and since then multiple synthetic permanent and absorbable suture materials have been developed that are both monofilament and braided.

The ideal suture is nonreactive, inexpensive, easy to handle, retains its tensile strength until its surgical purpose is served, has a high degree of knot security, and is absorbed only after its purpose has been served. Because most patients will have either skin staples or subcuticular stitches on the skin, and the use of any material in this area is merely to approximate the wound edges, the emphasis in this section is on selection of suture material for hysterectomy or other pelvic operations. Selection of suture materials for wound closure is discussed in Chapter 12. It is worth keeping in mind that even perfect suture material will not compensate for poor surgical technique and inability to tie knots properly.

Plain and chromic catgut suture materials have a long track record in gynecology and are favored by many "senior" operators who appreciate their ease of use. In situations in which wound strength is not a priority and rapid absorption is desired, catgut suture is an acceptable choice. Because vascular pedicles need to be maintained for only 96 hours, chromic catgut is adequate as it retains significant tensile strength for 4 to 5 days. When tissue reaction should be minimized, as in pelvic surgery, or when tensile strength should be maintained for many weeks, as in fascial closure, catgut suture is less than ideal. Vicryl or Dexon are preferable for pelvic surgery because of minimal tissue reaction and retention of tensile strength for several weeks. Vicryl has been shown to minimize the amount of vaginal vault granulation tissue after hysterectomy when compared with chromic catgut.[12] Table 5–5 is a list of some of the commonly available permanent and absorbable suture materials.

CLOSURE, DRAINAGE, AND DRESSINGS

Once the operation is completed, the incision must be reapproximated. "Reperitonealization" of the pelvic floor is a time-honored tradition that has never been prospectively studied in a randomized trial. The incidence of postoperative intestinal obstruction is higher when reactive suture materials such as plain or chromic catgut are used to close the pelvic peritoneum.[13] Whether reperitonealization with Dexon or Vicryl is associated with an increased risk of postoperative small bowel obstruction has not been evaluated. There are no data to prove that closing the peritoneum prevents adhesions of intestine to the pelvic floor or the vaginal cuff. Moreover, there is always the possibility that the ureter may be kinked or occluded by poor suturing technique.

Routine drainage of the retroperitoneal spaces by passive or active closed-suction methods is not recommended for benign, uncomplicated gynecologic surgery.[14] The same recommendation can be made for routine drainage of the abdominal incision.[15] Routine retroperitoneal drainage after pelvic lymphadenectomy has also been abandoned by many gynecologic oncologists. Pelvic drainage does not decrease the incidence of pelvic lymphocyst or infection after radical pelvic surgery and may actually increase the incidence of these complications.[16]

Active closed-suction drainage may be indicated in certain situations associated with an increased risk of postoperative infection such as a ruptured tubo-ovarian abscess, although copious irrigation at the time of surgery followed by broad-spectrum antibiotic therapy postoperatively may be adequate. Drainage is recommended after primary ureteral reanastomosis or ureteroneocystotomy. The retroperitoneal drain must be carefully positioned to avoid avulsing the ureter when the drain is removed.

INTRAOPERATIVE MANAGEMENT

With the exception of problems with patient intubation, the management of anesthesia, and the administration of blood products and anti-

---

TABLE 5–5
Characteristics of Different Suture Materials

Nonabsorbable Suture

Natural fiber—silk, cotton
Stainless steel

Synthetic Nonabsorbable Suture

Multifilament polyester (Dacron, Mersilene)
Coated multifilament polyester (Ti-Cron, Ethibond)
Nylon monofilament (Dermalon, Ethilon)
Nylon multifilament (Surgilon, Neurilon)
Polypropylene monofilament (Surgilene, Prolene)

Synthetic Absorbable Suture

Polyglycolic acid (Dexon)—90 days to absorption
Polyglactin 910 (Vicryl)—72 days to absorption
Polydioxanone (PDS)—180 days to absorption
Polyglyconate (Maxon)—180 days to absorption

Natural Absorbable Suture

Plain catgut—70 days to absorption
Chromic catgut—90 days to absorption

biotics, virtually all other intraoperative problems encountered during gynecologic surgery are the direct or indirect result of actions by the surgeon. These problems generally arise out of three situations: (1) difficulty completing the operation due to limited surgical exposure or unexpected pathology; (2) injury to adjacent nongynecologic structures (e.g., small or large intestine, bladder, ureter, major blood vessel); and (3) injuries to gynecologic structures (ovary, oviduct, uterus) that may necessitate unplanned resection. Some general comments about gynecologic pelvic surgery and practical guidelines for the management of intraoperative injury will facilitate the development of surgical strategies to counter intraoperative difficulties when they arise.

The difference between mediocre and excellent gynecologic surgery (and surgeons), and between uncertainty and confidence in management of complications, is the ability to operate in the pelvic spaces, particularly the retroperitoneum. Understanding the anatomy of the retroperitoneal space is essential to enter the spaces safely and to operate with confidence in the pelvis. Any manner of complicated pelvic surgery—extensive endometriosis involving the pararectal area or ureter, resection of malignant ovarian tumors, or control of pelvic bleeding—is performed more safely using a primary retroperitoneal approach. Moreover, safe dissection of the ureter, control of uterine artery or paravaginal bleeding, and repair of

injury to pelvic structures are all predicated on the ability to enter the retroperitoneum safely.[17, 18]

The retroperitoneal spaces are all potential spaces in the pelvis that are avascular and that may be developed by careful blunt and sharp dissection (Fig. 5–3). The boundaries of several of these potential spaces are structures—ureter, large vessels, rectosigmoid, bladder—that the surgeon must identify to decrease the risk of injury (Table 5–6).

The lateral boundary of the retroperitoneum is the pelvic sidewall. The safest way to enter the retroperitoneum on either side of the pelvis is to visualize a "triangle" with the round ligament at its base, infundibulopelvic ligament with the ovarian vessels as the near side, and the pelvic sidewall with the psoas muscle as the far side. The retroperitoneum is safely entered by opening the peritoneum far lateral to the infundibulopelvic ligament and extending the incision cephalad. The incision may begin by transecting the round ligament at least halfway to the pelvic sidewall either with suture ligatures or Bovie cautery, and extending the incision along the middle of the triangle formed by the pelvic sidewall and infundibulopelvic ligament. It is important to stay lateral to the infundibulopelvic ligament. Once the peritoneum is incised, the loose areolar tissue of the retroperitoneum may be bluntly dissected medial to the vessels; *never* dissect between the vessels and the pelvic sidewall. The

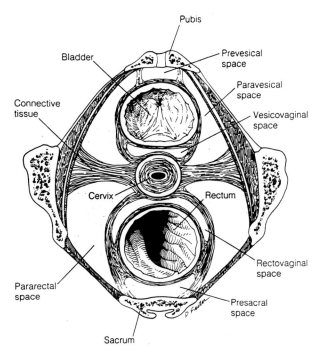

FIGURE 5–3
The retroperitoneal spaces are depicted. The cardinal ligament or "web" separates the pararectal and the paravesical spaces.[19]

TABLE 5-6
Boundaries of the Retroperitoneal Spaces

Pararectal space—bounded medially by the superior vesical artery, laterally by the external iliac vessels and obturator nerve, posteriorly by the uterine artery, and inferiorly by the levator ani

Paravesical space—bounded medially by the ureter and rectum, laterally by the hypogastric artery and pelvic wall, anteriorly by the uterine artery, posteriorly by the sacrum, and inferiorly by the levator ani

Prevesical space (e.g., retropubic space or space of Retzius)—bounded by the posterior surface of the symphysis pubis and inferiorly by the dome of the bladder

Presacral space (e.g., retrorectal space)—bounded posteriorly by the sacrum, anteriorly by the rectum, and laterally by the uterosacral ligaments

Vesicovaginal space—bounded posteriorly by the cervix and vagina, anteriorly by the bladder, and laterally by the bladder pillars

Rectovaginal space—bounded anteriorly by the vagina, posteriorly by the rectum, and laterally by the uterosacral ligaments and rectal pillars

ureter is identified on the medial leaf of the broad ligament.

After the pararectal space is developed, the ureter is identified on the medial leaf of the broad ligament. A word of caution is needed about identifying the ureter: remarks about the characteristic rubbery feel or "snap" of the ureter or its supposed identifying circular vascular pattern on its surface notwithstanding, distinguishing the ureter from the hypogastric artery or even on occasion the ovarian vessels may be difficult to do by simple palpation or even visual inspection. This is particularly true when the anatomy is distorted or hemostasis is less than optimal. The only "foolproof" way to identify the ureter conclusively is to identify the following structures systematically in the retroperitoneum in the following order:

1. Enter the retroperitoneum as just described.

2. Identify the psoas muscle on the lateral border of the retroperitoneal space and then find the external iliac artery adjacent to the psoas muscle.

3. Follow the external iliac artery up to the bifurcation of the common iliac artery. The hypogastric artery may be identified coming off the common iliac artery and the ureter identified as it crosses over the bifurcation of the common iliac artery from lateral to medial. The ureter may thus be correctly distinguished from the iliac vessels and the ovarian vessels.

When hypogastric ligation is required to control pelvic hemorrhage, the anatomic ap-proach is the same as described earlier, that is a retroperitoneal dissection. The goal of hypogastric ligation is to allow a stable clot to form by diminishing arterial "pulse pressure." Because of vascular anastomoses in the pelvis, bilateral ligation is required. It is essential that the internal iliac artery be ligated (so as not to lose blood) as opposed to the external iliac (so as not to lose the leg) or the ureter (so as not to lose a kidney). The same steps described for identification of the ureter must be followed in the same order to verify that the correct structure is being ligated. A right-angled clamp is passed under the hypogastric artery using gentle dissection. A lateral to medial dissection decreases the likelihood of injury to the underlying hypogastric vein. In most patients, the posterior branch of the hypogastric comes off immediately after the bifurcation of the common iliac artery, and attempting to isolate it to avoid ligating it only increases the likelihood of a significant injury to the iliac veins. Once positively identified, the hypogastric may be either singly or doubly tied with 2-0 silk or Vicryl.

INTRAOPERATIVE COMPLICATIONS

In this section the focus is on two issues: (1) management of unexpected pelvic pathologic processes at the time of planned surgery for a less extensive or benign gynecologic condition and (2) management of specific intraoperative complications such as urinary tract or small or large intestinal injury or vascular problems.

Unexpected pathologic processes encountered during a "routine" gynecologic pelvic operation for presumed benign disease may either be unexpected malignancy (gynecologic or otherwise), unexpected benign pelvic pathology (e.g., extensive endometriosis, dense adhesions, chronic pelvic inflammatory disease with obliteration of normal tissue planes), or unexpected difficulty because of limited surgical exposure.

Shown in Table 5–7 are five examples of unanticipated pathologic processes that gynecologists may encounter, strategies to "avoid" them, and how to manage them intraoperatively. Problems of a general surgical nature discovered during routine gynecologic surgery that the gynecologist is not trained to perform require appropriate intraoperative consultation. In general, situations in which the uterus or pelvic mass appears to be too large to be safely removed occur as a consequence of a

T A B L E 5 - 7
Strategies to Avoid and Manage Unexpected Intraoperative Pathology

Type of Problem	To Avoid	To Manage Intraoperatively
Mass larger than anticipated	Pelvic exam preoperatively Pelvic ultrasound	Convert incision to a Maylard or extend the vertical incision
Ovarian cancer	Radiographic evaluation of mass to detect characteristics suggestive of cancer; preoperative CA 125 test	Frozen section for confirmation of clinical importance Intraoperative consultation with gynecologic oncologist
Endometrial cancer	Endometrial biopsy in high-risk patients	Intraoperative consultation with gynecologic oncologist
Cervical cancer	Preoperative Papanicolaou test	Intraoperative consultation with gynecologic oncologist
Severe endometriosis	Bowel preparation; review of prior operative notes if applicable	Use retroperitoneal approach to minimize risk of ureteral injury; avoid blunt dissection

transverse incision; in such cases the rectus muscle may be divided and the incision converted to a Maylard. If this maneuver is unsuccessful, a vertical incision is made. An enlarged uterus may fill the pelvis from sidewall to sidewall, and efforts to achieve traction on the uterus with lateral clamps placed at the uterine cornua may not be useful and may increase bleeding. Placement of a "corkscrew" in the uterine fundus provides cephalad and maximizes lateral exposure. When unexpected pelvic adhesions (e.g., bowel to pelvic viscera, bladder to uterus) are encountered, it is important to handle tissues gently and to dissect sharply with a knife or Metzenbaum scissors. Blunt dissection with a sponge stick or index finger is a poor technique that increases the risk of organ damage and excessive blood loss.

The issue of whether to use indwelling ureteral catheters before laparotomy is debated. There is no literature to document that the use of indwelling catheters lowers the incidence of ureteral injury and may give the surgeon a false sense of security in terms of how close to the ureter the dissection may progress. Putting in a ureteral catheter is not an acceptable substitute for being able to enter the retroperitoneum and identify the ureter intraoperatively, and should be required by an experienced gynecologic surgeon in only the most extraordinary circumstances.

Intraoperative injury to the bladder, rectosigmoid, small bowel, ureter, or a large pelvic blood vessel is a bridge that every busy gynecologic surgeon will eventually cross if he or she does enough cases. In fact, injuries to the aforementioned structures are, within limits, accepted complications of major gynecologic surgery and should be discussed as part of the informed consent process for every patient.

What is not generally acceptable, however, is failure to recognize and appropriately correct these complications. Gross injuries to the bowel, bladder, ureter, or vessels are not difficult to recognize (e.g., stool or intestinal contents in the operative field, urine or the Foley bulb in the operative field, hemorrhage). In contradistinction, small injuries to the bladder or bowel may be subtle and the complication only recognized during an eventful postoperative recovery. Whenever there is a question of a complication and the surgeon is unsure either if it exists or how to fix it, intraoperative consultation should be sought immediately. Anticipating the higher probability of certain problems in select cases ensures that intraoperative management of such complications is less problematic.

Table 5–8 identifies several of the more common intraoperative problems that may be encountered, what may be done before surgery to minimize their occurrence, and how to manage them intraoperatively. Certain caveats merit emphasis. For clamp or crushing injuries of the ureter, insertion of a ureteral stent may be sufficient if the clamp was in place for less than 30 minutes. If the ureter was clamped for a longer period of time, necrosis is likely and it is safer either primarily to reanastomose normal ureteral tissues or to perform a ureteroneocystotomy. It is vital not only to identify the ureter before clamping and cutting the infundibulopelvic ligament but also to trace the course of the ureter on the medical leaf of the broad ligament if there is any disease process such as a broad ligament fibroid or severe endometriosis that might alter the course of the ureter. It is necessary to do this before clamping and cutting the uterine vessels. When drains are placed for ureteral injury, they

TABLE 5–8
Intraoperative Complications: Recognition and Management

Organ	To Avoid Injury	To Diagnose and Correct Injury
Bladder	Insert Foley catheter before making skin incision	Flush bladder with sterile milk to detect cystotomy; repair injury with running 3-0 absorbable suture; Foley drainage for 5–7 days
Ureter	Visual identification by opening the retroperitoneal space	Use intravenous indigo carmine to identify extravasation; intraoperative consult with gynecologic oncologist or urologist for repair
Rectosigmoid	Sharp dissection	Irrigate wound; freshen edges; reapproximate with 3-0 Vicryl, followed by second layer of interrupted Prolene
Small bowel	Sharp dissection	Small injuries can be repaired like rectosigmoid injury; more extensive injuries require resection and reanastomosis; avoid compromise of bowel lumen
Bleeding from vaginal cuff	Meticulous surgical technique	Identify ureter and bladder; isolate bleeding site and ligate
Bleeding from ovarian vessels		Open retroperitoneum and identify ureter; then isolate ovarian vessels and suture ligate
Bleeding from uterine vessels		Open retroperitoneum and identify ureter; then isolate uterine artery from hypogastric and clip or suture
Bleeding from pelvic sidewall		Apply immediate pressure; crossmatch blood; open retroperitoneum, identify bleeding vessel, and suture ligate

should be positioned carefully so that removal will not avulse the ureter.

With resection of some pelvic tumors, it may facilitate the dissection to intentionally open the bladder when a tissue plane cannot be established, particularly with difficult hysterectomy. This method facilitates dissection and provides a single, simple, controlled cystotomy to close instead of multiple lacerations at different levels near the bladder base and ureteral orifices. (For additional discussion of management of operative injuries to the urinary tract, refer to Chapter 9.)

Of intestinal injuries on a gynecology service, 37% occurred during incisions into the peritoneal cavity, 35% during lysis of adhesions in the pelvis, 10% during laparoscopy, and 18% during either dilatation and curettage or vaginal surgery.[20] One third of lacerations were major and required resection, and almost two thirds of the intestinal injuries occurred during what would have been otherwise uncomplicated gynecologic operations in which intestinal damage was neither expected nor planned for. Entering the abdomen above the superior limit of prior incision, as well as meticulous sharp dissection and gentle handling of tissue, were all believed to be time-honored techniques that would decrease but could not prevent all intestinal injuries. Injuries to the small intestine should be repaired immediately. Small bowel enterotomies should be closed at right angles to the long axis of the bowel to avoid stenosis. Drains are not necessary for small bowel injuries and repair.

Pelvic bleeding may be difficult to control during extensive operations for gynecologic malignancy such as debulking procedures or during extensive dissection for endometriosis or chronic pelvic inflammatory disease. Much has been written about methods to control postoperative (usually post-hysterectomy) bleeding. Without overstating the obvious, the best way to treat postoperative bleeding is to *avoid* the situation. This requires careful inspection to ensure that the pelvis is dry before wound closure. Although the decision as to when persistent oozing from raw pelvic peritoneal surfaces may be safely ignored is one that is a function of surgical experience, some general guidelines are useful.

There is no substitute for identification of the bleeding vessels. Almost any bleeding from any area in the pelvis may at least be initially controlled by direct pressure with a sponge stick or a laparotomy pack. After the initial control of the bleeding, blood products should be requested, consultation sought as indicated, special instruments obtained if needed, and the patient's condition stabilized hemodynamically. Control of bleeding from the infundibulopelvic ligament or the uterine vessels often requires a retroperitoneal approach to control hemorrhage and to avoid injury to the ureter. Persistent bleeding from diffuse areas in the pelvis or in veins too deep to ligate safely may respond to direct pressure with a hot pack and hypogastric ligation if simple pressure is not sufficient. Bilateral hypogastric artery ligation alone will control pelvic hemorrhage approximately 50% of the time.[21]

In unusual cases, pelvic hemorrhage will not be controlled by pressure, hot packs, or vessel ligation. It is imperative to recognize this situation. A large pelvic pack (15 feet of thick gauze) or a series of such packs tied together should be pushed hard into the pelvis against the pelvic surfaces and brought out through a stab incision made in the patient's lower abdominal wall.[22] This is a variation on the umbrella or mushroom pack first described by Logothetopulos in 1926.[23] The patient should be moved out of the operating room and into surgical intensive care as quickly as possible. The patient's coagulation studies must be checked immediately and fresh frozen plasma made available. MAST trousers may be of benefit.[24] Radiographic embolization of bleeding vessels may also be attempted.[25]

UNINTENTIONAL INJURY TO REPRODUCTIVE ORGANS

Good judgment comes from experience; some experience comes from bad judgment.

B. Patsner, M.D.

Unintentional injury to nonreproductive pelvic viscera such as bladder are unpleasant possible complications of any pelvic surgery but if properly managed should not produce any long-term alteration in the patient's quality of life. This is not the case for unintentional injury to reproductive organs that are to be preserved, such as the unplanned loss of an ovary in a patient with only one ovary or loss of a uterus during myomectomy. Gentle handling of tissue and performing surgery in a planned, unhurried manner when benign disease is at issue goes a long way to minimizing the likelihood of surgical error or mishap that may significantly alter or destroy the patient's fertility status.

Unplanned loss of an ovary may occur if ovarian cystectomy is poorly performed or if efforts to eradicate surface disease such as endometriosis result in injury to the vascular supply. Although the bulk of ovarian blood supply is through the infundibulopelvic ligament, there is collateral circulation through the uterine vessels through the broad ligament, and the ovary may be preserved even if the ovarian vessels are cut. Patients undergoing cystectomy must be informed of the possibility that the amount of remaining ovarian tissue may be small after a "conservative operation." Use of needle tip cautery, small scalpel (No. 15 blade), and small needle and suture material (4-0, 5-0 Vicryl on small, atraumatic needles) lessens the likelihood of injury to the remaining ovary that might necessitate resection.

A patient scheduled for myomectomy only will interpret hysterectomy as a sign that the operation was not a success.[26] Myomectomy instead of hysterectomy may be considered in a variety of circumstances (Table 5–9). Preoperative hysteroscopy to diagnose and resect submucous fibroids as well as evaluate tubal patency is recommended. Gonadotropin-releasing hormone agonists, such as leuprolide acetate, may be administered preoperatively to decrease the size of fibroids and potentially lessen blood loss associated with the surgical procedure.

A variety of different techniques have been proposed to lessen intraoperative blood loss at the time of myomectomy, among them clamps for the uterine and ovarian vessels, tourniquets or tape through the broad ligament to constrict the uterine vessels, and the injection of dilute vasopressin solution (1 ampule in 20 mL of normal saline) into the myometrium. Although there are no randomized, controlled series that compare these techniques, many gynecologists indicate that the use of vasopressin provides the driest operative field and minimizes the likelihood of uncontrolled bleeding or uterine artery injury, either of which would increase the likelihood of unplanned hysterectomy though the potential for delayed or unrecog-

TABLE 5–9
Indications for Myomectomy

Desire to retain childbearing status
Retention of uterus desired
Correction of infertility
Evaluation of rapidly enlarging myoma (e.g., rule out cancer)
Correct bleeding problems

nized bleeding from the suture line after the vasopressin effects wear off remains an uncommon but real risk.

THE DIFFICULT ABDOMINAL HYSTERECTOMY

On occasion even the most experienced gynecologic surgeon has difficulty completing an abdominal hysterectomy; the same may be said for total vaginal hysterectomy or even laparoscopic assisted hysterectomy. As with all surgery, proper patient selection and preoperative evaluation goes a long way toward avoiding some of these difficulties. Removing the uterus in patients undergoing surgery for advanced gynecologic malignancy or extensive endometriosis may be particularly challenging. In these situations, modifications of the standard approaches described in textbooks for simple abdominal hysterectomy may be useful. Three alterations in technique are suggested: (1) intentional cystotomy to facilitate anterior dissection; (2) "reverse hysterectomy" with entrance into the vagina followed by lateral and posterior dissection; and (3) supracervical hysterectomy.

Massive infiltration of the anterior leaf of the broad ligament or extensive scarring or fibrosis from multiple cesarean sections may make development of the bladder flap impossible.

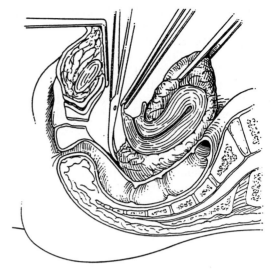

FIGURE 5–5
After incision of the posterior vaginal wall, the cul de sac mass can be sharply dissected from the rectosigmoid.

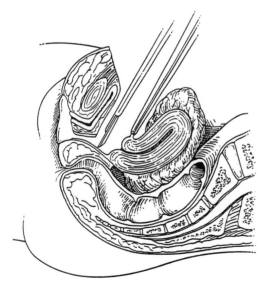

FIGURE 5–4
After ligation of the ovarian and uterine vessels and sharp dissection of the bladder from its attachments to the lower uterine segment and upper vagina, the anterior vagina is sharply entered.

Rather than create multiple unintentional bladder openings in an attempt to advance the bladder blindly, the dome of the bladder may be opened and the wall of the bladder held upward between thumb and forefinger to maximize traction and allow sharp dissection of the bladder off the lower uterine segment and cervix. Blunt dissection should not be used. On occasion, when lateral dissection is difficult, after the bladder has been advanced, the vagina may be entered anteriorly first and the cardinal ligaments then clamped upward toward the uterine vessels instead of from the uterine vessels down (Figs. 5–4 and 5–5). The surgeon should note that in situations in which this technique is used it will still be necessary to enter the retroperitoneum and identify the ureter to prevent the ureter from being cut when the uterine vessels are cut from below. Once the vagina has been entered anteriorly and the cardinal ligament transection begun it will then be easier to cut the posterior wall of the vagina and allow the uterus to be removed without lacerating the rectosigmoid. The technique is particularly useful when the normal tissue planes of the posterior pelvis are distorted or the cul de sac is obliterated by endometriosis, pelvic inflammatory disease, or tumor.

When extensive difficulty is encountered or the patient's condition is unstable, the hysterectomy may be concluded by either cutting through the cervix or amputating the specimen above the cervix (supracervical hysterectomy). So long as the cervix is known to be free of any pathologic process there is no medical contraindication to leaving the cervix. One must keep in mind that the patient may develop problems with abnormal bleeding or abnormal cervical cytologic findings that may prove challenging to evaluate. Removal of the cervix at a later date (trachelectomy) is difficult for the same reasons it was not removed at the first operation. Thus the cervix should be removed routinely, with exceptions made only in the most unusual surgical circumstances.

REFERENCES

1. Duff P, Park RD. Antibiotic prophylaxis in vaginal hysterectomy: a review. Obstet Gynecol 1980;55 (suppl):193.
2. Mittendorf R, Aronson MP, Berry RE, et al. Avoiding serious infections associated with abdominal hysterectomy: a meta-analysis of antibiotic prophylaxis. Am J Obstet Gynecol 1993;169:1119–1124.
3. Cruse PJE, Foord R. A five-year prospective study of 23,649 surgical wounds. Arch Surg 1973;107:206–214.
4. Orr JW Jr, Taylor PT Jr. Wound healing. In: Orr JW Jr, Shingleton HM, eds. Complications in Gynecologic Surgery: Prevention, Recognition and Management. Philadelphia, JB Lippincott; 1994, p 174.
5. Masterson BJ. Skin preparation. In: American College of Surgeons: Care of the Surgical Patient. New York, Scientific American, 1991.
6. Orr JW Jr, Orr PF, Barrett JM, et al. Fascial closure: continuous or interrupted? A prospective evaluation of #1 Maxon suture in 402 gynecologic procedures. Am J Obstet Gynecol 1990:163:1485–1489.
7. Morrow CP, Hernandez WL, Townsend DE, DiSaia PJ. Pelvic celiotomy in the obese patient. Am J Obstet Gynecol 1977;127:335–339.
8. Edlich FR, Rodeheaver GT, Thacker JG, Edgerton MT. Fundamentals of Wound Management in Surgery: Technical Factors in Wound Management. South Plainfield, NJ, Chirurgecom, 1977.
9. Johnson JC, Barnes WA. How to choose the right abdominal incision. Cont Obstet Gynecol 1993;3:56–73.
10. Patsner B. Abdominal hysterectomy: does type of clamp affect the incidence of postoperative pelvic infection? Obstet Gynecol Surv 1993;48:26506.
11. Sowe DE, Masterson BJ, Nealon N, von Fraunhofer JA. Effects of thermal knives on wound healing. Obstet Gynecol 1985;66:436–439.
12. Kenney A, Thomas DJ. The use of polyglycolic acid sutures to prevent vaginal vault granulations after total abdominal hysterectomy. JR Coll Surg Edinburgh 1978;23:230–233.
13. Callaghan P. Hands of the peritoneum. Lancet 1986;1:849–850.
14. Moss JP. Historical and current perspectives on surgical drainage. Surg Gynecol Obstet 1981;152:517–527.
15. Lubowski D, Hunt DR. Abdominal wound drainage: a prospective, randomized trial. Med J Aust 1987;146: 133–135.
16. Patsner B. Closed suction drainage versus no drainage following radical hysterectomy with pelvic lymphadenectomy for stage IB cervical cancer. Gynecol Oncol 1995;57:232–234.
17. Knapp RC, Donahue VC, Friedman EA. Dissection of paravesical and pararectal spaces in pelvic operations. Surg Gynecol Obstet 1973;137:758–762.
18. Hill EC. Exploring the anatomy of the retroperitoneum. Cont Obstet Gynecol 1986; pp 64–72.
19. Barnes WA, Delgado G. Retroperitoneal approaches to pelvic surgery. Cont Obstet Gynecol 1986; pp 83–92.
20. Krebs H-B. Intestinal injury in gynecologic surgery: a ten-year experience. Am J Obstet Gynecol 1986;155: 509–514.
21. Clark SL, Phelan JP, Yeh S, et al. Hypogastric artery ligation for obstetrical hemorrhage. Obstet Gynecol 1985;66:353–356.
22. Cassels JW, Greenberg H, Otterson WN. Pelvic tamponade in puerperal hemorrhage. J Reprod Med 1985;30:689–692.
23. Logothetopulos K. Eine absolut sichere Blutstillungs methode bei vaginalen under abdominalen gynakologischen operationen. Zentralbl Gynakol 1926;50:3203–3204.
24. Guerre EF, O'Keefe DF, Eliot JP, et al. Uncontrollable intra-abdominal hemorrhage treated with packing and use of a MAST suit. J Reprod Med 1987;32:230–232.
25. Greenwood LH, Glickman MG, Schwartz PE, et al. Obstetric and nonmalignant gynecologic bleeding: treatment with angiographic embolization. Radiology 1987;164:155–159.
26. LaMorte AL, Lalwani S, Diamond MP. Morbidity associated with abdominal myomectomy. Obstet Gynecol 1993;82:897–900.

Edward R. Kost
David G. Mutch

6

C H A P T E R

Hemorrhage

To expire by successive hemorrhage is perhaps the least painful of deaths, and yet it is the most awful. The repeated loss of blood so directly intimates approaching dissolution, and the patient feels his spirit and strength ebbing so perceptibly at each return of hemorrhagy, that he clings to life. Those of the most resolute mind are overcome with anxiety which they cannot conceal, and look round for some one to delay at least the fatal: and the surgeon feels himself so responsible, that with him it is truly an anxious scene.

John Bell, *The Principles of Surgery*[1]

Certainly one of the most stressful situations faced by the gynecologic surgeon is intraoperative or postoperative hemorrhage. A systematic, expedient, and technically proficient response is often necessary to reverse a clearly life-threatening situation. The gynecologic surgeon must be able to visualize the anatomic components of the abdomen and pelvis with a keen understanding of the various surgical planes and spaces as well as be familiar with the conventional measures used to control operative bleeding. When confronted with unanticipated hemorrhage the surgeon should be able to predict which vessels are injured and have a specific plan for managing the situation. This includes an understanding of the criteria for the intraoperative administration of blood products.

ANATOMY

An understanding of the anatomic distribution of the blood supply to the pelvis is central to safe gynecologic surgery. The vascular supply to the pelvis is derived predominately from the internal iliac (hypogastric) artery (Fig. 6–1). However, the collateral circulation of the female pelvis is extensive and provides a variety of intercommunicating sources of arterial blood from various sources along the arterial tree, a fact that often makes control of hemorrhage difficult. The internal iliac artery divides into an anterior and posterior division or trunk. The posterior division gives rise to three major vessels: the iliolumbar, lateral sacral, and superior gluteal arteries. These arteries provide important collateral circulation to the pelvis after selective ligation of anterior division of the hypogastric artery. The anterior division is the main visceral vascular supply to the organs of the pelvis. The pattern of branching of the anterior division is quite variable with as many as nine different major branching patterns with 49 different subtypes of branchings being described.[2] The anterior division includes five visceral and three parietal branches. The visceral branches include the uterine, superior vesical, middle hemorrhoidal, inferior hemorrhoidal, and vaginal, while the parietal branches include the obturator, inferior gluteal, and internal pudendal. Specific anatomic relationships are discussed in detail in reference to specific types of vascular injuries.

ARTERIAL BLEEDING

The arterial system is composed of vessels that deliver blood from the heart to the tissues. The

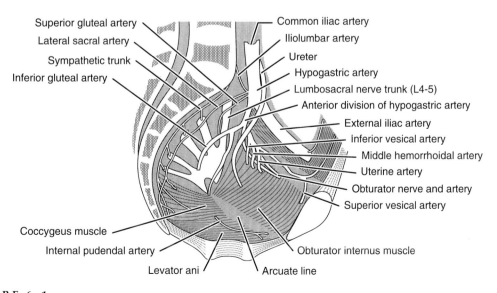

Superior gluteal artery
Lateral sacral artery
Sympathetic trunk
Inferior gluteal artery
Common iliac artery
Iliolumbar artery
Ureter
Hypogastric artery
Lumbosacral nerve trunk (L4-5)
Anterior division of hypogastric artery
External iliac artery
Inferior vesical artery
Middle hemorrhoidal artery
Uterine artery
Obturator nerve and artery
Superior vesical artery
Coccygeus muscle
Internal pudendal artery
Levator ani
Obturator internus muscle
Arcuate line

FIGURE 6–1
Anatomy of the pelvic floor, showing relationships of pelvic musculature, divisions of hypogastric artery, the pelvic ureter, and nerve plexuses.

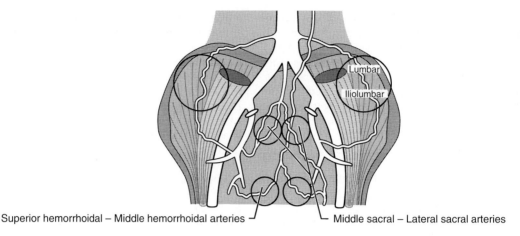

Superior hemorrhoidal – Middle hemorrhoidal arteries ⌐   ⌐ Middle sacral – Lateral sacral arteries

FIGURE 6–2
Principal anastomosis of the pelvic vessels. Lumbar-iliolumbar, middle sacral–lateral sacral, and superior hemorrhoidal–middle hemorrhoidal arteries.

histologic characteristics depend on the size of the vessel. Large vessels that must withstand stress and pressure contain large amounts of elastic tissue, whereas medium and small vessels contain less elastic tissue and more smooth muscle. Arterial bleeding is generally high pressure, pulsatile, and bright red. Because arteries do not possess intraluminal valves, blood flow can be bidirectional depending on the intra-arterial pressure gradient. The ability of blood to flow according to pressure gradients forms the basis for collateral circulation of the pelvis. Using aortograms obtained after internal iliac artery ligation, Burchell demonstrated the pathways of collateral flow.[3] Radiopaque material reached all arteries of the pelvis even after internal iliac artery ligation. Ligation alters the pathways and reverses the direction of flow in some arteries but does not prevent flow to any pelvic artery. The main collateral supply comes from the middle sacral, superior hemorrhoidal, and lumbar arteries (Fig. 6–2). An understanding of the various extrapelvic arteries that communicate with the pelvic circulation is important during a difficult hysterectomy because these vessels may create problems in achieving adequate hemostasis.

ARTERIAL INJURIES

Arterial injuries occurring during gynecologic surgery generally result from injury to the branches of the hypogastric artery. In general, treatment involves ligation of the involved vessel without resulting ischemic injury, owing to the extensive collateral circulation in the pelvis. However, injury to the common or external

iliac arteries requires surgical repair because these vessels provide blood supply to the lower extremity. Injury to these vessels may result from damage during placement of lateral trocar during laparoscopy, injury during lymph node dissection, or injury during difficult sidewall dissection. In most cases, the site of injury is readily apparent as pulsatile hemorrhage and the injury is repaired as described later. If there is unrecognized vascular compromise at the time of surgery, the patient may present in the postoperative period with evidence of compromise of the blood supply to the lower extremity manifested by the five Ps: *pulselessness, paresthesia, paralysis, pallor,* and *pain* at least one major joint below the site of injury. Other signs of damage to the external iliac artery include pallor, bluish mottling, coolness, and venous distention of the extremity.

Treatment of arterial injuries requires a well-planned sequence of actions.[4] Depending on the complexity of the injury, consultation with a vascular surgeon is recommended. Initially, the patient is stabilized with appropriate fluid and blood product administration. Antibiotic prophylaxis is given. A wide operative field is necessary to localize efficiently the site of arterial injury. Dissection is performed along the pathway of the involved vessels to gain proximal control of bleeding. Subsequently, an effort is made to gain distal control of bleeding. Inspection of the site of injury is made to determine the extent of repair. Bleeding is controlled with vascular clamps placed 2 to 3 cm proximal and distal to the site of bleeding. The proximal clot is removed by flushing with heparin, while the distal clot is removed manually or by passing a Fogarty balloon catheter. Local heparinization is performed to inhibit further clot formation. If greater than 1 to 2 cm of artery will need to be resected, a graft should be used. Excess adventitia and detached or injured intima is excised. The injury is repaired using a continuous, fine monofilament suture of 5-0 or 6-0 polyethylene placed 2 mm from the cut ends with bites 2 mm apart. Sutures should be everting. If a saphenous vein graft is used, it should be in reversed direction so that the valves do not obstruct blood flow. After the sutures are placed the proximal clamp is removed first, allowing air and blood to exit through the suture line. After the distal clamp is removed, gentle pressure is applied over the suture line. Pulses are checked in the distal extremity. Attempts should be made to cover the artery with fascia.

VENOUS BLEEDING

The venous system functions to return blood to the heart, as well as to regulate the vascular capacity and as a peripheral pump mechanism during exercise. Veins possess muscle and collagen but have considerably less elastic tissue than arterioles. Veins are thin-walled, low-pressure vessels. In contrast to arteries, veins have intraluminal valves that restrict bidirectional flow. Large veins such as the external iliac, common iliac, and vena cava lack valves. The veins that drain the pelvis originate from an extensive venous plexus before ending in the same named branches as the arteries. The exiting branches of the internal iliac vein are thin-walled, fixed, and fragile. The major veins in this area are a branching system that may have smaller veins entering their lateral and inferior surfaces, making visualization and repair extremely difficult.

VENOUS INJURIES

A thorough knowledge of the venous anatomy of the abdomen and pelvis enables the gynecologic surgeon to anticipate potential areas of venous injury. During lymph node dissection for gynecologic malignancy the surgeon is frequently operating in close proximity to the common, internal, and external iliac veins, as well as the vena cava. During dissection of the lymphatics of the right common and external iliac vessels the thin walls of the iliac veins may be traumatized if their precise boundaries are not delineated. The right common iliac artery courses on the medial side of the common iliac vein near its proximal portion but deviates to the lateral side of the external iliac vein as it approaches the femoral canal. The left common and the external iliac arteries remain on the lateral side of the corresponding iliac vein throughout the entire course of the left iliac vessels. Therefore, the lateral aspects of the

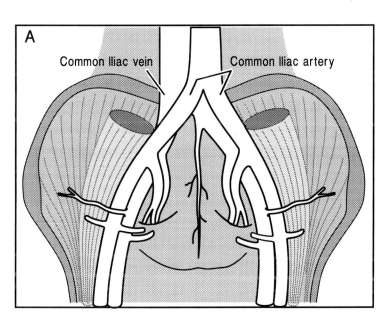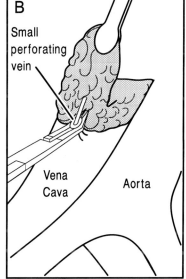

FIGURE 6–3
(A) Relationship of the iliac arteries and veins. *(B)* The small vein is identified as one elevates the nodal tissue off the vena cava.

left common and external iliac arteries can be dissected without danger of trauma to the vein, which will always be medial to the arteries (Fig. 6–3A).

The inferior vena cava can be easily injured in the process of performing a para-aortic dissection. Damage to the vena cava may cause massive hemorrhage, which if not initially managed correctly may result in having to resort to inferior vena caval ligation. To avoid injury to the vena cava during lymph node dissection, one should look for a rather constant small vein existing in the nodal bundle and entering the vena cava just above its bifurcation (see Fig. 6–3B). Generally, as one elevates the nodal tissue the vein is either avulsed or, worse, tears a small strip in the wall of the vena cava. Injury to the vena cava may also occur as a result of Veress needle puncture during laparoscopy.

The repair of venous injuries is difficult and at times impossible. Thrombosis at the site of repair commonly occurs and is associated with the risk of pulmonary embolism. Certain authorities believe that reconstruction of the innominate, common femoral, and popliteal veins is especially important and should be attempted because of the demonstrable inadequacies of the collateral flow.[4] On the other hand, the entire internal iliac venous tree may often be ligated with impunity, as may any of its branches. One need not preserve the integrity of this vein to continue vascular function of the pelvis. Often the precise location of the venous bleeding is difficult to recognize, owing to the low pressure of the venous system. Venous injury is frequently characterized by dark, steady bleeding and may be difficult to differentiate from a hematoma or small arterial bleeding vessels.

While treatment of pelvic venous bleeding frequently involves ligation of the involved vessel, ligation of the common or external iliac veins may result in significant venous congestion resulting in massive edema and a cool, blue extremity. Therefore, injuries of the vena cava, common iliac vein, and external iliac vein are best repaired. Treatment of venous injuries requires a well-planned sequence of actions.[5] The hemorrhage is initially controlled with judicious pressure or packing. This will also prevent air passage into the vein, preventing air embolus. The patient is stabilized with appropriate fluid and blood product administration. Appropriate antibiotic prophylaxis is initiated. Dissection is performed along the pathway of the involved vessels to gain proximal and distal control of bleeding. If a coexist-

ing arterial injury is found, the artery is repaired first. Due to the low pressure nature of the venous system, hemostasis can usually be obtained by applying direct pressure with a sponge stick. If the injury is large and repair is anticipated, vascular tapes can be encircled around the vein, serving as a temporary tourniquet. Methods of repair include ligation, lateral suture repair, end–end anastomosis, venous patch graft, and venous replacement graft.[6] The choice of repair depends on the type of vessel and its location. Specific strategies for management and repair of venous injury will be discussed later in this chapter. General principles of venous repair include exploration of the vein and removal of thrombus. Repairs are performed with fine synthetic suture and small needles. Continuous sutures are used, and less tension is applied than with arterial repairs.

CRITERIA FOR THE INTRAOPERATIVE ADMINISTRATION OF BLOOD PRODUCTS, FRESH FROZEN PLASMA, AND VOLUME EXPANDERS

Whole blood can be separated and stored as individual components, a process aided by the development of plastic bags. This allows the administration of only the specific components needed by the patient.

Each blood product needs to be correctly identified before being administered. Most hospitals require two individuals to independently check the identification of each unit before it is administered. The blood product should be transfused through a filter. Standard filters are found in blood administration sets. Special leukocyte depleting filters that remove most of the white blood cells may be used to prevent febrile episodes during transfusion. Only normal saline should be used with blood products to prevent damage to the blood components. Unless administration exceeds 50 mL/kg/h, blood products do not necessarily need to be warmed before transfusion.[7]

Red blood cells are replaced to increase oxygen-carrying capacity and in response to hypotension secondary to blood loss. Each unit of packed red blood cells will, on average, increase the hemoglobin by 1 g/dL. Oxygen-carrying capacity is adequate in most people when the hemoglobin is greater than 7 g/dL. Therefore, transfusion of packed red blood cells is appropriate when the patient has a hemoglobin of 7 g/dL or less or when the patient is symptomatic from ongoing bleeding.

Transfusions should be initiated at higher hemoglobin levels in patients with illnesses that decrease tissue oxygen delivery such as chronic lung or cardiovascular disease.

Volume expansion using packed red blood cells and normal saline or lactated Ringer's solution is appropriate for almost all cases of shock. Only when the total volume loss exceeds 25% should whole blood be considered for replacement. Even in this extreme situation, packed red blood cells, fresh frozen plasma, and crystalloid are generally considered to be comparable to whole blood.

Blood products are usually stored in solutions containing citrate-phosphate-dextrose or citrate-phosphate-dextrose adenine-1. The life of red blood cells stored in the former is 21 to 35 days and 35 days when stored in the latter. Occasionally, red blood cells may be frozen at $-80°$ C and can then be stored in glycerol for up to 3 years. Unfortunately, frozen blood is not very practical in the acute situation because of the time required to thaw and wash the cells.

Platelet transfusion may be required when there is a deficiency of circulating platelets, as might occur in an acute massive hemorrhage. One unit of platelets will usually increase the platelet count in the average woman by 5,000 to 10,000/mm³. Administration of platelets should always be performed through a blood filter. Platelets should never be given prophylactically even in the case of massive hemorrhage. Rather, the platelet counts should be followed and the patient transfused when clinically indicated. In general, the platelet count should be above 50,000/mm³ before and during operative procedures. Fresh frozen plasma and platelets should be adequate to correct most coagulopathies. Coagulation studies should be obtained after every 5 to 10 units of blood loss to assess the need for these blood products. Fresh frozen plasma should be administered only when indicated by coagulation studies that show a prothrombin time or partial thromboplastin time of one and one-half times normal.

THE USE OF THE CELL SAVER

Intraoperative blood salvage can be accomplished by a device known as the cell saver, which can harvest, clean, and readminister autologous blood to the patient during a surgical procedure. In theory, one could avoid transfusions by using the cell saver in all patients. Unfortunately, this technique is not appropriate in many surgical cases, including most cases of pelvic surgery. Practical reasons for not using the cell saver in pelvic surgery include (1) the cell saver requires at least 500 mL for priming; (2) it is expensive to use and maintain; and (3) it is contraindicated in bowel cases or other surgical procedures where there may be bacterial contamination such as the violation of the vaginal cuff. Some centers also discourage the use of the cell saver in cancer patients, especially in cases in which there may be direct contamination from malignant cells.

KEYS FOR THE CONTROL OF INTRAOPERATIVE BLEEDING

Packs

Control of bleeding from the vaginal cuff and the surrounding tissues of the pelvic floor is a major concern to gynecologists. The use of direct pressure to stop bleeding is a basic maneuver in surgical practice, enhancing the body's intrinsic coagulation cascade. In circumstances in which bleeding persists despite standard hemostatic maneuvers (e.g., direct vessel suturing or clipping, ligation of the hypogastric and ovarian vessels) the pelvis can be packed, thus applying direct pressure to the pelvic sidewalls and floor. Several techniques have been described.

The Logothetopulos vaginal pack, first described in 1926, was designed to be of assistance in compressing the retracted, bleeding vessels in the pelvis.[8] The pack, prepared and sterilized before surgery, consists of 6 yards of 4-inch-wide gauze roll laminated into a 2-ply gauze veil measuring 24 × 24 inches. This can be used in an umbrella fashion within the pelvic cavity by bringing the four corners of the opened gauze together with one end of the gauze roll protruding. This is marked with a suture for identification. The body of the pack is then shaped like a ball and the distal ends of the pack are twisted to form a stalk and tied with a ligature. The ligature is attached to an eyed probe, which is passed through the vaginal cuff or perineal defect. The ureters are placed over the pack. Traction is applied on the free margins of the pack as it is pulled through the vaginal vault. Traction is maintained by placing a large ring pessary over the stalk flush against the perineum. After 48 hours, the stalk is soaked in saline and hydrogen peroxide; and the inner roll of gauze, which had been previously marked, is pulled out. The veil may be pulled out at the same time or 24 hours later. Analgesia may be necessary before removing the pack. This approach attempts to compress the bleeding vessels against the bony and fascial resistance of the pelvis. A further advantage is that the packing can be removed through the vagina without the need for reopening the abdomen. The effectiveness and safety of the Logothetopulos pack have been well documented.[9, 10] To avoid the potential complications of provoking fresh hemorrhage and the adherence of the pack to intestines and ureter with the potential for subsequent fistula formation, Parente and coworkers employed a nonwet polyethylene sheet rather than gauze as the external veil.[10]

Masterson described an alternative technique for control of pelvic hemorrhage.[11] In this procedure the pelvis is tightly packed with a large breast roll gauze and the gauze is layered into the pelvis in such a way that its removal will not produce knots, causing difficulty in its extraction from the wound. Before placement the upper portion of the roll is soaked in povidone-iodine (Betadine) and brought out the edge of the abdominal wound. The wound is then closed with retention sutures and a 4- to 5-cm defect is left for pack removal. If bleeding is controlled, the patient is brought back to the operating room in 48 hours. A light anesthetic is administered, and the pack is removed. The wound is gently irrigated to remove any superficial hematoma. Retention sutures are placed, and care is taken not to manipulate the area of old venous injury. Although hernias are increased when packs are used through the incision, little other morbidity has been noted.[11]

Drains

The history of surgical drains begins with the writing of Hippocrates (circa 406 BC), but their postoperative use, indications, and efficacy remain controversial.[12] The dictum "when in doubt, drain" from Lawson Trait is well known to most gynecologic surgeons.[13] Although most surgeons agree that drainage of obvious collection of pus or blood is appropriate, their prophylactic use is still debated. Halsted suggested that "no drainage at all is better than the ignorant employment of it."[12] Unfortunately, tradition, institutional, and individual bias too often determine the current practices of the type and duration of pelvic drainage. Prophylactic drainage is intended to prevent the accumulation of blood, pus, and bile, and rarely to

permit the early detection of surgical complications. Drainage is not a substitute for good surgical technique and meticulous hemostasis. Complications that have been reported from drains include site sepsis, bleeding from abdominal wall vessels, incisional hernia, and evisceration of small bowel. Predisposing factors included general debility, corticosteroid administration, increased intra-abdominal pressure, and stab incisions for drains that had external diameters of more than 1 cm.[13]

At the time of radical surgery for gynecologic malignancy, venous oozing may occur from tumor beds, raw peritoneal surfaces, and various dissection beds. The use of closed suction drains may be used in these cases both to remove accumulated blood and as a sentinel drain to follow the amount and concentration of the bloody drainage. The method of drain placement consists of a separate stab incision made with a scalpel well away from the incision. A clamp is than passed through the stab incision and passed through the abdominal wall with care to puncture the fascia far enough away from the incision that the drain will not be included in the fascial closure. Care is taken to avoid damage to bowel, bladder, and blood vessels as the clamp is passed through the abdominal wall. The surgeon may place a hand on the posterior aspect of the abdominal wall at the site of puncture, thus protecting the abdominal contents. The drain is secured to the skin with silk suture. The amount of drainage is closely followed in the postoperative period, and if it is grossly bloody a hematocrit can be obtained on the fluid. If the amount of drainage and the hematocrit of the fluid reflect active bleeding, the patient is stabilized by appropriate volume resuscitation. Coagulopathy, if present, should also be corrected. If after these measures the patient continues to show evidence of active bleeding, consideration is given to reexploration. Removal of the drain depends on the initial indication for drainage. If the drain is placed as a sentinel drain to detect blood accumulation in the abdominal cavity, then once the surgeon is assured that the patient is hemodynamically stable, the drain may be removed.

Thumbtacks

The use of thumbtacks for the control of hemorrhage from the presacral plexus is described in the gynecologic literature.[14] Situations in which the use of thumbtacks have been reported include the control of presacral hemorrhage resulting from presacral neurectomy, abdominal sacral colpopexy, cytoreductive surgery for ovarian cancer, pelvic exenteration, proctectomy, abdominoperineal resection, and low anterior resection.[14–18] When bleeding is not controlled by packing, clips, bone wax, or ligature, the application of a steel thumbtack on the points of active bleeding has been reported to result in immediate cessation of the bleeding (Fig. 6–4). It is important that the thumbtacks are made of a metal such as stainless steel that will not corrode. If difficulty is encountered in pushing the pointed end into the hardened sacrum, a flat instrument, such as a retractor, can be used as a lever. Alternatively the thumbtack may be placed using a Kelly clamp. Timmons and coworkers have described an instrument designed to afford easier and more precise anterior sacral application of thumbtacks.[16] The instrument consists of a 12-inch long stainless steel rod with a recess in one end, the diameter of which precisely accommodates the head of the thumbtack. The recession terminates with a small magnet fixed into the rod that effectively holds the thumbtack. The stainless steel rod can be constructed with various bends to enable greater flexibility for thumbtack placement. Regardless of the method of application, the thumbtack should be pushed in so that the flat top rests flush against the presacral fascia and bone. Three additional points deserve mention. First, the risk for subsequent development of sacral osteomyelitis from this technique is not known but must be kept in mind during patient follow-up. Second, there has been a case in which several of the thumbtacks used in the presacral space detached. It was not known whether injury to the internal viscera and organs occurred secondary to the loose thumbtacks. Third, both surgeons and pathologists must use caution when exploring the pelvic or abdominal cavities after pelvic procedures in which thumbtacks were used owing to the considerable danger posed by these sharp objects.

Hypogastric Artery Ligation

One of the most effective and rapid methods of controlling severe pelvic hemorrhage is by ligation of both hypogastric arteries. The hemodynamics of this procedure were studied by Burchell.[3] Bilateral ligation of the internal iliac artery decreased the mean arterial pressure by 24%, the mean blood flow by 48%, and the pulse pressure by about 85%. The reduction in pulse pressure is clearly the most important reason for the hemostatic effect of internal iliac artery ligation. The high-pressure arterial system is converted to a relatively low-pressure system, and compression alone is sufficient to permit thrombosis of the bleeding vessel to occur. Burchell did not report adverse effects from ligation of the internal iliac artery proximal to the posterior division; however, others have reported necrosis of the tissue in the buttock region resulting from occlusion of the posterior division.[19] Because of the important collateral circulation with the femoral and aortic systems, it is recommended to ligate the anterior division of the hypogastric artery distal to the posterior parietal branches.

Ligation of the internal iliac artery is a relatively simple procedure that may well be life-saving (Fig. 6–5). It is considered essential that all residents in obstetrics and gynecology be trained to perform this operation. In ligating the hypogastric artery, the peritoneum is opened on the lateral side of the common iliac artery near its bifurcation. The ureter is identified and left attached to the medial peritoneal reflection to avoid disturbing its blood supply. The common, internal, and external iliac arteries must be clearly identified because inadvertent ligation of the common or external iliac artery results in vascular compromise to the lower extremity. The posterior branch of the hypogastric artery originates near the origin of the hypogastric artery on its posterior surface. This division must be clearly identified before the selection of the point of ligation. Good exposure is essential. Development of the pararectal and paravesical spaces improves exposure of the operative field and better defines the anatomic structures. The two structures at greatest risk are the ureter and the hypogastric

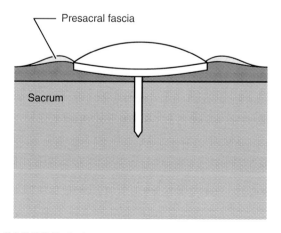

FIGURE 6–4
Cross section of thumbtack tamponading presacral vessel.

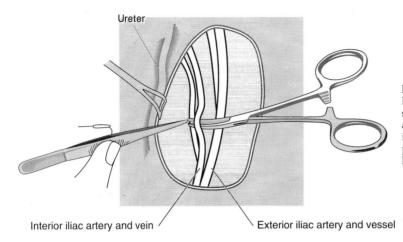

Ureter

Interior iliac artery and vein

Exterior iliac artery and vessel

FIGURE 6–5
Ligation of hypogastric artery, showing peritoneal reflection with attached ureter and bifurcation of iliac artery and vein. Silk suture is placed around anterior division of hypogastric artery.

vein. The hypogastric vein is deep and lateral to the artery and may be damaged as instruments and ties are passed around the artery. The artery may be gently grasped with a medium-sized Babcock clamp, then gently mobilized by blunt dissection with the use of a blunt-tipped right-angled clamp. After the artery is dissected and mobilized free from the vein, nonabsorbable suture (1-0 silk) is passed around the artery with a right-angled clamp, always passing the tips of the clamp from lateral to medial under the artery to avoid damage to the hypogastric vein. A second free-tie is placed distal to the initial ligature to avoid recanalization. Transection of the vessel is not essential or desirable in this procedure. Hypogastric artery (anterior division) ligation is performed bilaterally.

Use of Microfibrillar Collagen, Oxidized Regenerated Cellulose, Absorbable Gelatin, Thrombin Preparations, and Fibrin Glue

In situations in which venous oozing persists despite standard measures, several hemostatic materials are available to the surgeon that can be locally applied to areas of bleeding. Microfibrillar collagen preparations consist of purified bovine collagen (Avitene, MedCheur Products, Inc., Woburn, MA 01801; Instat, Johnson and Johnson Medical, Inc., Arlington, TX 76004-0130). Hemostatic activity, which is an inherent property of collagen, is largely dependent on the basic helical structure of collagen. When collagen comes into contact with blood, platelets aggregate on the collagen and release coagulation factors that, together with plasma factors, result in the formation of fibrin, and

finally in the formation of a clot. Microfibrillar collagen cannot control bleeding due to systemic coagulation disorders. Appropriate therapy to correct the underlying coagulopathy should be instituted before use of the product. Indications for the use of microfibrillar collagen include its use as an adjunct to hemostasis when control of capillary, venous, and arteriolar bleeding by pressure, ligature, and other conventional methods is ineffective or impractical. It should not be used in instances of pumping arterial hemorrhage. The surgeon should not rely on any agent for control of a significant amount of arterial or venous bleeding. Every effort should be made to identify the bleeding vessel and to occlude it with either a hemoclip or a ligature. Microfibrillar collagen should not be used in the closure of skin incisions because it may interfere with the healing of skin edges. In addition, it should not be employed on bony surfaces because it may significantly reduce bond strength for methylmethacrylate adhesives. As with any foreign substance, use in contaminated wounds may enhance infection. It is recommended that the excess material should be removed after hemostasis is obtained because reported cases of bowel adhesion or mechanical pressure sufficient to compromise the ureter have been reported. Microfibrillar collagen should be applied with pressure directly to the bleeding surface. Surfaces to be treated are blotted to remove excess blood, and pressure should be applied between 2 to 5 minutes, depending on the type of bleeding. Although microfibrillar collagen may be left in situ whenever necessary, it is recommended that the excess material be removed for the previously stated reasons. Animal studies have shown that absorption occurs in 8 to 10 weeks.

Oxidized regenerated cellulose (Surgicel,

Johnson and Johnson Medical, Inc., Arlington, TX 76004-0130) is an absorbable hemostatic. Its mechanism of action is not completely understood, but it appears to be a physical effect rather than an alteration of the normal physiologic clotting mechanism. After it has been saturated with blood, it swells into a black or brown gelatinous mass that aids in the formation of a clot, thereby serving as a hemostatic adjunct in the control of local hemorrhage. The indications for use are similar to those of microfibrillar collagen. Minimal amounts of Surgicel in appropriate size are laid on the bleeding site or held firmly against the tissues until hemostasis is obtained. In contrast to the microfibrillar collagen compounds, oxidized regenerated cellulose is strong and can be sutured or cut without fraying. In addition to its local hemostatic properties, Surgicel is bactericidal in vitro against a wide variety of gram-positive and gram-negative organisms.[20] Animal studies show that it does not tend to enhance experimental infections.[21, 22] Although Surgicel may be left in situ when necessary, it is advisable to remove it once hemostasis is achieved. It must always be removed from the site of application when used around areas of bony confines, such as the obturator space, because Surgicel, by swelling, may exert pressure, resulting in paralysis or nerve damage.

Absorbable gelatin sponge, Gelfoam (Upjohn, Kalamazoo, MI) is a water-soluble, hemostatic product prepared from purified pork skin gelatin USP granules. The mechanism of action is not completely understood, but it appears to be a physical effect rather than any alteration of the normal physiologic clotting mechanism. The indications for use are similar to those of microfibrillar collagen. The Gelfoam is cut to the desired size, is saturated with sterile saline or left dry, and is applied with pressure directly to the bleeding site. It should be held in place with moderate pressure until hemostasis results. A second application can be performed if necessary. Once hemostasis is attained, excess Gelfoam should be carefully removed. When not used in excessive amounts, Gelfoam is completely absorbed without inducing excessive scar formation.[23–25] Barnes reviewed experiences with Gelfoam in gynecologic surgery.[25] No excessive scar tissue, attributable to the absorption of Gelfoam, could be palpated at postoperative examination. Although Gelfoam has been used during intravascular catheterization for the purpose of producing vessel occlusion, this application is not recommended by the manufacturer.

Topical thrombin (Thrombogen, Johnson and Johnson Medical, Inc., Arlington, TX 76004-0130) is indicated as an aid in hemostasis wherever oozing blood from capillaries and small venules is accessible. Thrombogen is a protein substance produced by a conversion reaction in which prothrombin of bovine origin is activated by tissue thromboplastin in the presence of sodium chloride. Thrombin requires no intermediate physiology for its action because it clots the fibrinogen of the blood directly. Failure to clot blood occurs in the rare cases where the clotting defect is the absence of fibrinogen itself. It is imperative that Thrombogen not be injected or otherwise be allowed to enter large blood vessels. Extensive intravascular clotting and even death may result. Topical application may be performed using the dry powder or a spray form, or the surface may be flooded using a sterile syringe and small-gauge needle. The most effective hemostasis results when the Thrombogen mixes freely with the blood as soon as it reaches the surface. Thrombogen may be used in conjunction with absorbable gelatin sponges.

Fibrin glue is a natural adhesive that duplicates and enhances the final stages of normal coagulation. In the presence of calcium chloride, a fibrin monomer is formed when fibrinogen is mixed with thrombin. This is then transformed into a strong polymer in the presence of cryoprecipitate that contains factor XIII. The use of fibrin glue has been reported to be highly effective in controlling surface, especially venous, bleeding as well as bleeding that is not suitably managed by suturing due to the location of the bleeding, friable tissues, or adhesions.[26, 27] An additional advantage is that the mechanism by which fibrin glue acts is not dependent on host intrinsic clotting factors. It therefore may be used to successfully control local hemorrhage in the presence of severe coagulopathy. Several delivery systems are described in the literature.[28, 29] Ten milliliters of cryoprecipitate is thawed and allowed to come to room temperature. Thrombin is reconstituted in 10 mL of sterile saline to a concentration of 1000 units/mL. The two substances are simultaneously and slowly injected onto the site of bleeding such that the solutions mix in situ. A fibrin coagulum is formed instantaneously and is gently compressed with gauze if possible. Multiple applications can be performed if necessary to obtain hemostasis.

Intra-Arterial Embolization

In patients who are considered too ill to tolerate surgery, or those with extensive malignant disease in the pelvis, embolization of the hypogastric arteries has been advocated as an alternative therapy.[30, 31] Furthermore this technique has been shown to be of great value in cases where bleeding persists after ligation of the internal iliac arteries.[32] Embolization is performed with the use of special catheters under radiologic guidance. Percutaneous catheterization of the femoral artery under local anesthesia provides direct access in a retrograde manner to the hypogastric artery or one of the other collateral vessels if prior hypogastric artery ligation had been performed. It is important to identify the bleeding site accurately and to embolize the vessel at that level. When the site of bleeding is identified by angiography, the vessel is cannulated and hemostatic material is injected. The choice of material used for the embolization depends on the desired duration of the occlusion and the size of the vessel. Gelfoam soaked in saline or contrast media can be used in small vessels, whereas wire coils are more suitable for larger vessels where they cause a severe inflammatory reaction in the vessel with clot formation.[33] Where occlusion is not wanted permanently, autogenous blood clot can be used that will recanalize within 36 to 48 hours.[31] Reported complications of intra-arterial embolization include allergy to the contrast medium, hematoma or abscess formation at the puncture site, infarction of the target site, and embolization of nontarget organs.[34] However, no significant complications have been reported as a direct result of embolization in the pelvis.[30, 35]

SPECIFIC SITUATIONS

Rectus Muscle Hematoma and Bleeding Secondary to Avulsion of the Inferior Epigastric Vessel

Introduction of the trocar/cannula into the lower quadrants of the abdomen during laparoscopic procedures may result in damage to abdominal wall vessels. While diagnostic laparoscopy involves placement of predominantly midline trocars, operative laparoscopy usually involves the lateral placement of at least one large-diameter trocar. The blood vessels at risk for injury depend on the level of placement (Fig. 6–6). Immediately above the pubic crest, both the superficial and inferior epigastric vessels are at risk for injury. In thin patients the superficial epigastric vessels may be visualized by transillumination of the anterior abdominal wall via the laparoscope. In contrast, the inferior epigastric vessels may often be visualized directly through the laparoscope. The risk of vessel injury may be minimized by placing trocars medial to the obliterated umbilical artery or lateral to the round ligament insertion. As one approaches the umbilicus, both the medial vessels (superficial and deep epigastric) and the lateral vessels (superficial and deep circumflex iliac) are at risk for injury. The inferior epigastric vessels originating from the external iliac vessels run from the pelvic side wall to course deep to the rectus muscle. Placement of trocars at what are estimated to be the

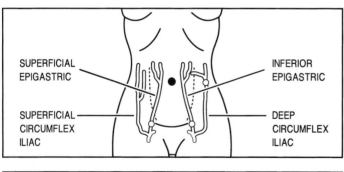

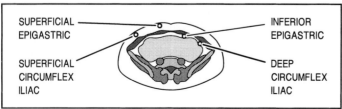

FIGURE 6–6
Approximate location of the superficial and deep vessels of the anterior abdominal wall, frontal and axial views. In the frontal view, dashed lines indicate relative location of the lateral margin of the rectus abdominis muscle. In the axial view, taken at 1 cm below the umbilicus, rectus muscles are indicated in dark gray.

lateral margins of the rectus muscle should minimize vessel injury. Injuries to the inferior epigastric vessels above the pubic crest are particularly troublesome because the vessels are tethered to the anterior abdominal peritoneum and are unable to retract.

Predisposing factors for vessel injury include lateral trocar placement, the use of large-caliber trocars, and repeated reinsertion of trocars. Therefore, when it is necessary to place lateral trocars, one should consider using those with the smallest diameter possible. When larger trocars are needed, they should be placed in the relatively avascular midline. Trocar sleeves should be secured in place either by suturing to the skin or by use of a trocar sleeve with a coarse screw profile that effectively locks the trocar in place.

Vessel injury may result in severe bruising of the anterior abdominal wall, which may track around the lateral wall and extend into the thighs. Abdominal wall hematoma or, rarely, significant intra-abdominal hemorrhage may also occur. If a vessel of significant size is damaged, the bleeding may leak from the incision or from the trocar site, being visible intra-abdominally as drainage around the shaft of the cannulae. Such bleeding is often tamponaded by the time the procedure is completed. Unless the bleeding is obviously from a large arterial vessel, the cannulae should not be removed but steps taken to control the bleeding. For bleeding that persists, a fairly simple laparoscopic approach consists of passing a heavy-gauge suture (1-0 Maxon or PDS) on a large straight needle through the full thickness of the abdominal wall under laparoscopic visualization.[36, 37] Once the needle has penetrated the peritoneum, it is grasped with self-locking forceps through a second port, then passed through the abdominal wall again. The suture is subsequently tightly knotted on one side of the trocar. Once the laparoscopic procedure is completed, the trocar is removed under direct visualization and the site is carefully inspected for bleeding. Unfortunately because the injured vessels are not selectively ligated, patient movement during the postoperative period may result in significant bleeding. If the surgeon is not certain that adequate hemostasis has been achieved, consideration should be given to widening the incision, selectively grasping the injured vessel with fine vascular forceps, and occluding the vessel by appropriate means. The trocar should be left in place until immediately before repair to help localize the site of vessel injury. Alternatively, tamponade using a Foley catheter placed into the tro-

car site for 24 hours has been suggested to control hemorrhage after abdominal wall vessel injuries.[38]

When a rectus muscle hematoma develops after an unrecognized vascular injury, the patient may present in the postoperative period with bleeding from a trocar site with associated swelling and tenderness to palpation. Acute evaluation should focus on determining the extent of bleeding. If the patient is hemodynamically stable, initial management is direct pressure at the puncture site. The patient is observed for a minimum of several hours. If the size of the hematoma is stable, she is sent home with strict precautions and is seen back in the office within 24 hours. No attempt should be made to aspirate or open a stable hematoma, because this may increase the risk of abscess formation.[39] If there is evidence that the hematoma is enlarging despite the application of direct pressure, it should be opened and drained.

The following is an approach to the scenario of a rectus muscle hematoma. A midline vertical skin incision is made to allow adequate exposure to the proximal and distal aspect of the hematoma. The anterior rectus sheath is incised, and the superior extent of the hematoma is identified. The rectus muscle is gently retracted laterally, and the inferior epigastric vessels are identified coursing on the inferior aspect of the muscle. As soon as one has reached the superior aspect of the hematoma the inferior epigastric vessels are dissected out and ligated under direct visualization. The hematoma is removed, and the dissection bed is carefully inspected for venous contributors. The area is copiously irrigated and a No. 7 Jackson-Pratt closed suction drain is placed in the area of the hematoma. The use of prophylactic antibiotics may be considered, but there are no data to suggest that this decreases the incidence of abscess formation.

Presacral Venous Plexus Bleeding

On rare occasions, hemorrhage from the presacral venous plexus derived from the middle sacral veins can be life threatening. The explanation for the difficulty in obtaining hemostasis lies in the anatomy of the region. Qinyao and colleagues studied the morphologic features of venous passage on the pelvic surface of the sacrum in 100 pieces of randomly selected sacrum.[18] The presacral veins were found to be formed not only by the lateral and medial sacral veins and their tributaries (the presacral venous plexus) but also by the sacral basivertebral veins. The thin-walled basivertebral veins freely communicate with the presacral plexus. The majority of the sacral basivertebral veins originated as open canals in the spongiosa of the sacral body before emerging from their foramina. The adventitia of these veins are blended with the sacral periosteum at the margin of the openings of their foramina, forming an anatomic "anchor structure." During surgery when the presacral fascia is lifted together with the periosteum on the sacrum, the sacral basivertebral veins are easily lacerated near their foramina with the ruptured ends retracting into their foramina. Because the bleeding vessels are frequently retracted into the bony foramina, conventional hemostatic measures including cautery, suture ligation, hot packs, hypogastric artery ligation, use of absorbable gelatin sponge or microfibrillar collagen, or packing with bone wax may not be sufficient.

When bleeding occurs from the presacral area, laparotomy sponges are immediately placed and held by compression for several minutes. If this does not effectively stop the bleeding, additional hemostatic maneuvers are initiated. Exposure of the bleeding points may be enhanced by maintaining pressure over the lower bleeding points. Starting at the superior aspect of the dissection individual bleeding points are defined. Two hemostatic measures have proved effective for bleeding from the sacral basivertebral vein foramina: packing with bone wax and the use of thumbtacks.[40] In the first technique the foramen is broken with a blunt-ended instrument and the vessel is packed with bone wax. In the second technique stainless steel thumbtacks are pressed into each

bleeding foramen as previously described (Fig. 6–7). Ligation of the bilateral internal iliac arteries will have no effect on the hydrostatic pressure of the sacral venous pool because this is not a major blood supply to the sacral region. Furthermore, ligation of the bilateral internal iliac veins may actually aggravate presacral bleeding because the normal venous blood flow of the pelvic venous plexus will be completely obstructed, and consequently more blood coming from these veins will be directed to the injured presacral venous plexus veins through the lateral sacral veins.

Obturator Foramen and Bleeding

The obturator vessels and nerve course on the pelvic sidewall, exiting the pelvis through the obturator foramen. These structures are intimately involved with the lymph node–bearing tissue commonly removed during surgery for gynecologic malignancy. The anatomy of the obturator space is somewhat variable. In a study of 283 limbs, the obturator artery arose from the internal iliac artery in 70%, from the inferior epigastric in 25.4%, and nearly equally from both in 4.6%.[41] In the majority of patients the obturator artery and vein course deep to the obturator nerve. Once identified, the obturator nerve serves as the inferior boundary of lymph node dissection and the surgeon stays above the vessels. However, in cases in which accessory or aberrant obturator vessels arise from the inferior epigastric vessels, these vessels must be carefully identified and either ligated or avoided. Injury to the vessels may result in significant arterial and venous bleed-

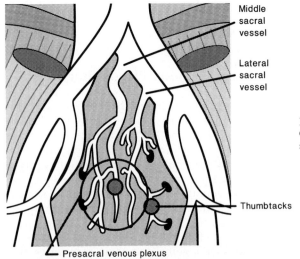

Middle
sacral
vessel

Lateral
sacral
vessel

Thumbtacks

Presacral venous plexus

FIGURE 6–7
Control of presacral venous plexus bleeding with stainless steel thumbtacks.

ing. Visualization of the operative field should be optimized. If not already developed, the paravesical space should be opened and the course of the obturator nerve clearly identified. Injury to the obturator artery in most cases is readily identified by its pulsatile blood flow. Once identified, the artery is either ligated or clipped. Control of venous bleeding may be more problematic, particularly if the vein has retracted into the obturator foramen. Initially, pressure is applied at the obturator foramen with a sponge stick for several minutes. Care should be taken not to avulse the obturator nerve, which is also coursing through the foramen. If one is fortunate, hemostasis will be obtained with pressure alone. The blind placement of suture ligatures or hemostatic clips in the area of bleeding is to be avoided. The obturator foramen is formed from the fascia covering the obturator internus muscle and is not a bony structure. With the obturator nerve under direct visualization, the foramen may be enlarged and careful dissection of the area performed. Individual bleeding vessels are clipped or ligated. Inferior dissection should be avoided because one will encounter an extensive plexus of pelvic veins. The patient should be checked in the postoperative period for evidence of obturator nerve injury.

Pelvic Floor Hemorrhage

Bleeding encountered in the pelvic floor often arises from damage to the extensive plexus of veins originating in the pelvis. An expedient and technically proficient response is often necessary to reverse a potentially morbid situation. In managing damage to the internal iliac vein or its branches, the surgeon is faced with the control of bleeding in a structure that frequently cannot be mobilized. The exiting branches of the internal iliac vein are fixed, fragile, and may produce almost uncontrollable hemorrhage if injured. A stepwise approach is helpful. The initial response to such bleeding should be prompt pressure directly applied on the defect against the pelvic wall. An assistant is directed to maintain pressure on the vein by pressing it gently against the pelvic wall. The vein is exposed by lifting the round ligament on the side of the injury strongly upward. A retractor is placed above the femoral artery and dissected upward to the bifurcation of the common iliac artery. The ureter is identified along the medial leaf of the broad ligament. The pararectal and paravesical spaces are developed, and the obliterated um-

bilical or superior vesical artery and the obturator nerve are identified. Two suction tips are placed in the wound, and the sponge stick pressed against the venous defect is gently removed. As soon as the surgeon has clearly identified the defect and its size, the sponge stick is replaced. A sucker is put directly near the defect. If the defect is small, a small clip may be all that is needed to close the hole in the vein and control the bleeding. It should be noted that the presence of a clip on the defect makes its suture infinitely more difficult, because the clip will be incorporated in the suture and the defect will not close. If the defect is large, one may divide the vein by placing large clips on each side of the defect. An alternate approach that may better control bleeding from veins entering laterally or inferior to the venous trunk is to place a running vascular suture in the vein and control bleeding. If the laceration is large and several venous trees have been torn where several perforators enter, two maneuvers remain. The entire area is sutured with a 1-0 chromic suture in a continuous fashion, realizing that some of the pelvic plexus of nerves may sustain injury. As a last resort, the pelvis may be tightly packed by one of the several techniques previously mentioned.

Bleeding and Hematoma from the Infundibulopelvic Ligament

Bleeding from the ovarian vessels can result from crush injuries due to the use of crushing clamps, particularly the less desirable double clamp technique. A second type of situation occurs when the ligature securing the infundibulopelvic ligament is lost. The following is an approach to the scenario described previously. The lower end of the vein is grasped with a small clamp, the ureter is identified, and the dissection is done sharply upward in the retroperitoneal space while the ureter is observed. Additional exposure can be obtained by incising up either gutter and reflecting the peritoneum. As soon as one has reached the top of the hematoma as identified by resumption of the veins into a more normal caliber, a right-angled clamp is placed on them. A tie is passed around the veins at this point, again while carefully identifying the ureter. One may perform either suture ligature, noted earlier, or occasionally a large clip may be placed below the vein. The hematoma, thus isolated, should be removed. Any small venous contributors to this hematoma should be clipped with small clips, or the electrocautery may be used. The distal end of the veins near the hysterectomy site should be inspected to make sure that they are not contributing to the hematoma formation. A dry pack should be placed with some pressure over the site where the hematoma had been removed. One rarely will encounter difficulty in controlling such bleeding where sharp dissection and precise vessel ligation are performed. If necessary, the ovarian artery of either side may be ligated near its origin from the aorta just below that of the renal arteries, proximal to the hematoma.

REFERENCES

1. Bell J. The principles of surgery. In: Baue AE, et al, eds. The Classics of Surgery Library, special ed. Birmingham, AL, Gryphon Editions, 1989, p 43.
2. Gould SF. Anatomy. In: Gabbe SG, Niebyl JR, Simpson JL, eds. Obstetrics, Normal and Problem Pregnancy. New York, Churchill Livingstone, 1986, p 26.
3. Burchell RC. Physiology of internal iliac artery ligation. J Obstet Gynaecol Br Commonw 1968;75:642–651.
4. Freeark RJ, Baker WH. Arterial injuries. In: Sabiston DC, ed. Textbook of Surgery, the Biological Basis of Modern Surgical Practice, 13th ed. Philadelphia, WB Saunders, 1986, pp 1895–1897.
5. Rich NM. Venous injuries. In: Sabiston DC, ed. Textbook of Surgery, the Biological Basis of Modern Surgical Practice, 13th ed. Philadelphia, WB Saunders, 1986, pp 1954–1955.
6. Rich NM, Hobson RW II, Wright CB, Swan KG. Techniques of venous repair. In: Swan KG, Hodson RW II, Reynolds DG, et al, eds. Venous Surgery in the Lower Extremity. St. Louis, Warren H. Green, 1975.
7. Blood component therapy. ACOG technical bulletin No. 199. Washington, DC, American College of Obstetricians and Gynecologists, November 1994.
8. Logothetopulos K. Eine absolut sichere Blutstillungsmethode bei vaginalen. Und Zentralbl Gynakol 1926;50:3202.
9. Logothetopulos K. Antwort auf die Bemerkung von Max Stickel ueber meine tamponaden Methode. Zentralbl Gynakol 1933;57:2679.
10. Parente JT, Dlugi H, Weingold AB. Pelvic hemostasis: a new technic and pack. Obstet Gynecol 1962;19:218–221.
11. Masterson BJ. Intraoperative hemorrhage. In: Nichols DH, ed. Clinical Problems, Injuries, and Complications of Gynecologic Surgery. Baltimore, Williams & Wilkins, 1988.
12. Moss JP. Historical and current perspectives on surgical drainage. Surg Gynecol Obstet 1981;152:517–527.
13. Loh A, Jones PA. Evisceration and other complications of abdominal drains. Postgrad Med J 1991;67:687–688.
14. Patsner B, Orr W Jr. Intractable venous sacral hemorrhage: use of stainless steel thumbtacks to obtain hemostasis. Am J Obstet Gynecol 1990;162:452.
15. Mann WJ. A comment on thumbtacks for hemorrhage control. Am J Obstet Gynecol 1990;163:1092–1093.
16. Timmons MC, Kohler MF, Addison WA. Thumbtack use for control of presacral bleeding, with description of an instrument for thumbtack application. Obstet Gynecol 1991;78:313–315.
17. Khan FA, Fang DT, Nivatvongs S. Management of presacral bleeding during rectal resection. Surg Gynecol Obstet 1987;165:275–277.
18. Qinyao W, Weijin S, Youren Z, et al. New concepts in severe presacral hemorrhage during proctectomy. Arch Surg 1985;120:1013–1020.
19. Marsden DE, Cavanagh D. Hemorrhagic shock in the gynecologic patient. Clin Obstet Gynecol 1985;28:389.
20. Dineen P. Antibacterial activity of oxidized regenerated cellulose. Surg Gynecol Obstet 1976;142:481–486.
21. Dineen P. The effect of oxidized regenerated cellulose on experimental intravascular infection. Surgery 1977; 82:576–579.
22. Dineen P. The effect of oxidized regenerated cellulose on experimental infected splenectomies. J Surg Res 1977;23:114–116.
23. Treves N. Prophylaxis of post mammectomy lymphedema by the use of Gelfoam laminated rolls. Cancer 1952;5:73–83.
24. Rarig HR. Successful use of gelatin foam sponge in surgical restoration of fertility. Am J Obstet Gynecol 1963;86:136.
25. Barnes AC. The use of gelatin foam sponges in obstetrics and gynecology. Am J Obstet Gynecol 1963;86:105–107.
26. Walterbusch G, Haverich A, Borst HG. Clinical experience with fibrin glue for local bleeding control and sealing of vascular prostheses. Thorac Cardiovasc Surg 1982;30:234.
27. Kram HB, Nathan RC, Mackabee JR, et al. Clinical use of nonautologous fibrin glue. Am Surg 1988;54:570.
28. Salvino CK, Esposito TJ, Smith DK, et al. Laparoscopic injection of fibrin glue to arrest intraparenchymal abdominal hemorrhage: an experimental study. J Trauma 1993;35:762–766.
29. Rousou JA, Engelman RM, Breyer RH. Fibrin glue: an effective hemostatic agent for nonsuturable intraoperative bleeding. Ann Thorac Surg 1984;38:409–410.
30. Smith DC, Wyatt JF. Embolization of the hypogastric arteries in the control of massive vaginal hemorrhage. Obstet Gynecol 1977;49:317.
31. Dehaeck CMC. Transcatheter embolization of pelvic vessels to stop intractable hemorrhage. Gynecol Oncol 1986;24:9–16.
32. Heaston DK, Mineau DE, Brown JB, et al. Transcatheter arterial embolization for control of persistent massive puerperal haemorrhage after bilateral surgical hypogastric artery ligation. AJR 1979;133:152–154.
33. Gianturco G, Anderson J, Wallace S. Mechanical devices for arterial occlusion. AJR 1975;124:428.
34. Johnmide IS, Jackson DC. Therapeutic catheterization. In: A Practical Approach to Angiography. Boston, Little, Brown, & Co, 1980.
35. Brown BJ, Heaston DK, Poulson AM, et al. Uncontrollable postpartum bleeding: a new approach to haemostases through angiographic arterial embolization. Obstet Gynecol 1979;54:361–364.
36. John M. Complications of laparoscopic surgery. In: Phipps JH, ed. Laparoscopic Hysterectomy and Oophorectomy: A Practical Manual and Colour Atlas. New York, Churchill Livingstone, 1993, pp 61–62.
37. Semm K. Operative Manual for Endoscopic Abdominal Surgery. Chicago, Year Book Medical Publishers, 1987, pp 150–151.
38. Hurd WW, Pearl ML, DeLancy JOL, et al. Laparoscopic injury of abdominal wall blood vessels: a report of three cases. Obstet Gynecol 1993;82:673–676.
39. Majeski JA. Rectus sheath abscess. South Med J 1986;79:1311.
40. Wang QY, Wu S, Shi WJ, et al. On the cause, prevention and treatment of presacral massive hemorrhage during rectectomy. Chung Hua Wai Ko Tsa Chih 1980;18:562–563.
41. Anderson JE. Grant's Anatomy Atlas, 8th ed. Baltimore, Williams & Wilkins, 1983, plate 3–54.

7

Alton V. Hallum III

CHAPTER

Gastrointestinal Tract Complications

Major gynecologic surgery carries an inherit risk of injury to associated abdominal and pelvic viscera. An intimate understanding of anatomy is the foundation of managing surgical complications. This understanding, along with adequate preoperative evaluation and preparation, enables the well-trained gynecologist to manage most surgical complications. In this chapter the pertinent anatomy of the gastrointestinal tract is reviewed and the surgical management of bowel injury and of unanticipated pathologic processes is discussed.

ANATOMY

The small bowel is 6 meters long in the adult and is divided into two segments: the jejunum and ileum. The jejunum comprises the first two fifths of the small intestine and has a larger lumen than the ileum, which comprises the distal three-fifths of the small intestine. The mesenteric fat does not reach the mesenteric border of the jejunum, and the terminal vasa recta are long in the jejunum. In the ileum, in contrast, the mesenteric fat is above the jejunal wall and the vasa recta are short. The small bowel mesentery is suspended from the dorsal body wall from the left lateral aspect of the second lumbar vertebrae to the right lateral aspect of the fourth lumbar vertebrae. Through this structure traverse the blood supply, the autonomic nerves, and the lymphatics of the small intestine.

The vascular supply of the small intestine arises from the superior mesenteric artery. This originates from the aorta immediately above the neck of the pancreas (Fig. 7–1). After coursing beneath the pancreatic neck, this artery passes over the ventral surface of the left renal vein and third portion of the duodenum. It then divides into 12 or more branches to supply the jejunum and ileum (Fig. 7–2). These vessels anastomose, and multiple arcades and the vasa recta pass from these arcades to the submucosa of the gut. Collateral blood supply can be established from the celiac axis through the superior pancreatoduodenal artery and from the inferior mesenteric artery through the marginal artery of Drummond and the arch of Riolan, which connect the left colic to the middle colic artery. The venous drainage of the small intestine is by means of the superior mesenteric vein. This vein joins with the inferior mesenteric vein and splenic vein to form the portal vein. This union occurs at the inferior margin of the pancreas.

The colon is 1.5 meters long. The ascending and descending portions of the colon are retroperitoneal, whereas the sigmoid and transverse colon are intraperitoneal structures. The colon is characterized by three distinct longitudinal muscular strips, known as the *teniae coli*, that meet at the base of the appendix. The colon appears to have multiple segments, termed *haustra*, that are separated by internal folds called plicae semilunares. The serosa has multiple fatty appendages called *appendices epiploicae*, which are most numerous in the sigmoid colon. The greater omentum arises from the greater curvature of the stomach and is loosely attached to the transverse colon mesentery and drapes over the transverse colon proper.

The origin of the blood supply to the colon and rectum is from the superior mesenteric artery, the inferior mesenteric artery, the inter-

FIGURE 7–1
Arterial supply to the stomach, duodenum, and spleen. The stomach has been reflected superiorly with the posterior surface in view. (From Gershenson DM, DeCherney AH, Curry SL. Operative Gynecology. Philadelphia, WB Saunders, 1993.)

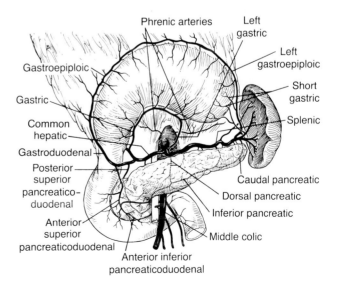

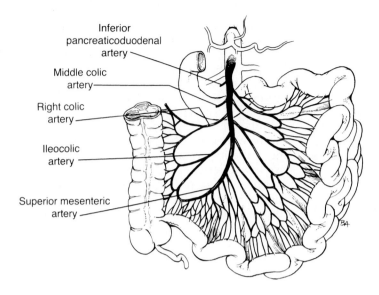

FIGURE 7-2
Distribution of the superior mesenteric artery. (From Gershenson DM, DeCherney AH, Curry SL. Operative Gynecology. Philadelphia, WB Saunders, 1993.)

nal iliac artery, and the pudendal arteries. The superior mesenteric artery, after providing branches to the jejunum and ileum, further divides into the ileocolic, right colic, and middle colic arteries (Fig. 7–3). The inferior mesenteric artery divides into the left colic artery, the sigmoid artery, and the superior hemorrhoidal artery. The middle hemorrhoidal artery is a branch of the internal iliac artery, and the inferior hemorrhoidal artery arises from the pu-

dendal artery. All of these arteries interconnect in anastomotic arcades. The richest arcade is between the left colic and the middle colic arteries, by the previously mentioned marginal artery of Drummond and the arch of Riolan.

The bowel wall is divided into four layers. The serosa is the outermost layer and is formed by a layer of peritoneum. The muscularis contains an outer longitudinal and inner circular layer of smooth muscle. These muscle groups

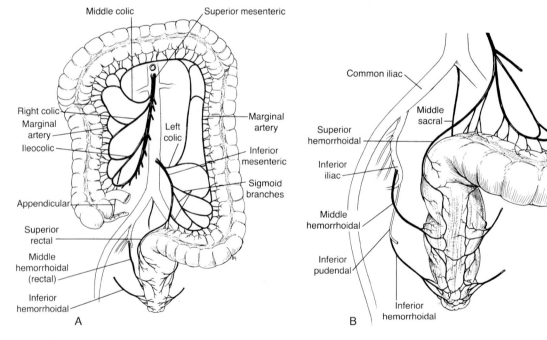

FIGURE 7-3
A, Arterial supply to the colon. *B,* The superior, middle, and inferior rectal arteries supply the sigmoid colon and rectum.

are separated by lymphatics and nerve fibers known as Auerbach's plexus. The submucosa is composed of connective tissue with a rich vascular and lymphatic network as well as Meissner's nerve plexus. The mucosa creates characteristic folds in the small intestine known as valvulae conniventes. These convolutions in the smaller villi greatly increase the surface area and, therefore, the absorptive capacity of the small intestine. In the large intestine, a single columnar layer of epithelium is found without villi. Many crypts are present with goblet cells that secrete mucus.

INTESTINAL INJURY

The general gynecologist should understand predisposing factors that lead to intestinal injury, as well as steps in the surgical procedure that are prone to intestinal injury. Krebs reviewed a 10-year experience of gastrointestinal injuries in 17,650 patients undergoing gynecologic operations.[1] One hundred twenty-eight intestinal lacerations were encountered in this study. Thirty-seven percent of the intestinal injuries occurred on entry into the abdominal cavity, 35% during lysis of adhesions and visceral dissection, 10% during laparoscopy, 9% during vaginal surgery, and 9% during dilatation and curettage or dilatation and evacuation. Three fourths of the injuries involved the small intestine, and 25% occurred in the large intestine. Roughly three fourths of the injuries were incurred during uncomplicated gynecologic operations. Thirty-six of the 128 lacerations (28%) were deemed preoperatively or intraoperatively to involve the risk of bowel injury because the patients had adhesions, neoplasms, infection, or endometriosis. Obesity and prior abdominal incision were associated with a threefold higher risk of intestinal injury.

Recognizing these risk factors, several preventative measures are recommended. First, in patients at risk of adhesive disease, a thorough bowel preparation should be performed. This will minimize infectious morbidity and allow an easier repair as the bowel is evacuated. In patients with prior abdominal incisions, entry into the abdominal cavity should take place at a site higher than the previous skin incision to minimize the risk of bowel adhesions to the interior abdominal wall.[2] A sharp entry into the abdominal cavity with a scalpel or scissors minimizes the risk of bowel injury. When scissors are used for peritoneal entry, the peritoneum can be grasped with forceps or hemostats and placed on tension. The peritoneum is then rolled between the thumb and index finger to assess for adherent viscera. When this is ruled out, the peritoneum can then be cut with confidence.[3] To use a scalpel for a sharp entry into the abdominal cavity, a layer-by-layer dissection with the scalpel blade is performed to the level of the fascia. With the fascia incised, the rectus muscles can then be sharply separated and the peritoneum exposed. The wound edges should then be elevated and retracted laterally to tent the peritoneum. With the use of only the weight of the blade, the scalpel is run across the peritoneum. The traction generates an effective negative pressure in the peritoneal cavity. When the peritoneum is then cut, air enters the peritoneal cavity and the underlying bowel drops away. If the bowel is densely adherent to the peritoneum, this layer-by-layer method allows the surgeon to identify the bowel wall. The surgeon can then continue the opening of the peritoneum in a portion of peritoneum without adhesions. When this is not possible, the fascial edges should then be grasped and placed on upward and lateral traction. A moist laparotomy pack is used to place gentle countertraction on the bowel, and enterolysis should then be undertaken with Metzenbaum scissors. Blunt dissection should be avoided. Although blunt dissection is occasionally effective in filmy adhesions, sharp dissection is recommended even in this situation, because it serves as an opportunity to hone dissection skills that are absolutely necessary in dense adhesions or when tissue planes are obliterated.

Successful enterolysis is accomplished with rigid adherence to the following fundamental surgical techniques:

1. *Traction and countertraction.* The surgeon and assistant should place the tissue plane for dissection on traction by pulling in opposite directions. The tissue plane can then be separated with the least surgical effort. When scissors are used, it is recommended that the tips be placed perpendicular to the dissection plane. Brief snips of the scissor tips across the dissection plane will accomplish a gradual cutting action. Pushing and spreading with the scissor tips can be an effective tool with loose, filmy adhesions. However, this frequently causes bowel injury with tenacious adhesions. Speed and skill are gained with experience. Therefore, practicing sharp dissection in filmy adhesions increases the surgeon's comfort and success when particularly dense adhesive disease is encountered.

2. *Keep dissection on the same plane.* The trac-

tion and countertraction generated by the surgeon and the assistant should create a flat surface for dissection. The adhesions are then released in a systematic manner that avoids creation of a deep hole. Dissecting in a deep hole greatly increases the risk of injury. If such an injury is vascular, the location makes its management extremely difficult.

3. *If stuck, go elsewhere.* Enterolysis requires patience, meticulous technique, and good decision-making. When difficulty with dissection is encountered, it is prudent to move to a different area or approach the adhesion from a different angle. One should always perform the easy dissection first. This philosophical choice of dealing with all simple aspects of dissection first generally renders the difficult portion of the dissection simple.

ENTEROTOMY MANAGEMENT

Injury to the bowel is classified into three categories: (1) serosal injury, (2) seromuscular injury, and (3) full-thickness injury. The repair of a bowel injury is dictated by the category of injury and method of injury. Surgical injuries include sharp and thermal (electrical). Understanding the type of intestinal injury and the method of surgical injury dictates the type of repair needed.

An injury confined to the serosa of the intestine, whether large or small, does not require surgical repair. When a seromuscular injury is present, it should be checked by compressing the bowel proximal and distal to the injury site. If the mucosa bulges through the defect, multiple vertical Lembert sutures should be placed to oversew the defect. The axis of closure should be perpendicular to the length of the intestine to minimize the reduction of the intraluminal caliber of the intestine.

Frank enterotomy with disruption of the serosa muscularis and mucosa is generally managed with a multiple-layer closure. The edges of the injury, especially if caused by an electrosurgical source, should be checked for adequate blood supply. When a coagulative type of electrosurgical injury is encountered, the true extent of necrosis is beyond the visible injury. With this in mind, the edge of a thermal injury should be freshened until good blood supply is demonstrated by brisk bleeding from the edge. Once blood supply has been evaluated, manipulation of the bowel wall should be limited to avoid additional injury. The edges of the wound that serve as the apices of the closure should be tagged with 3-0 absorbable

polyglycolic suture. These edges are then placed on traction that is perpendicular to the axis of the bowel. This traction delineates the line of closure. The edges are then approximated with sequential interrupted seromucosal stitches using 3-0 polyglycolic or silk sutures that invert the edge. It is recommended that all sutures be placed before tying knots in this interrupted fashion to maintain an open space to place the sutures without tissue trauma. The knots are then tied in a sequential fashion and cut. The thickness of each bite should be 3 to 5 mm apart, with each bite taking 3 to 5 mm of tissue. The closure is then reinforced with a second seromuscular Lembert closure (Fig. 7–4). If one closes the bowel in a perpendicular axis and uses interrupted sutures, the diameter of the bowel lumen should not be compromised. If significant narrowing is noted, a segmental bowel resection should be performed with an end-to-end anastomosis.

Many methods of bowel closure exist, including interrupted two-layer closure as described earlier, as well as continuous one-layer closure, or continuous two-layer closures, all with acceptable results. The two-layered closure is recommended here because this method has more uniform acceptance as a method of closure.[4-8]

The open closure begins with an assessment of the bowel edges with particular attention at the mesenteric border. Excellent hemostasis at this site minimizes the risk of hematoma for-

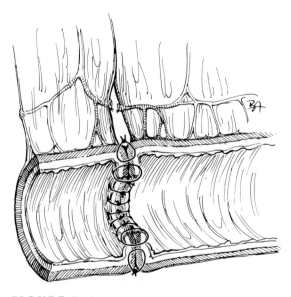

FIGURE 7–4
Two-layer inverting intestinal anastomosis. (From Gershenson DM, DeCherney AH, Curry SL. Operative Gynecology. Philadelphia, WB Saunders, 1993.)

mation that can impair wound healing. Inspection of the bowel should also examine for the luminal diameter of each segment to be approximated. In the setting of an acute obstruction, there is usually a significant discrepancy in the size. This difference can be corrected by making a linear incision in the antimesenteric border of the smaller segment of intestine. This is called a Cheatle incision (Fig. 7–5). This will effectively increase the diameter and allow more uniform approximation. When the discrepancy is so large than an end-to-end anastomosis cannot be readily performed, an end-to-side or side-to-side anastomosis may be necessary. Invariably, the two-layer technique is similar to all of these approximations. The posterior walls of the bowel segments are approximated with serial interrupted Lembert seromuscular sutures of 3-0 silk. The lateralmost sutures are tagged for traction. The posterior mucosa is then approximated using a full-thickness interrupted or running 3-0 polyglycolic suture using the Connell or Cushing suture. This mucosal suture is carried around to the anterior bowel wall to complete the mucosal closure (Fig. 7–6). The anterior wall is then oversewn with interrupted vertical Lembert sutures to complete this second layer. The luminal caliber is not significantly reduced if attention to detail is paid during the closure.

A single-layer closure can also be safely performed and minimize the luminal decrease.[8]

Another popular method for bowel resection and anastomosis is the use of surgical stapling devices (Fig. 7–7). Three classes of staplers are commonly used: (1) GIA, gastrointestinal anastomosis (Fig. 7–8); (2) TA, thoracoabdominal (Fig. 7–9); and (3) EEA, end-to-end anastomosis (Fig. 7–10).

In principle, these instruments supply a staggered double or triple row of staples across the intestine. The GIA and EEA devices also contain a knife within the instrument that is used to divide two separately placed lines of staples. This allows division and anastomosis of bowel, depending on the manner in which these instruments are used.

Stapled bowel resection is usually accomplished with a GIA stapler. A window is made under the mesenteric border of the intestine (Fig. 7–11). The smaller arm of the GIA is passed through this window and the stapler is clamped. The length of the GIA is variable, and one must ensure that an adequate staple line is placed by examining the markings on the instrument. The bowel is then divided (Fig. 7–12). This is performed on either side of the segment to be removed. The mesentery is then divided close to the mesenteric border of the bowel to minimize the risk of adjacent mesen-

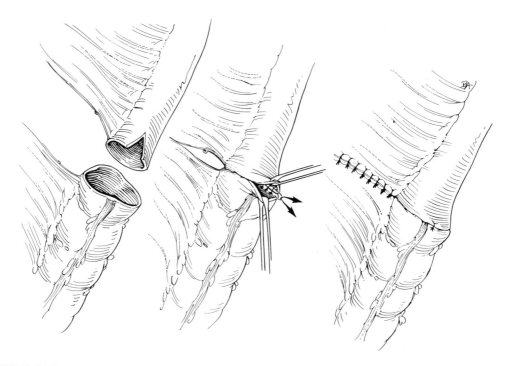

FIGURE 7–5
A Cheatle cut is used to allow for disparity in luminal size. The mesenteric defect is sewn closed. (From Gershenson DM, DeCherney AH, Curry SL. Operative Gynecology. Philadelphia, WB Saunders, 1993.)

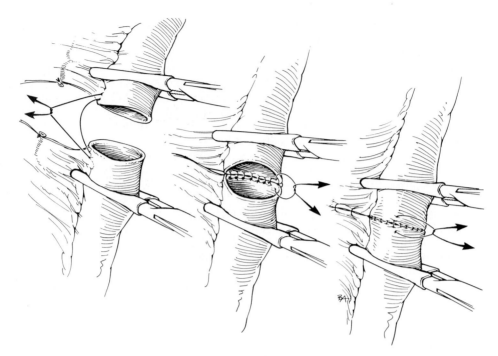

FIGURE 7-6
With rubber-shod clamps applied to prevent intestinal spillage, the intestinal segments are sewn together. (From Gershenson DM, DeCherney AH, Curry SL. Operative Gynecology. Philadelphia, WB Saunders, 1993.)

teric vessels to the segments that will be anastomosed. The anastomosis most frequently used is a side-to-side functional end-to-end anastomosis (Fig. 7–13). The antimesenteric end of the staple lines is approximated, and the segments of intestine are run parallel to one another. A distal antimesenteric seromuscular stitch is also placed 5 to 6 cm distal to the staple line. The antimesenteric corners of the staple line are then excised with Mayo scissors. The arms of the GIA stapler are then passed into the bowel lumen. The antimesenteric borders of the intestine are then clamped together. Particular attention should be made to ensure the mesentery is not incorporated in this clamping. The staple line is then fired. Intraluminal inspection after removal of the stapling device should be performed to ensure no bleeding of the staple line has occurred. The remaining defect is then closed using a TA stapler. The mesentery is then reapproximated with interrupted 3-0 sutures.

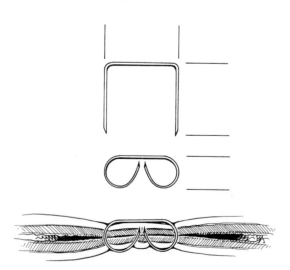

FIGURE 7-7
Wire staple is bent into a "B" figure, allowing for secure tissue approximation without compromise of blood supply. (From Gershenson DM, DeCherney AH, Curry SL. Operative Gynecology. Philadelphia, WB Saunders, 1993.)

VASCULAR COMPROMISE

Vascular compromise to a segment of intestine can be incurred in a number of ways. Injury to the mesentery, extensive seromuscular damage, and anastomosis extending beyond the blood supply of the attendant mesentery are the most frequent surgical reasons for vascular compromise. Incarcerated hernia, torsion, and intussusception are the spontaneous methods of vascular compromise to segments of bowel. Advanced age, atherosclerotic vascular disease,

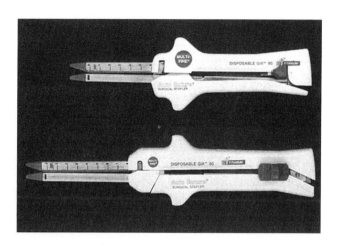

FIGURE 7–8
The GIA stapler is used to divide a segment of intestine (United States Surgical Corporation. All rights reserved.) (From Gershenson DM, DeCherney AH, Curry SL. Operative Gynecology. Philadelphia, WB Saunders, 1993.)

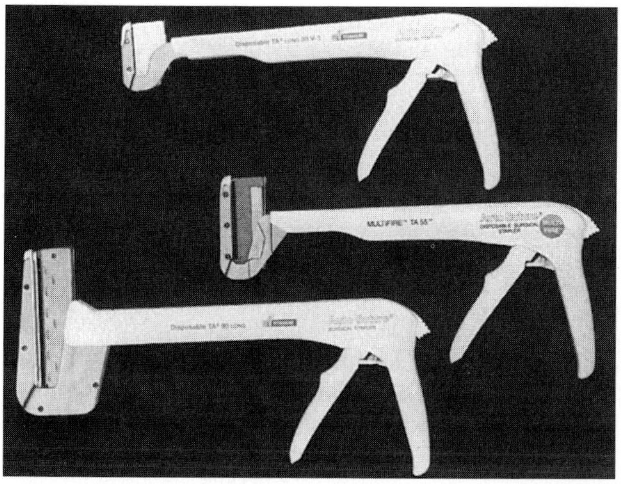

FIGURE 7–9
The TA stapler, shown here in three available sizes, places a double row of staples across an intestinal segment (United States Surgical Corporation. All rights reserved.) (From Gershenson DM, DeCherney AH, Curry SL. Operative Gynecology. Philadelphia, WB Saunders, 1993.)

FIGURE 7–10
The EEA device is most useful for the creation of a low rectal anastomosis (United States Surgical Corporation. All rights reserved.) (From Gershenson DM, DeCherney AH, Curry SL. Operative Gynecology. Philadelphia, WB Saunders, 1993.)

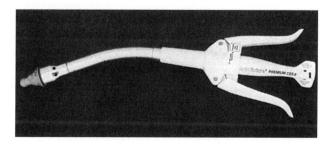

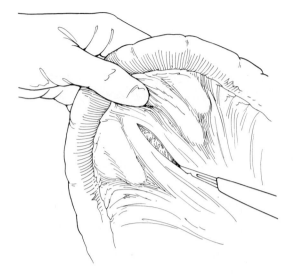

FIGURE 7–11
The mesentery is scored using a knife. (From Gershenson DM, DeCherney AH, Curry SL. Operative Gynecology. Philadelphia, WB Saunders, 1993.)

and prior radiation are all predisposing factors for vascular injury during intestinal surgery. Recognition of vascular insufficiency must be recognized intraoperatively rather than develop into a postoperative emergency.

Several steps can limit the risk of vascular compromise when performing bowel anastomosis. If a bowel resection is performed, the luminal margin should be tipped toward the supplying mesentery. This maneuver increases the diameter of the bowel lumen as well as decreases the possibility of vascular compromise to the antimesenteric portion of the intestine.

The bowel, in the setting of decreased blood flow, usually appears dusky or mottled with a purple-gray hue. This may be misleading because of venous engorgement rather than arterial insufficiency. If one is considering leaving a segment of bowel in place with these visible changes, the vascular integrity can be assessed by injecting 1000 mg of fluorescein. After the intravascular injection of this dye, the bowel is then viewed under the illumination of a 360-nm ultraviolet Wood lamp. With arteriolar insufficiency, the bowel segment will not fluoresce. Lack of fluorescence is an indication for bowel resection and reanastomosis or a revision of an anastomosis. Similarly, larger arteriolar integrity can be assessed intraoperatively with a Doppler device at the mesenteric margin of the bowel. When an arterial Doppler signal is present within 1 cm of the anastomosis, adequate healing occurs.[9]

Preexisting bowel edema can increase the development of a dusky appearance to the bowel. The resolution of the edema improves the blood supply. Consequently, if the blood supply is deemed adequate by the aforementioned techniques or demonstration of brisk bleeding of bowel edges before anastomosis, then many surgeons tolerate focal dusky changes as long as they are not intense.

MANAGEMENT OF UNEXPECTED PATHOLOGIC PROCESSES

Meckel's Diverticulum

Meckel's diverticulum is the most common congenital abnormality of the gastrointestinal tract. It occurs in 2% to 3% of patients.[10] The length of the diverticulum is usually 3 to 5 cm, and it is typically found 1.5 to 2 feet from the ileocecal valve.[11]

The lifetime risk of developing a problem from Meckel's diverticulum is approximately 4%.[12] The majority of problems associated with Meckel's diverticulum occur in the pediatric

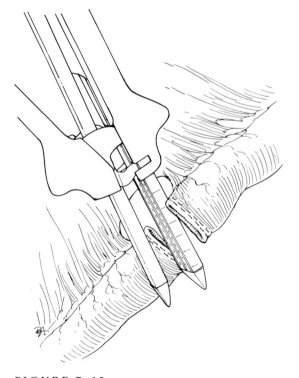

FIGURE 7–12
The GIA stapler is used to divide the small intestine, simultaneously sealing the proximal and distal limbs with a double row of staples. (From Gershenson DM, DeCherney AH, Curry SL. Operative Gynecology. Philadelphia, WB Saunders, 1993.)

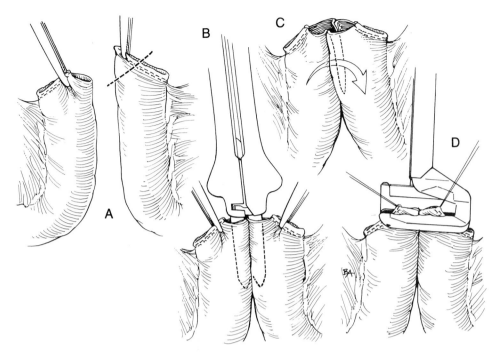

FIGURE 7–13

A, The two segments of small intestine are approximated by the antimesenteric aspect. A small nipple of tissue is trimmed off as shown. *B,* The jaws of the GIA stapler are placed, one in each intestinal segment. *C,* After the GIA is fired, the two segments are now connected with a lumen between. *D,* A TA stapler is used to seal the remaining defect. (From Gershenson DM, DeCherney AH, Curry SL. Operative Gynecology. Philadelphia, WB Saunders, 1993.)

age group. The management of asymptomatic Meckel's diverticulum at laparotomy depends on several factors. If a persistent vitelloumbilical chord is encountered, this may cause an internal hernia with obstruction. Therefore, this is an indication for resection of the diverticulum. The length of the diverticulum as well as the opening into the ileum can influence the risk of complications. A narrow opening and a length of greater than 2 cm may increase the risk of intussusception and obstruction by foreign body or concretion. Palpation of the diverticulum should be performed to assess for foreign body or calculus as well as to detect inflammation. Heterotopic mucosa is not reliably identified by palpation. Mackey and Dineen identified 16 instances of heterotopic mucosa in 140 cases of asymptomatic Meckel's diverticula removed at laparotomy.[13] In this same series, in patients with symptomatic Meckel's diverticulum requiring surgery, the incidence of heterotopic mucosa was 34%. The majority of these patients had gastric mucosa, which can give rise to a peptic ulcer within the diverticulum or adjacent to its stoma. This can cause intestinal hemorrhage and, occasionally, perforation.

Meckel's diverticulum should be considered when exploratory surgery is being done in a patient with acute pelvic pain or in whom the suggestion of appendicitis is high. An investigation for this abnormality should be undertaken when the appendix or the pelvic viscera appear normal. In a manner similar to acute appendicitis, an acutely inflamed Meckel diverticulum may progress to perforation.

A rare finding of a Meckel diverticulum is its presence in a hernia, which is classically known as Littré's hernia. Neoplasms arising in Meckel's diverticulum are also exceedingly rare. Weinstein and associates reported a series of 106 cases of neoplasms occurring in Meckel's diverticula. One fourth of these cases were benign. Sarcoma and carcinoid were the two most frequently reported malignancies in this series.[14]

Resection of an asymptomatic, unattached, thin-walled diverticulum with a wide stoma is not necessary.[11] When resection is required, the diverticulum should be inspected for a vitelloumbilical cord, and this should be isolated, clamped, divided, and ligated. The artery supplying the diverticulum must be isolated and divided on the mesenteric side of the adjacent ileum. This minimizes the risk of a subsequent fibrotic band, which can narrow the lumen.

The diverticulum may then be excised and the adjacent ileum then reapproximated in two layers in a transverse axis to avoid narrowing the caliber of the ileum. A segmental resection can be performed in the setting of inflammation, gangrene, or frank ulceration.

UNEXPECTED CARCINOMA

A surgeon is invariably crestfallen when carcinomatosis is encountered in an operation for a presumed benign process. The surgeon must collect his or her thoughts to determine the proper management of this complication. A meticulous exploration should be done to determine the origin of the tumor. A sample of the tumor should be sent for frozen section diagnosis. If the patient has a previous history of malignancy, this information should be provided to the pathologist. The intestines should be examined from the stomach to the rectum by visible and manual palpation. Likewise, the pancreas, kidneys, liver, and gallbladder should also be palpated. The uterus, ovaries, and tubes should next be assessed. If the frozen section diagnosis is consistent with ovarian cancer, every effort at maximum cytoreductive surgery should be undertaken. Consultation with a gynecologic oncologist or general surgeon is strongly advised, especially if intestinal resection is required. If carcinoma other than ovary is diagnosed, then cytoreductive surgery is not indicated. In those patients who cannot achieve debulking to less than 1 cm, the surgery should be directed to palliating symptoms. This may often require intestinal resection with reanastomosis if the bowel compromised is *focal*. If the risk of obstruction is high at *multiple* sites, then resection is not indicated. A diverting ileostomy or colostomy should be done, depending on the location of highest pending obstruction in frankly obstructed patients. This measure can be saved as a second procedure in patients with progression or chemotherapy. Approximately 80% of patients will respond to platinum-paclitaxel chemotherapy.

If an adnexal mass is detected and found on frozen section to contain a primary ovarian tumor, a systematic staging laparotomy should be performed. Preferably, a vertical skin incision is used when the risk of cancer is high. Washings from the pelvis, paracolic gutters, and hemidiaphragms should be collected at the outset of the case. The upper abdomen is explored, with particular attention addressed to the hemidiaphragms, omentum, stomach, pancreas, liver parenchyma, and retroperitoneal node sites. The reproductive desires of the premenopausal patient should be known before surgery is undertaken. If the contralateral ovary appears benign in a woman wishing to conserve her fertility and there is no evidence of spread outside the ovary, then the uterus and normal-appearing ovary may be conserved while obtaining the other biopsy samples necessary for a complete staging. If the mass has adhesions to adjacent organs, these adhesions should be collected for histologic inspection. Multiple random peritoneal biopsy samples are then collected from the lateral pelvic walls, bladder and cul-de-sac, paracolic gutters, and hemidiaphragms. An omentectomy is then performed. Pelvic and para-aortic lymph node biopsy samples should be taken to the level of the insertion of the ovarian veins. Lymph node dissection is the most technically demanding aspect of this staging procedure. One should have experience with this procedure and an ability to manage its complications. Otherwise, this portion of the operation should be performed by a consulting gynecologic oncologist or general surgeon.

APPENDICEAL PATHOLOGY

Gynecologists invariably encounter unexpected appendiceal pathologic processes in the course of their surgical career. One should have an understanding of the anatomy of the appendix as well as the pathologic processes associated with this vestigial organ. The appendix is found at the confluence of the teniae. This is usually 2.5 cm below the ileocecal junction with the base on the inferomedial side of the cecum. The origin of the appendiceal base from the confluence of the teniae is universally conserved; however, the location of the appendiceal tip is highly variable. The location of the tip of the appendix often determines the symptoms and signs of the patient presenting with appendiceal inflammation. The appendix tip that hangs in the true pelvis often mimics adnexal disease when inflamed. Consequently, a gynecologic surgeon who explores a patient for pelvic pain should be prepared to manage appendiceal disease.

Appendicitis usually occurs in young patients and has a natural history normally less than 36 hours from onset to perforation. Young women are also at greatest risk for pelvic inflammatory disease. The physician must consequently temper the early surgical management necessary for appendicitis with the knowledge that many other processes may cause a similar presentation. Appendicitis usually starts because of obstruction of the appendiceal lumen. As intraluminal pressure rises, capillary profusion decreases and the integrity of the mucosa is disrupted with this vascular compromise. Localized infection and muscular degradation weaken the appendiceal wall. The appendix can swell and perforation may develop. The adjacent tissue becomes secondarily inflamed. Frequently, the small bowel and omentum form a mechanical barrier to isolate this inflammatory process. With perforation, if the area is localized (walled off), the peritonitis will be localized. However, if this perforation allows free pus to leak in the abdominal cavity, frank peritonitis and rapid progression to septic shock occur.

Taking a detailed history is very important in patients who present with early or advanced appendicitis. In early appendicitis, patients complain of vague periumbilical pain. This vague pain is visceral and due to the stretching of the appendiceal wall. This is indicative of a localized process limited to the appendix. As the appendicitis progresses and the adjacent tissues become inflamed, the parietal peritoneum becomes irritated and causes localized (lateralized) pain. This parietal (somatic) pain can be influenced by the location of the appendix tip. When the appendix is in a retrocecal or paracecal region, appendicitis must be considered, along with cholecystitis, duodenal ulcer, pyelonephritis, and nephrolithiasis. When the appendix tip is in the iliac fossa, one must consider other differential diagnoses, which can include Meckel's diverticulum, duodenal ulcer, ureterolithiasis, regional enteritis, mesenteric adenitis, and *Yersinia* infection.

The difficulty in discriminating between appendicitis and gynecologic processes occurs when the appendix tip is within the true pelvis. Irritation of the pelvic peritoneum occurs much in the same manner as can happen with an ectopic pregnancy, ovarian torsion, tubo-ovarian abscess, or ruptured corpus luteum cyst.

Invariably, appendicitis is associated with anorexia and nausea. If high-pressure distention of the appendix tip is noted, the patient may also experience vomiting. Occasionally, patients may have diarrhea. An urge to bear down is often a sensation felt in patients with early appendicitis.[15] Physical signs noted on examination include localizing deep tenderness and associated muscle rigidity. Again, depending on the appendiceal tip, this deep tenderness may be found in the right lower quadrant or in the pelvis by examination. If the appendix tip is irritating the anterior lower quadrant peritoneum, then classic McBurney's point tenderness and local rigidity are found. If a retrocecal appendix is noted, then the patient frequently has irritation of the psoas and quadratus lumborum, which causes muscle, flank, or iliac pain. When the tip is in the pelvis, the obturator fascia may be inflamed. Unfortunately, abdominal wall rigidity may be absent and mislead one's suspicion away from appendicitis. An inflamed appendiceal tip may also irritate the rectosigmoid or bladder peritoneum and cause perturbation of these organ sites. Similarly, irritation of the adnexa may lead to cervical motion tenderness and confusion with a gynecologic process.

The duration of acute appendicitis from onset to perforation is usually 36 hours or less. Most patients seek medical attention within the first 12 to 18 hours.[16] Because of this rapid progression, observation of the patient with an otherwise nonacute abdomen is frequently recommended. Evolution of this process over 4 to 6 hours will make an uncertain diagnosis more clear if appendicitis is present. Once a decision is made to operate, then exploration should be undertaken to identify the appendix and other structures that may mimic the presentation, including the distal ileum (Meckel's diverticulum), ovaries, and fallopian tubes. With evolving appendicitis, the omentum frequently envelops the appendix, as will adjacent loops of small intestines. In a nonperforated appendix, loose fibrinous adhesions may occasionally anneal these structures in an effort to isolate the appendix from the other intraperitoneal structures. These adhesions separate easily. When a phlegmon occurs after appendiceal perforation, these adhesions of the regional viscera and omentum become more tenacious. Careful sharp dissection is necessary to minimize the risk of injury of these inflamed organs. If an abscess has formed, one should limit the spread of this pus intraoperatively, during the dissection. Resection of the appendix involves division of the mesoappendix and ligation of the appendiceal tip. With a nonadherent appendix, the appendix is grasped and the mesoappendix is placed on gentle traction. In this manner, the mesoappendix can be divided into several pedicles that are individually clamped and ligated with self-ties. Particular attention is addressed to the appendiceal artery, which is a terminal branch of the ileocolic artery. This inserts into the appendix most prominently at the base. Particular attention needs to be made in developing this lower pedicle of the mesoappendix. When the mesoappendix is inflamed and edematous, these blood vessels can often be difficult to manage. If a vessel retracts into the mesoappendix, frequently carefully placed figure-of-eight sutures along the cut edge or just proximal cut edge control the bleeding. Gentle, firm pressure is recommended when securing knots. This allows the inflamed tissue to squeeze together. Rapid, jerking motion frequently tears the inflamed tissue, resulting in more bleeding. Ligation of the appendiceal base is performed with two sutures of 2-0 silk or 1-0 chromic suture. The ligation should occur approximately 5 mm from the junction of the appendix with the cecum. The ligatures are often placed in a crush zone made by applying a straight hemostat. The crush maneuver displaces feces out of the ligated base. The appendix is then cut above the ligatures. The appendix stump can be buried with a pursestring suture of 2-0 silk placed approximately 1 cm lateral to the appendix base in a seromuscular fashion. When the cecum is inflamed, this pursestring suture is usually not recommended. The appendix tip, when not buried, is then brushed with electrocautery to sterilize the mucosa. Copious irrigation is then carried out by instillation and aspiration of small amounts of fluid. Dumping large volumes of fluid into the operative field, then aspirating, may contribute to dissemination of contaminated material into the abdominal cavity.

With a perforated appendix, the tip is frequently bound down in the phlegmon. Because of the extensive inflammation, mobilization of the tip may risk tearing the appendix base or cecum. When this is encountered, the mesoappendix and appendix base should be divided first before mobilizing the tip. If a large pelvic abscess is encountered and the appendix cannot be readily identified, evacuation of the abscess is undertaken without removal of the appendix. Antibiotics are given postoperatively for 5 to 7 days. A delayed, staged appendectomy can then be performed 6 to 8 weeks after this initial drainage. If preoperative radiographic studies suggest an abscess that is isolated from the abdominal cavity, the abscess may be drained under ultrasonographic or computed tomographic guidance. This potentially allows a single definitive operation because the antibiotics and drainage reduce the local inflammation. If the appendix is not visualized during the primary procedure or not removed after antibiotic medical management, recurrent appendicitis may evolve. To minimize this risk, a staged appendectomy is recommended.

Rarely, the appendix can give rise to neoplas-tic processes. The most common malignancies are carcinoid tumors and adenocarcinoma. Carcinoid tumors are usually benign in behavior even if frankly malignant under histologic examination. They frequently are brown-tan grossly. Simple appendectomy is usually the only procedure necessary. A caveat must be addressed for tumors larger than 2 cm or when mesenteric lymph node metastases are evident. These patients usually require a right ileocolectomy. Adenocarcinoma of the appendix is rare; and because of the vestigial nature of the organ, it usually presents as advanced disease. Again, a right colectomy is performed with resection of the regional mesentery. When intra-abdominal spread and liver metastases are present, a palliative bypass is usually performed.

Pseudomyxoma peritonei can arise with both ovarian and appendiceal origin. In this situation, both the pathologic ovary and the appendix should always be removed. The pseudomyxoma peritonei can present as mucoid, jelly-like fluid in the abdomen or as a very desmoplastic, styrofoam-like process with malignant pseudomyxoma. The former material can be loosened for evacuation by instilling 10% dextrose. This will effectively melt the gelatinous material. The anesthesiologist should be warned to check for increased glucose levels during the operation. If an adnexal mass is removed and the pathologist gives a diagnosis of a mucinous cystadenoma or mucinous adenocarcinoma, the appendix should be removed because of the rare synchronous tumors that can arise in the appendix and ovary. This is more common in right-sided ovarian masses.

A mucocele of the appendix may arise with obstruction of the appendix and no secondary infection or vascular compromise. These masses may evolve into a signficant size if the process develops slowly. Resection of the mass is similar to the simple appendectomy.

Increasing use of laparoscopy in the management of lower abdominal pain has led to increasing use of laparoscopic appendectomy. Most clinicians, however, use laparoscopy to render a diagnosis and convert to the appropriate open procedure necessary to address the disease present. With acute appendicitis, a lateral port may be placed that is 12 mm in size and used to grasp the inflamed appendix with a laparoscopic Babcock clamp and to deliver the appendix through the port site for open resection. Particular care must be taken with this management to adequately irrigate the incision site and to obtain adequate fascial closure to minimize the risk of a postoperative hernia. Pure laparoscopic appendectomies can be performed in a number of ways. The manner used is based on the experience of the surgeon and instrument preference. Laparoscopic appendectomy requires advanced video laparoscopic skills and is usually limited to nonadherent, nonperforated appendices. Because most surgeons require more time to perform a laparoscopic appendectomy, a complicated appendicitis should not be managed by most surgeons laparoscopically. The video laparoscope is usually placed in the umbilical port. Five-mm ancillary ports are placed under direct visualization in the right and left lower quadrants with a 12-mm port in the suprapubic region. The appendix tip is grasped and placed on gentle traction. The mesoappendix can then be divided with an endoscopic stapling device, bipolar electrocautery, sequential hemoclip application, or sequential pre-tied chronic loop ligatures. I prefer the use of pre-tied chromic loops because this is the least expensive method. The mesoappendix is developed using blunt dissection with endoshears into sequential pedicles that are secured with an endoloop. The method of application involves passing the endoloop through the ipsilateral lower-quadrant port. A 5-mm grasping instrument is then passed through the loop and used to grasp the pedicle. The pedicle is then cut distal to the grasper, and the loop is then secured over the pedicle base. A trained surgical team can accomplish this maneuver more rapidly than bipolar cautery of the entire mesoappendix can be done. Frequently, the entire mesoappendix can be secured with an endoloop in one pedicle. The appendix base is then ligated twice with an endoloop. A third distal endoloop is placed, and the appendix is cut between the distal loop and the base ligatures. When a perforated appendix or very inflamed appendix base is encountered and the risk of laceration of this structure near the cecum is high, endoscopic stapling is recommended to minimize the risk of tearing with manipulation. After laparoscopic appendectomy, the appendix is removed through a 10- or 12-mm port. A perforated or gangrenous appendix should be placed in the bag before removal. Again, copious irrigation is carried out.[17, 18]

DIVERTICULAR DISEASE

The large bowel may give rise to outpouchings at the site of vessel perforation through the longitudinal bands of the colon (teniae). These outpouchings are more common with advancing age and weight of the patient. They are more frequent in the left colon, especially the sigmoid. Obstruction of these diverticula by feces or particulate matter may cause inflammation. Symptoms elicited by this inflammation include lower abdominal pain (left greater than right), changes in bowel habit, and diarrhea and narrowing caliber of stools. With a diverticular abscess, extrinsic compression of the colon may cause constipation and tenesmus. Fever and leukocytosis are frequently present. Rectovaginal examination may reveal a palpable pelvic mass when an abscess is present. Preoperative imaging should include contrast-bearing enema or computed tomography with rectal contrast medium enhancement. Computed tomography also provides an assessment of the ureter. Development of fistulas can occur with diverticular abscesses. Communication with the small intestine, ureter, bladder, and vagina may occur, and computed tomography is beneficial in demonstrating these processes.

Conservative management is initially used and is composed of intravenous antibiotics and nasogastric suction. Chronic diverticulitis without an abscess usually improves with this therapy. If the patient does not improve, computed tomography with water-soluble rectal contrast medium should be obtained. If the abscess is localized, it can be drained percutaneously and eliminate the need for staged surgical management.

Patients requiring emergency surgical exploration for diverticulitis have generalized peritonitis and occasionally hemorrhage. These patients will not have adequate bowel preparation. There is considerable debate as to the optimal management.[19] The traditional management is a two- or three-stage procedure, beginning with a transverse colostomy and drainage of the abscess. This may be the initial surgery in those patients too medically compromised to undergo resection of the involved segment of colon with diverticulitis. A second-stage operation may then be performed if the patient improves, which would include resection of the involved colon with colostomy and either mucous fistula or closure of the rectal stump to create a Hartmann pouch (Fig. 7–14). The third stage in this traditional management would then be reanastomosis 2 to 3 months after the second-stage operation. Performing a simple transverse colostomy and drainage may not remove the cause of sepsis and, therefore, most surgeons attempt resection of the involved colon with the initial surgery if the patient is medically stable. Initial surgery with

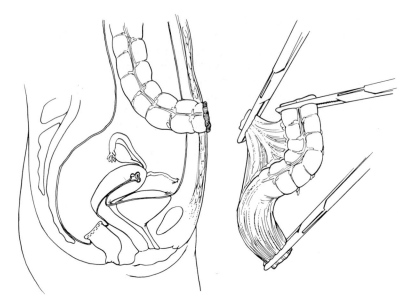

FIGURE 7–14
End-descending colostomy with Hartmann pouch. (From Gershenson DM, DeCherney AH, Curry SL. Operative Gynecology. Philadelphia, WB Saunders, 1993.)

resection of the involved colon and end colostomy in Hartmann's pouch is the most commonly practiced management. Some surgeons have recommended lavage with primary reanastomosis and no colostomy.[20]

A gynecologist exploring an abdomen in a patient with pelvic pain and with a mass is faced with a management dilemma when encountering a diverticular abscess. If the gynecologist does not have substantial experience in bowel surgery, a consultation with a general surgeon or gynecologic oncologist should be obtained. Resection of the mass should be undertaken if the patient is not medically compromised. In those rare instances in which a colon cancer has not been ruled out preoperatively, a frozen section of the resected segment of colon should be performed to ensure the adequate mesenteric resection is obtained if cancer is present. When the bowel is unprepared, most surgeons would recommend end colostomy and creation of a Hartmann pouch with a second-stage anastomosis.

LARGE BOWEL OBSTRUCTION AND CECOSTOMY VERSUS TRANSVERSE COLOSTOMY

Rarely, a gynecologist explores the abdomen for a large bowel obstruction. The most common causes are colon cancer, diverticular disease, Crohn's disease, inflammatory bowel disease, and extrinsic compression by ovarian carcinoma.

Radiographic findings of large bowel obstruction include a dilated colon. The diameter of the cecum should be measured to assess the risk of perforation. When the cecum measures greater than 10 cm, the risk of perforation is extremely high. This warrants surgical exploration. In a medically compromised patient, a right lower quadrant incision to deliver the cecum for a tube cecostomy is the most expedient procedure to decompress the patient. However, the irrigation of the obstructed colon is difficult with this procedure. In Ogilvie's syndrome (pseudo-obstruction) a tube cecostomy is preferable to a skin level cecostomy or transverse colectomy because simple decompression is the treatment. This syndrome can occur after recent surgery and has been described after vaginal delivery and cesarean section. Ogilvie's syndrome may also be managed by endoscopic evacuation of gas, but the right colon may be difficult to access and the risk of perforation may increase with this procedure. When an obstructing lesion is present, especially in the left colon, a transverse loop colostomy or skin level cecostomy can more easily remove stool between the colostomy and the obstruction site with irrigation. A potential problem with a transverse loop colostomy to manage a large bowel obstruction is that large cecal dilatation may cause segmental ischemia and necrosis in the cecum. Therefore, the cecum should be inspected if a transverse loop colostomy is performed.

A cecostomy is performed by making an incision over McBurney's point through the skin external oblique, internal oblique, and transverse muscles. Because of the caliber of the cecum, a muscle-splitting technique, used in an appendectomy, should be avoided and the muscle should be directly divided to deliver the cecum for inspection and cecostomy. Once the peritoneum is incised, the cecum should be inspected for areas of necrosis. If necrosis is identified, this should be used as the site for cecostomy by resection of this portion of the cecal wall. A 16-gauge needle decompression can be performed to more thoroughly complete the inspection. The defect can then be oversewn with an imbricating suture. For a tube cecostomy, pursestring sutures are made approximately 2 cm in diameter using 3-0 silk or polyglycolic acid suture. A stab incision is then made in the center of the pursestring and a 32 F to 34 F mushroom catheter is inserted into the cecum and advanced into the ascending colon. The pursestring sutures are then tied. The tube is then brought out through a separate stab incision. The peritoneum of the cecum is then attached to the parietal peritoneum using interrupted Lembert sutures in a manner consistent with a Stamm gastrostomy to isolate the opening from the rest of the abdominal cavity.

For a skin-level cecostomy, the cecum is sutured with interrupted 3-0 polyglycolic seromuscular stitches to the external oblique fascia. This isolates the cecal opening from the peritoneal cavity. The cecum is then opened parallel to the longitudinal bands. This is then matured to the skin. The fascial defect and skin defect should be no more than 4 to 5 cm long. If the fascial or skin opening is greater than this before maturing the cecostomy, these incisions can be reduced with interrupted sutures. The cecostomy is then sewn to the skin with interrupted 3-0 or 4-0 sutures.

A transverse loop colostomy can also be performed for obstructing lesions (Fig. 7–15). Typically, the mid or right portion of the transverse colon should be used. Vascular compromise in the left transverse colon may occur if problems with the middle colic tributaries or the marginal artery of Drummond tributaries are insufficient. A 5- to 6-cm incision (longitudinal) is made in the abdomen. The peritoneum is entered, and the transverse colon is grasped. The omentum is dissected off the colon and displaced cephalad. If greater than 10 cm of dilation of the cecum is present, the incision should be lengthened to inspect the cecum. The transverse colon should be mobile enough to allow the loop of selected transverse colon to be delivered easily out of the field without tension. A window is made in the mesentery under the loop of colon. This is isolated with a Penrose drain and tagged. The abdominal

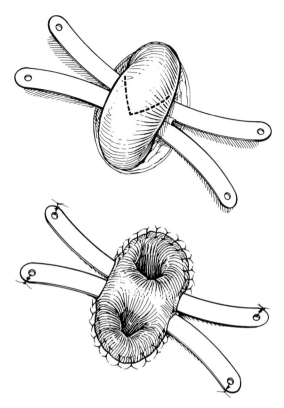

FIGURE 7–15
Loop colostomy is matured. (From Gershenson DM, DeCherney AH, Curry SL. Operative Gynecology. Philadelphia, WB Saunders, 1993.)

incision is then closed to permit only 2 to 3 fingerbreadths. The serosa of the transverse colon can be secured to the anterior fascia with interrupted sutures. With a dilated colon, this is often not permissible. In a manner similar to cecostomy, if marked dilation is present and needle decompression can be performed, a glass rod or plastic bridge can then be inserted through the mesenteric window (Fig. 7–16). A

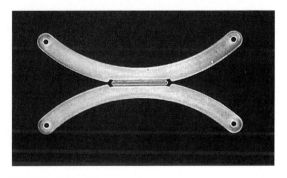

FIGURE 7–16
Hollister bridge. (From Gershenson DM, DeCherney AH, Curry SL. Operative Gynecology. Philadelphia, WB Saunders, 1993.)

semilunar transverse incision is made in the entire mesenteric portion of the colon. The stoma is then matured by sewing full-thickness bowel to skin with interrupted sutures to secure a mucocutaneous approximation. An atraumatic needle with 3-0 or 40 polyglycolic suture is used. The bridge is left in place for 2 weeks. After this time, fixation of the stoma to the anterior abdominal wall is adequate. A frequent complication with transverse loop colostomy is a hernia, which can be minimized with attention at the time of approximating new fascia intraoperatively.

GASTROSTOMY

Tube gastrostomies are typically performed as a secondary procedure during an intra-abdominal operation. Tube gastrostomies may also be placed without a laparotomy by use of percutaneous endoscopic-guided placement or by an invasive radiologist under fluoroscopic guidance. Gynecologists use intraoperative gastrostomy when patients are at risk for prolonged gastric decompression (i.e., extensive carcinomatosis with impending small bowel obstruction, multiple bowel resections). This is most commonly encountered in patients undergoing debulking surgery for ovarian carcinoma. Those patients with suboptimal debulking who are at high risk for proximal small bowel obstruction can benefit postoperatively from the gastrostomy tube. The gastrostomy tube can be used for decompression and for low-rate enteral feedings. It may also be left in place in these patients during chemotherapy. If bowel function returns, the gastrostomy tube may be clamped. Because approximately 40% of patients will rapidly progress in this setting, high-grade obstruction due to carcinomatous obstruction can be relieved if the gastrostomy tube is maintained for intermittent drainage.

Several techniques have been developed for open tube gastrostomy placement. The most popular is the Stamm gastrostomy. The anterior wall of the stomach is exposed, and a pursestring suture approximately 1.5 cm in diameter is circumscribed with a seromuscular 2-0 polyglycolic or silk suture. The stomach is then opened with electrocautery in the middle of the pursestring site. A 24 F or greater Foley catheter or mushroom catheter is inserted. The pursestring suture is then secured. A stab wound is then made in the left upper abdomen through the rectus muscle. The rectus fascia at the level of the midline incision is grasped and placed on medial traction to allow appropriate

location. A Péan clamp is passed through the incision and used to grasp the distal end of the catheter. This is then withdrawn through the created defect in the anterior abdominal wall.

A second imbricating pursestring suture can then be placed around the catheter to further bury the gastric opening. The anterior wall of the stomach around the gastrostomy tube is then approximated to the anterior parietal peritoneum with interrupted 2-0 sutures. The catheter is placed on traction to approximate the anterior stomach wall against the abdominal wall and isolate the opening from the abdominal cavity. A second gastrostomy method, known as the Witzel technique, involves placement of the catheter into the stomach wall in an identical fashion as the Stamm procedure, using a pursestring suture. However, to isolate the gastrostomy opening from the abdominal cavity, the gastrostomy tube is laid parallel to the anterior wall of the stomach and serial imbricated sutures are used to bury the gastrostomy tube with overlying adjacent anterior gastric wall. A similar anterior abdominal wall stab opening is created, and the gastrostomy tube is passed through this defect. The anterior stomach wall is not secured to the anterior abdominal wall peritoneum. These are equally effective techniques, but most surgeons use the Stamm method.

A third gastrostomy method can be performed using a linear GIA stapling device. This Janeway gastrostomy does not require a chronic indwelling tube because a segment of stomach is brought through to the skin level. The anterior stomach wall is grasped with Babcock clamps in the mid body, closer to the greater curvature than the lesser curvature. This segment of anterior stomach wall is elevated, and a linear GIA is used to staple, ligate, and divide the anterior stomach wall and create a nipple measuring 4 to 5 cm in length. This nipple is then oversewn along the staple line to decrease the caliber and minimize potential reflux through this site and also isolate the staple line. The nipple is then drawn through a stab incision made immediately above this site. The nipple of the anterior stomach wall is then brought up through the abdominal wall and the tip is opened. A 16 F or 18 F catheter is inserted into the stomach through this opening. The nipple is then sewn to the skin using full-thickness 3-0 polyglycolic sutures. This site is excellent for intermittent tube feedings and also for intermittent gastric decompression. Due to the limitation of catheter size, particulate matter cannot be easily drained through this catheter method.

POSTOPERATIVE CARE

Patients undergoing gastrointestinal surgery require some period of bowel rest after their surgery. For a simple appendectomy or uncomplicated colostomy, bowel function can be initiated quickly, in 1 to 2 days. With extensive enterolysis or with extensive bowel edema, a more prolonged period of bowel rest with gastric decompression is warranted. The old dictum of nothing by mouth until bowel movement or passage of flatus has been abandoned in an effort to shorten hospital stays. Resumption of normal bowel sounds and less than 1 L of nasogastric secretions in a 24-hour period are adequate to begin a trial of nasogastric tube clamping and periodic measurement of residual volumes. If adequate gastric emptying is evidenced by less than 150 mL of aspiration every 6 hours, then the nasogastric tube can be removed. Prolonged nasogastric suction is recommended when large bowel resection and anastomosis or small bowel resection and anastomosis is performed. Dilation of the anastomoses can increase the risk of leakage and subsequent breakdown, as well as impede blood flow to the healing anastomotic site. This is especially important when the patient has a preexisting history of atherosclerosis, diabetes, or prior abdominal or pelvic irradiation that predisposes to poor wound healing.

Baker long-tube placement has been advocated in patients with extensive small bowel adhesions.[21] This relatively stiff tube is passed through the entire small intestine to minimize the risk of kinking of the small intestine, which can become fixed with the re-formation of adhesions. This is frequently used in patients requiring multiple operations for small bowel obstructions. A tube is advanced through a small gastrostomy or jejunostomy opening that is secured by a pursestring suture and subsequently buried in a manner consistent with a Witzel imbrication as described earlier. The tube is advanced through the entire small intestine by milking the catheter tip along through the intestine. The tip is passed through the ileocecal valve, and the balloon tip is inflated with 5 mL of mercury or contrast medium. The small intestine is then arranged so the loops of intestines take gentle curves. The tube is then passed through a separate stab incision. Nasogastric decompression is also performed in the postoperative period. The Baker tube is left in place for 14 to 21 days. The balloon is then decompressed, and the tube is gradually withdrawn over 6 to 12 hours. No more than 6 to 8 inches is withdrawn at a time to minimize the risk of intussusception.

STOMAS

Location and size of intestinal stomas are critically important for patient satisfaction and to minimize the complication rate after surgery. Consequently, the surgeon should preoperatively counsel and mark patients for stoma sites. Right and left sites should be marked. The patient should be questioned and examined about the types of clothing she wears and where her clothing waistline is located. A stoma site that occurs in a skinfold or underneath a patient's waistline increases the risk of appliance leaking and consequent patient misery. Locating a stoma too close to an incision, a bony prominence, or umbilicus may make uniform faceplate application difficult. This is especially problematic in gastrostomy and ileostomy stomas that have secretions that can be very caustic to the skin.

In selecting a stoma site, the segment to be brought to the skin level should be mobilized sufficiently to allow delivery through the ab-

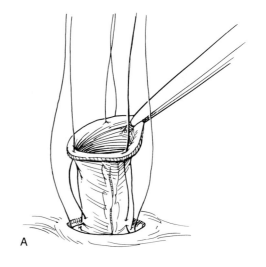

A

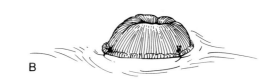

B

FIGURE 7–17
A and *B*, Rosebud stoma formation. (From Gershenson DM, DeCherney AH, Curry SL. Operative Gynecology. Philadelphia, WB Saunders, 1993.)

dominal wall defect without tension. The mesentery should not be on traction nor should it be excessively constricted by the opening through the fascia and rectus muscles. Too large an opening increases the risk of peristomal hernias. Inadequate mobilization increases the risk of sloughing of the end of the stoma or retraction of the stoma. Both of these may require reoperation for revision or tedious faceplate measures to optimize stoma appliance function. Preoperative consultation with a trained enterostomal therapist provides the patient with information and helps smooth her postoperative management of the stoma. Elevation of the stoma opening above the skin level helps minimize the risk of leaking underneath the faceplate of the stoma appliance. This can be accomplished by rosebudding the stoma when securing the intestinal edge to the skin (Fig. 7–17). A full-thickness pass through the intestinal edge is made with the 3-0 or 4-0 suture. Approximately 2 cm below this a seromuscular stitch is passed in the intestinal wall. The stitch is then passed through the skin. When securing this suture, a fold of intestine is elevated above the level of the skin.[22] This helps the bowel contents to fall out of the lumen and into the bag without tracking under the faceplace. This is most important with ileostomy stomas. Likewise, the size of the stoma is important. Two-cm stomas should be created for ileostomies. A greater diameter stretches the lumen and minimizes the height of the rosebud effect. Three- to 4-cm openings for colostomies are generally recommended. Loop colostomies require a larger opening. A greater risk for postoperative peristomal hernia formation occurs with a larger fascial opening. Stoma results are a direct reflection of the surgeon's familiarity with the procedure and attention to detail. Careful preoperative assessment and intraoperative technique ensures a minimum of postoperative complications.

REFERENCES

1. Krebs HB. Intestinal injury in gynecologic surgery: a 10-year experience. Am J Obstet Gynecol 1986;155:509–513.
2. Alvarez RD. Gastrointestinal complications in gynecologic surgery: a review for the general gynecologist. Obstet Gynecol 1988;72(3, part II):533–539.
3. Hurt WG, Dunn LJ. Complications of gynecologic surgery and trauma. In: Greenfield LJ, ed. Complications in Surgery and Trauma. Philadelphia, JB Lippincott, 1984, pp 790–799.
4. Gambee LP. A single-layer open-intestinal anastomosis applicable to the small as well as the large intestine. West J Surg Obstet Gynecol 1951;59:1–5.
5. DeAlmelda AC. A modified single-layer suture for use in the gastrointestinal tract. Surg Gynecol Obstet 1971;132:985.
6. Irvine TT, Edwards JP. Comparison of single-layer inverting, two-layer inverting, and everting anastomoses in the rabbit colon. Br J Surg 1973;60:453.
7. Goligher JC, Lee PWG, et al. A controlled comparison of one- and two-layer techniques of suturing for high and low colorectal anastomosis. Br J Surg 1977;64:49.
8. Gambee LP, Garnjobs TW. Ten years' experience with a single-layer anastomosis in colon surgery. Am J Surg 1956;92:222.
9. Dresner LS, MacArthur S, Wait RB. Small intestine. In: Davis JH, Sheldon GF, eds. Surgery, a Problem-Solving Approach, 2nd ed, vol. II. St. Louis, Mosby–Year Book, 1995, p 1334.
10. Soderlund S. Meckel's diverticulum: a clinical and histologic study. Acta Chir Scand 1959;248:1.
11. Ellis H. Meckel's diverticulum, diverticulosis of the small intestine, umbilical fistulae and tumors. In: Schwartz SI, Ellis H, eds. Maingot's Abdominal Operations, 8th ed. Norwalk, CT, Appleton-Century-Crofts, 1985, pp 833–837, 839.
12. Soltero MJ, Bill AH. The natural history of Meckel's diverticulum and its relation to incidental removal. Am J Surg 1976;132:168.
13. Mackey WC, Dineen T. A 50-year experience with Meckel's diverticulum. Surg Gynecol Obstet 1983;156:56.
14. Weinstein EC, Dockerty MB, et al. Neoplasms of Meckel's diverticulum. Surg Gynecol Obstet 1963;16:103.
15. Silen W. Cope's Early Diagnosis of the Acute Abdomen, 16th ed. New York, Oxford University Press, 1983, p 65.
16. Lewis F, Hunter JG. Appendix. In: Davis JH, Sheldon GF, eds. Surgery, a Problem Solving Approach, 2nd ed, vol II. St. Louis, Mosby–Year Book, 1995, p 1365.
17. Pier A, Goütz F, Bacher C. Laparoscopic appendectomy in 625 cases: From innovation to routine. Surg Laparosc Endosc 1991;1:8.
18. Tate JJ, Dawson JW, Chung SCS, et al. Laparoscopic versus open appendicectomy: Prospective randomized trial. Lancet 1993;342:633.
19. Gordon PH, Nivatvongs S: Rectum and anus. In: Davis JH, Sheldon GF, eds. Surgery: A Problem-Solving Approach, 2nd ed. St. Louis, Mosby–Year Book, 1995, p 1421.
20. Krukowski ZH, Matheson NA. Emergency surgery for diverticular disease complicated by general and fecal peritonitis: a review. Br J Surg 1984;71:921.
21. Baker JW. Stitchless plication for recurring obstruction of the small bowel. Am J Surg 1968;116:316.
22. Turnbull RB Jr, Weakley FL. Atlas of intestinal stomas. St. Louis, CV Mosby, 1967.

8
Peggy A. Norton

CHAPTER

Urologic Complications

Injury to the urinary tract is often associated with gynecologic surgery because of the close proximity of the female pelvic organs to the ureter, bladder, and urethra. Gynecologists are often called on to operate in the pelvis in conditions that make identification of the urinary tract difficult, such as emergency bleeding, extensive adhesions, abnormal or distorted anatomy, and infection. It has been said that given enough surgical experience, any gynecologist is likely to encounter operative injury to the lower urinary tract. The relative infrequency of such injuries makes even the best surgeon unpracticed or inexperienced in their management. If urologic complications are suspected intraoperatively or postoperatively, consultation with other surgeons should be considered. Appropriate consultants may include urologists, gynecologic oncologists, urogynecologists, or others with special interest or experience in the lower urinary tract.

Some experience may be gained by reading textbooks and published reports of urologic complications, so that the surgeon is familiar with their management in theory, if not in practice. This chapter deals with complications to the lower urinary tract associated with gynecologic surgery. These complications may include operative injury and alterations in lower urinary tract function, such as a patient with obstructed voiding after anti-incontinence procedures. Individual complications are discussed according to the anatomic division of the lower urinary tract (bladder, ureter, and urethra). Principles for the prevention, recognition, and management of these complications are similar in each anatomic area and are discussed in the latter half of the chapter. Finally, tests that may be helpful in the evaluation of these complications are addressed separately.

COMPLICATIONS ASSOCIATED WITH THE URINARY BLADDER

When recognized and treated appropriately, bladder injury rarely leads to long-term complications. The urinary bladder is a unique organ well suited to its function of storage and emptying. The bladder wall is formed of alternating layers of smooth muscle, which can accommodate an increase in volume from empty to 600 mL with little increase in muscular tone. With overdistention, the bladder wall becomes thin and makes injury more likely; conversely, an empty bladder is less likely to be injured during pelvic surgery. Another important principle is that urine is contained in dependent

areas of the bladder: injuries to these areas must be drained longer than nondependent areas, where urine is less likely to rest and impair healing.

The urinary bladder lies in the retroperitoneal space of Retzius and rests on top of the anterior vaginal wall, cervix, and corpus uteri (Fig. 8–1). It is this intimate relationship with the pelvic organs that renders the urinary bladder prone to injury. When distended, the bladder is spherical. When empty, it is tetrahedral,[1] with a small posterior surface or base, a superior surface that expands with filling, and two inferolateral surfaces that receive the ureters. The posterior part of the superior surface rests on the corpus uteri, while the bladder base rests on the cervix and anterior vagina. The blood supply to the bladder is from the internal iliac arteries, with the superior vesical artery supplying the superior and lateral walls, and with contributions from the inferior vesical, obturator, and some components of the uterine and vaginal arterial supply, especially to the bladder base.

In the middle third of the anterior vaginal wall is the trigone, a triangular region defined by the ureteral orifices and the urethrovesical junction (bladder neck). Injury to this area affects bladder function and may also signal ureteral compromise. It is informative to identify the area of the trigone on vaginal examination. The bladder neck may be palpated easily if a Foley balloon is gently pulled down to the urethrovesical junction. The trigone rests in the anterior vaginal wall, with the ureteral orifices located some 2 cm lateral and cephalad from the bladder neck. This can be confirmed cystoscopically, using a finger to elevate the ureteral orifice and then noting this location vaginally.

Several factors are helpful in the dissection of the urinary bladder away from nearby pelvic organs. Identification of the muscular wall of the bladder is easier when the bladder is empty or may be facilitated in difficult dissections by intentional cystotomy at the dome of the bladder (see later). Excessive bleeding is one clue that the dissection may be too close to the bladder. In vaginal hysterectomy, the dissection should stay close to the midline with sharp scissors held with tips pointing away from the bladder (Fig. 8–2). In patients with previous cesarean sections, the bladder may be adherent to the lower uterine segment. In such cases, the addition of 2 mL of indigo carmine in 50 to 100 mL of sterile water or saline will stain bladder epithelium deep blue and may help to identify a dissection that has been carried into the bladder wall. In general, blunt

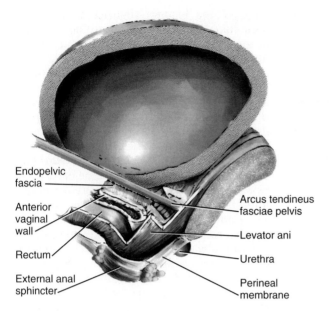

Endopelvic
fascia

Anterior
vaginal
wall

Rectum

External anal
sphincter

Arcus tendineus
fasciae pelvis

Levator ani

Urethra

Perineal
membrane

FIGURE 8–1
Relationship of the bladder to the vaginal
support structures. (From DeLancey JOL.
Structural support of the urethra as it relates to
stress urinary incontinence: the hammock
hypothesis. Am J Obstet Gynecol
1994;170:1713–1723.)

dissection with a sponge stick should be avoided in this area, especially if the bladder is adherent to the uterine wall.

Intraoperative Injury to the Urinary Bladder

Intraoperative injuries have been reported with abdominal hysterectomy (1.8%),[2] vaginal hysterectomy (0.4%),[2] cesarean section (less than 1%),[3] anti-incontinence procedures, surgery for pelvic organ prolapse, and laparoscopic procedures (approximately 1%).[4] Similar rates of bladder injury (2%–5%) are reported in general surgery procedures involving the pelvic organs.[5, 6]

UNINTENTIONAL CYSTOTOMY

Unintentional cystotomy is most likely to happen when the bladder wall is thinned or when the dissection has been difficult or very close to a poorly identified bladder wall.

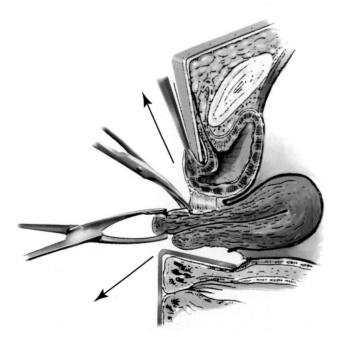

FIGURE 8–2
Dissection of the vesicovaginal space with the
points of the scissors directed away from the
bladder. (From Thompson J, Rock J, eds.
TeLinde's Operative Gynecology, 7th ed.
Philadelphia, JB Lippincott, 1992.)

Nondependent Unintentional Cystotomy

At the bladder dome, these injuries heal with short-term drainage and are unlikely to cause long-term sequelae. Such injury may occur during emergency cesarean or other situations of blunt dissection, particularly when there are adhesions from previous pelvic surgery. The greatest risk from nondependent unintentional cystotomy is that the injury may not be identified, especially if the injury is small and if urine is well drained away from this site. If any suspicion exists, 3 to 5 mL of intravenous indigo carmine should be given with 10 mg of furosemide; with the urethral catheter clamped, any compromise of the bladder wall can be visualized within 10 to 15 minutes.

These injuries should be closed in a double-layer closure and drained for 3 to 5 days. In general, a suprapubic catheter should not be placed through the unintentional site but located in a separate place at the bladder dome. Urethral drainage is an equally good option in the circumstance of nondependent injury, because the drainage time is anticipated to be limited. Do all unintentional cystotomies need repair and drainage? Bladder rupture from external trauma is sometimes managed with catheterization alone if the injury is known to be extraperitoneal.[5] After 10 days, the defect can be demonstrated as spontaneously closed on intravenous pyelography. In the case of cystotomy during gynecologic surgery, we would advocate immediate repair and appropriate drainage.

Dependent Unintentional Cystotomy

Urine may be present in dependent portions of the bladder even with adequate bladder drainage. Dependent cystotomy is an injury that may occur during vaginal surgery, in the posterior and lateral bladder walls in close proximity to the trigone. If any doubt exists, the cystotomy should be treated as dependent. Injuries at the bladder base may involve the ureters, and ureteral patency must be documented. A large defect in a dependent area of the bladder may require a second intentional cystotomy at the dome to repair the injury.

Dissection of the anterior vaginal wall is the one situation in which identification of bladder entry is facilitated by leaving a small amount of urine in the bladder, usually 50 mL or less. Because blue dye may be difficult to visualize, instillation of sterile milk (readily available from the nursery) may be useful to identify a small cystotomy. Otherwise, identification and management is similar to that for nondependent injuries, except that the bladder should be drained continuously for 7 to 10 days to allow healing in the presence of minimal urine. It may be more comfortable for these patients to use a suprapubic catheter.

SUTURE INJURIES TO THE BLADDER

Suture may enter the bladder wall during closure of the anterior vaginal cuff on hysterectomy, closure of a hysterotomy during cesarean section, placement of the elevating sutures of a retropubic or needle urethropexy, or anterior colporrhaphy. When the suture is tied, penetration of the bladder can be missed because there is no immediate leakage. Sutures that enter the bladder wall but not the bladder lumen may cause no long-term sequelae but can cause pain and irritable bladder symptoms. Permanent suture lying within the bladder is rarely asymptomatic and may lead to chronic cystitis or stone formation. Therefore, the surgeon who uses permanent suture near the bladder wall must ensure that perforation has not occurred, usually using cystoscopy. During needle urethropexy, a bladder perforation is easier to visualize using a 70-degree scope. Some surgeons prefer to perform cystoscopy with the needle in place before the suture is passed, because the metal instrument is easier to identify than the suture. There is no need to incorporate any bladder wall during anterior colporrhaphy, because this does not contribute any strength or volume reduction to the procedure and may produce urgency and frequency through irritation to the bladder trigone.

More troublesome is suture that incorporates the bladder wall and another structure: closure of low transverse hysterotomy during cesarean section or of the anterior vaginal cuff during hysterectomy. Once the suture is tied, the mistake may be more difficult to detect, and tissue necrosis ensues within 7 to 10 days. In healing, the necrotic bladder wall may develop into a vesicovaginal fistula. Identification of the bladder wall and sharp dissection away from the suture line is crucial to the prevention of these injuries. Cystoscopy, either urethral or suprapubic, may not identify these injuries if the lumen is not involved. Suture incorporation is treated intraoperatively by immediate release of the suture. The pinpoint perforation of the suture closes spontaneously and does not require prolonged drainage unless laceration of the bladder wall resulted from the suture and its removal. Fistula is further considered below.

BLUNT OR SHARP TRAUMA TO THE BLADDER

Intraoperatively, trauma is most likely to occur with the large straight "needles" used with the Pereyra, Stamey, or Raz urethropexy. Perforations with the needles used in these procedures can be treated by simply removing the needle. Other intraoperative trauma may occur with a laparoscopic trocar or urethral or cervical dilation and should be treated as cystotomy injuries described earlier. Occasionally, a hematoma may form in the wall of the bladder and may benefit transiently from compression by a filled bladder.

Postoperative Bladder Complications

Postoperative bladder complications can be divided into those from injuries that were not identified at the time of surgery and those associated with perivesical surgical procedures such as anti-incontinence operations.

POSTOPERATIVE IDENTIFICATION OF BLADDER INJURIES

It is fortunate to identify bladder injuries intraoperatively, because the repair is usually straightforward with few long-term sequelae. When the bladder injury is identified postoperatively, there has usually been considerable delay.

Vesicovaginal fistula is a dreaded sequelae of suturing of the bladder wall to other structures, usually the vaginal cuff at the time of hysterectomy. The patient presents with a new onset of continuous incontinence, somewhat better in the supine position and occasionally permitting partial bladder filling for voiding. The source of the leakage is not always easy to visualize per vagina or cystoscopically, especially if the site is minute. A triple tampon or swab test can be used (see later). Intravenous urography and voiding cystourethrography may be helpful in some cases, although the failure of these procedures to identify any fistula is nondiagnostic. However, postoperative loss of urine is more commonly due to severe urge, stress, or overflow incontinence. Urodynamic testing should be done if the symptoms of urine loss persist in the absence of a detectable fistula.

Post-hysterectomy vesicovaginal fistula is usually supratrigonal; that is, the connection between the bladder and vagina is at the top of the vault above the trigone and ureters. This is the most uncomplicated fistula to repair and is within the capabilities of most vaginal surgeons. The Latzko procedure uses partial colpocleisis to effect the repair and is successful in more than 80% of procedures. The connection between bladder and vagina is repaired by closing the top of the vagina (Fig. 8–3). The dissection is of the vaginal skin surrounding the fistula, and no attempt is made to excise the fistula tract. The top of the vaginal vault is then closed with progressive layers of delayed absorbable polyglycolic acid suture, testing for water-tightness with sterile milk after the second layer. Overlying suture layers should be avoided, and the tissue should be adequately mobilized for the suture line to be without tension. The use of local anesthesia with epinephrine is not recommended because this may impair healing. Although dyspareunia from shortening of the vagina is of theoretical concern, the actual shortening seen in these patients is minimal and appears to be less of a problem than shortening seen with overaggressive anterior colporrhaphy. Prolonged bladder drainage is not necessary and is even contraindicated after a Latzko repair of a supratrigonal post-hysterectomy vesicovaginal fistula—the bladder epithelium is untouched, and the catheter may actually prove irritating.

The timing of vesicovaginal fistula repair is an individual choice between surgeon and patient. No repair should be undertaken until inflammation and edema from the first procedure have resolved, usually after 6 weeks or more. The bladder should be continuously drained per urethra during this time. After initial healing, the choice is between immediate repair or delayed repair after 3 months. Thompson quotes a slightly higher reported success rate with delayed repair (95%) compared with immediate repair (80%).[7] However, these patients are miserable with the constant wetness, and immediate repair may save them months of discomfort.[8]

Larger fistula or second attempts at repair may necessitate the use of a bulbocavernosus fat graft if repaired per vagina or the use of an omental pedicle graft if repaired retropubically. These include the excision of the fistula tract and multiple-layer closure using delayed absorbable suture. The grafts are placed between the suture line and the vaginal epithelium, providing both increased vascular supply and intervening tissue to prevent recurrence. Fistulas may be difficult to manage in the case of radiated tissue, multiple fistulas, and fistulas close to the ureteral orifices and are best handled by an experienced specialist.

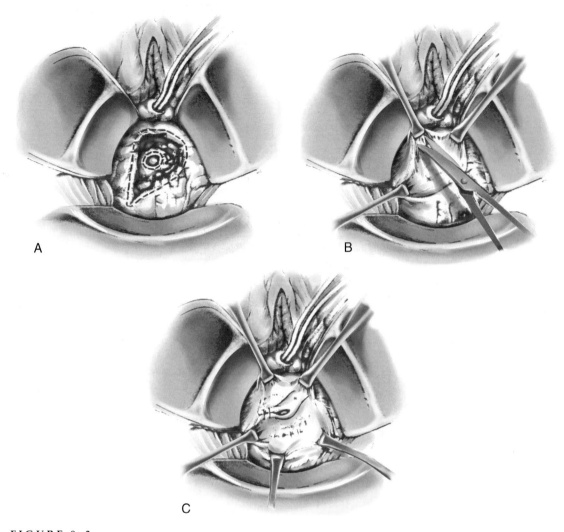

FIGURE 8–3
Latzko procedure for post-hysterectomy supratrigonal vesicovaginal fistula. *A,* Incision of vaginal epithelium 2 to 3 cm around fistula site. *B,* Excision of vaginal epithelium, mobilizing bladder wall. *C,* Parallel interrupted mattress sutures of 3-0 polyglycolic suture as an initial suture line, inverting tissue into the bladder. Two or three subsequent suture layers are added progressively closing the upper vagina. (From Thompson J, Rock J, eds. TeLinde's Operative Gynecology, 7th ed. Philadelphia, JB Lippincott, 1992.)

COMPLICATIONS ARISING FROM A SUTURE IN THE BLADDER

These complications depend on whether the suture is within the bladder lumen. Intraluminal sutures produce chronic cystitis, bladder pain and urgency, and, ultimately, stone formation (Fig. 8–4). Absorbable or delayed absorbable sutures may only cause transient symptoms that resolve within weeks as the sutures dissolve. Cystoscopy is the procedure of choice, because the diagnosis may be made and the suture possibly excised. A 70-degree scope must be used to ensure that all surfaces of the bladder have been explored. Permanent suture or suture with calculus is very difficult to cut using scissors passed through the scope, and the surgeon must be prepared to open the bladder retropubically to fully excise the suture. Extraluminal sutures (in the wall of the bladder) in theory may migrate into the lumen if under tension. Otherwise, these sutures cause bladder pain or are asymptomatic. Excision of suspected sutures in the bladder wall should be considered on an individual basis.

COMPLICATIONS ARISING FROM LEAKAGE OF URINE FROM THE BLADDER

If limited to the space of Retzius, undiagnosed bladder lacerations may cause persistent hema-

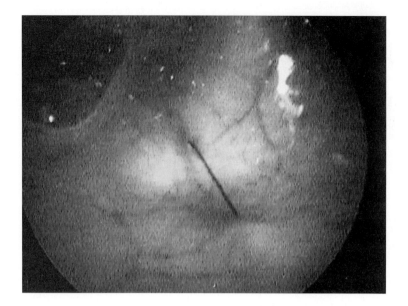

FIGURE 8–4
Intraoperative cystoscopy demonstrating suture through the bladder after needle urethropexy. The surgeon missed the suture using a 30-degree cystoscope; subsequent cystoscopy with a 70-degree scope demonstrated the perforation causing recurrent cystitis and urge incontinence. The bubble at the upper right hand corner identifies the dome of the bladder.

turia and even fat passed into the catheter. Intravenous pyelography can be used to identify the leakage of urine into the space of Retzius; cystoscopy is of limited use because the bladder often cannot be filled adequately to permit visualization. Leakage isolated in the space of Retzius eventually resolves with prolonged bladder drainage per urethra; the catheter should not be removed until 1 week after the hematuria resolves. If the laceration is through the peritoneum, leakage of urine into the abdomen will lead to ileus, distention, and possibly passage through the abdominal incision.

POSTOPERATIVE COMPLICATIONS OF SURGERY TO OR NEAR THE URINARY BLADDER

De Novo Detrusor Instability

This problem most commonly occurs after anti-incontinence procedures (up to 20%) and may be associated with overcorrection of bladder neck hypermobility. Some detrusor instability may be preexisting—the surgeon must carefully consider this diagnosis preoperatively, or the surgeon and the patient will misinterpret the urge incontinence as a complication of anti-incontinence surgery. Occasionally, women complain of urge incontinence after other procedures, such as anterior colporrhaphy or hysterectomy. The existence of sutures in the bladder must be considered, as should cystitis and inadequate voiding. Otherwise, much detrusor instability resolves within 2 to 6 weeks postoperatively. Urodynamic testing should be re-

served for those women in whom symptoms do not resolve after 6 to 8 weeks. Treatment may include improved bladder emptying or the judicious use of anticholinergic medications (which may compromise voiding).

De Novo or Exacerbation of Voiding Dysfunction

Up to 20% of women experience incomplete voiding a week or more after anti-incontinence procedures. Women with preoperative evidence of compromised voiding are routinely taught clean intermittent self-catheterization. Patients are more accepting of this technique when learned preoperatively. It is not uncommon after anti-incontinence procedures that women must use positional changes such as leaning forward to facilitate emptying. These patients should be monitored for significant residual urine. The voiding phase of a subtracted cystometrogram will demonstrate high detrusor voiding pressures with low or no flow. In any patient who has postvoid residuals (greater than 200 mL), irritative bladder symptoms, or flank pain with voiding, obstruction must be ruled out using urodynamic testing. If obstructed voiding is diagnosed, the patient may ultimately damage upper urinary tracts through increased intravesical pressures.

A takedown of the anti-incontinence procedure should be considered in the following scenarios that do not improve with time: women with obstructed voiding, women who are very symptomatic with altered voiding patterns, and women with large residuals leading to overflow incontinence, detrusor instability, or chronic cystitis.

The special case of radical hysterectomy for cervical carcinoma must be considered. Up to 50% of these patients have compromised voiding because of loss of autonomic fibers during resection of the uterosacral and cardinal ligaments. Such compromise may be minimized if the lowest one third to one half of the cardinal ligament is left intact. Inadequate voiding in these patients is due to atony, does not lead to upper tract damage, and is unlikely to benefit greatly from cholinergic stimulants such as bethanechol. Some improvement may be expected up to 1 to 2 years postoperatively.

Although pelvic irradiation is more commonly associated with urge incontinence, stress incontinence may develop in these women. Because anti-incontinence surgery depends on viable tissue healing and scar formation, retropubic procedures have been discouraged for these patients. Collagen injection at the bladder neck is a new therapy that offers some improvement in stress incontinence for these women.

COMPLICATIONS ASSOCIATED WITH THE URETERS

Ureteral injury occurs in 0.5% to 2.5% of gynecologic procedures.[9, 10] Gynecologic surgeons are most likely to operate near the ureter at its most vulnerable points. The ureters pass just below the blood supply to the ovary in the infundibulopelvic ligament and must be identified in the course of ovarian dissection in the medial reflection of the peritoneum. At the level of the internal os the ureters pass directly under the uterine arteries being clamped in the course of hysterectomy (Fig. 8–5). Finally, in the parametrium the ureters are within 1.5 cm of the cervix and at the lateral vaginal fornices (Fig. 8–6).

These are the types of lower urinary tract injury that mandate consultation with others who are more experienced in ureteral surgery. Expertise is required to judge situations such as whether a crush injury to the ureter should be managed with resection or with intraureteric catheterization. Because most gynecologists have little surgical experience in trauma to the ureters, they are wise to seek advice intraoperatively from urologists, gynecologic oncologists, or urogynecologists. The gynecologic surgeon should aspire to prevent such injuries, recognize them when they occur, and be familiar with the management of such injuries, even if he or she will not actually be performing the surgical procedure.

Intraoperative Injury to the Ureter

The type of injury influences the intraoperative management of these cases.

SUTURE LIGATION OR IMPINGEMENT

A suture around the ureter may occur in situations of emergency bleeding or obscured anatomy. One common scenario is the presence of severe endometriosis in which the path of the ureter may be altered and palpation of structure is difficult. The placement of ureteral stents is no guarantee that the ureters will not be injured. If significant inflammation or distortion of the anatomy exists, the stent is just as difficult to palpate as the ureter itself. A stent may make it more likely that the injury is discovered, but only if there is transection of the ureteral wall. Otherwise, the stent only has the benefit of preserving upper tract drainage, and only if the suture is not obstructive. Sutures placed near the ureters may produce a kinking effect. This is most commonly seen with a Moschcowitz plication of the cul-de-sac or anterior colporrhaphy.[11]

If the ligature is identified, it should be immediately removed and the ureter observed for peristalsis and patency. If the ligature was loose and the period of entrapment brief, no further therapy may be needed. If any doubt exists, or if the ureter appears dusky or without peristalsis, consultation should be made to decide whether to catheterize the ureter intra-abdominally or cystoscopically. If a nearby suture has produced kinking in the ureter, release of the suture is usually all that is required intraoperatively.

CRUSH INJURIES

Like suture ligation, these injuries occur with placement of clamps in times of emergency bleeding or obscured anatomy. The use of intraureteric catheters may not prevent these injuries, nor may the injury be recognized if the ureteric wall is intact. Crush injuries produce ischemia and local necrosis. Consultation should be obtained to decide whether the trauma is minimal and may be observed, is moderate and requires stenting, or is significant and necessitates resection and reimplantation.

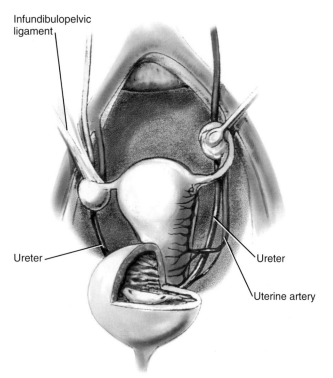

Infundibulopelvic ligament

Ureter

Ureter

Uterine artery

FIGURE 8–5
The most common sites of surgical injury to the ureter. (From Labasky R, Leach G. Prevention and management of urovaginal fistulas. Clin Obstet Gynecol 1990;33:385.)

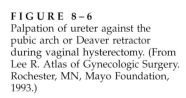

FIGURE 8–6
Palpation of ureter against the pubic arch or Deaver retractor during vaginal hysterectomy. (From Lee R. Atlas of Gynecologic Surgery. Rochester, MN, Mayo Foundation, 1993.)

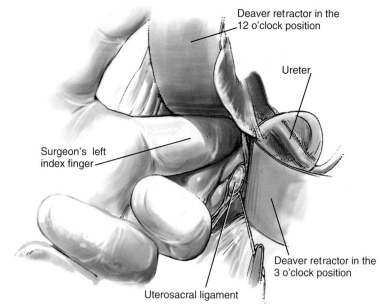

Deaver retractor in the 12 o'clock position

Ureter

Surgeon's left index finger

Deaver retractor in the 3 o'clock position

Uterosacral ligament

TRANSECTION INJURIES

Transection injuries are easier to recognize in theory, because extravasation of urine is seen or because ureteral catheterization reveals the injury. Nonetheless, transection of the ureter may go unrecognized and lead to urine in the abdomen and diagnosis postoperatively.

Transection injuries within 4 to 5 cm of the bladder are amenable to reimplantation. The proximal ureter is reimplanted without tension using a tunneling technique through the bladder wall to reduce reflux. In the case of a shortened ureter, two procedures can minimize the tension. A Boari flap uses a patch of bladder dome to reach the proximal ureter (Fig. 8–7). A psoas hitch procedure elevates the bladder (Fig. 8–8) by suturing the bladder wall

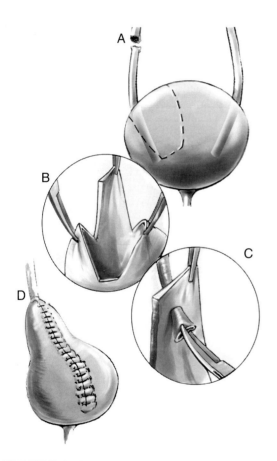

FIGURE 8–7
Boari bladder flap technique. *A*, Two converging incisions are created across the anterior bladder wall with the base posterior. *B*, Flap swung superiorly. *C*, Ureter is brought through opening 1 to 2 cm from the end of the flap, and an end-to-side anatomosis is performed. *D*, The anterior bladder wall is closed, and the flap is tubularized using absorbable suture. (From Kursh E. Injuries to urogenital organs. In: Kursh E, McGuire E, eds. Female Urology. Philadelphia, JB Lippincott, 1994.)

to the psoas muscle. Both will ensure that a ureter of compromised length can be reimplanted successfully without tension. If the transection occurs below the pelvic brim but farther than 5 cm from the bladder, the best course of action may be to resect any damaged area of ureter and perform a ureteroureterostomy (Fig. 8–9). The ends to be reanastomosed are spatulated to reduce the chance of local stricture. The ureter is stented for several weeks, and intravenous pyelography is used to document the patency of the ureter. These injuries should be drained retroperitoneally because the reanastomosis may take some time to become watertight. Injuries above the pelvic brim are uncommon and are managed exclusively by urologists and some gynecologic oncologists. A decision must be made between ureterotransureterostomy and diversion. In the first, the compromised ureter is reimplanted in the contralateral ureter. Because two kidneys are now draining into one ureter, high intraureteric pressure may lead to renal compromise, which is more common in the noninjured kidney.[12] Urinary diversion drains the injured ureter through a stoma; this is less acceptable to patients but less likely to compromise renal function.

DEVASCULARIZATION INJURY

The ureter receives its blood supply through the adventitial sheath. Compromise of this sheath and thereby the ureteral vasculature may occur in extensive pelvic dissection, such as during radical hysterectomy. Judgment should be used in deciding whether the injury is sufficient to warrant stenting. One special situation deserves special mention: injury due to laser or cautery at the time of laparoscopy. This technique requires visual identification of the ureter in its course through the abdominal cavity. Procedures such as laparoscopic uterosacral ligament ablation (the so-called LUNA procedure) are most likely to damage the ureter in its course just lateral to the uterosacral ligament.

Postoperative Complications of Ureteral Injury

Injury to the lower urinary tract should be discussed with every patient undergoing major gynecologic procedures. Most patients are grateful to wake up and find that although such injury occurred the problem was recognized and treated appropriately. Postoperative

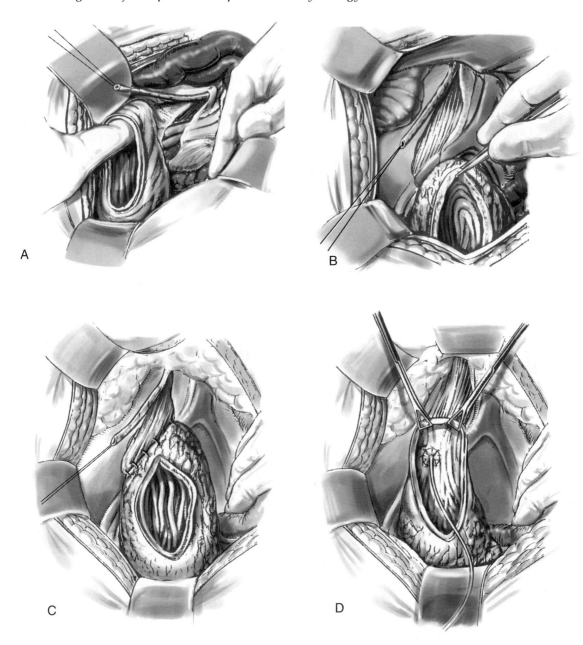

FIGURE 8–8
Psoas hitch procedure, mobilizing contralateral bladder *(A)* and exposing psoas tendon beneath the peritoneum *(B)*. The bladder is attached to the psoas *(C)* and the ureter tunneled into the bladder wall *(D)*, leaving stent in place. (From Mundy A. Urologic injury and how to cope. In: Stanton S, ed. Principles of Gynaecological Surgery. London, Springer-Verlag, 1987.)

identification of ureteral injury almost always results in the patient returning to the operative suite.

URETERAL OBSTRUCTION

If the injury results in obstruction of the ureter (ligation, kinking, or crushing), then dilation of the compromised ureter may lead to flank pain or fever. There may be minimal increases in blood urea and creatinine, and the obstruction may progress silently. Ultrasonography is a good screening test for ureteral and caliceal dilation. However, the use of ureteric catheters *in themselves* may lead to ureteral edema and atonic ureters.[13] If ureteric obstruction is recog-

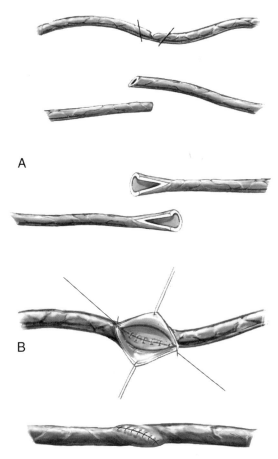

A

B

FIGURE 8–9
After ureteric injury near the pelvic brim there must be sufficient overlap to perform a ureteroureterostomy. *A*, The injured portion is excised and the ends spatulated to prevent stricture. *B*, Anastamosis end-to-end. (From Mundy A. Urologic injury and how to cope. In: Stanton S, ed. Principles of Gynaecological Surgery. London, Springer-Verlag, 1987.)

nized within 7 days, cortical damage may not occur. It is often practical to perform a percutaneous nephrostomy, a procedure that is widely available in the radiology department and effectively drains the bladder while more permanent treatment options are considered. After 1 week, an obstructed ureter may lead to cortical necrosis and a nonfunctional kidney.

URETERIC TRANSECTION OR LACERATION

If the injury leads to extravasation of urine into the abdomen, the patient may present with ileus, abdominal distention, decreased urine output, and even leakage through the abdominal wound. Although these sequelae are significant, transection injuries may be easier to

identify and more likely to result in repair before kidney damage can occur.

URETERAL EDEMA AND ATONY

This complication may result from handling of ureters during procedures or from intraureteric catheterization. The diagnosis of obstruction should be considered. This complication is usually self-limited, but is one argument against the routine use of intraureteric catheters. One study from the general surgery literature found that routine ureteric catheterization during posterior resection had an unacceptably high rate of ureteral edema and atony.[6]

URETEROVAGINAL FISTULA

This complication is most likely to occur after ligature around the ureter involving another structure, such as at the time of uterine artery ligation. The diagnosis may be made on intravenous pyelography or triple swab test with the ureteral output identified by dosing the patient with phenazopyridine (Pyridium) (urine stains orange). Retrograde ureteroscopy and retrograde ureterography may identify the precise location of the injury and dictate treatment as described in the intraoperative section previously. Urologists should be involved in the management of these patients.

COMPLICATIONS ASSOCIATED WITH THE URETHRA

The female urethra is 3 to 5 cm in length and composed of an epithelial mucosal layer, surrounding smooth muscle and vascular layer, and striated muscle from its midpoint to the defined external structure termed the *external urethral sphincter*. Complications associated with overcorrection of bladder neck hypermobility and compromised voiding are considered in the bladder section. The urethral mucosa has an important continence function in coaptation. Loss of connective tissue and vascularity may play a role in intrinsic sphincter deficiency, one cause of stress urinary incontinence.

Urethral complications in gynecologic surgery are uncommon and are usually associated with the repair of urethral diverticula. The normal urethra is surrounded in its dorsal (vaginal) aspect by numerous glands emptying into the urethral lumen. Some of these glands are complex in their relationship to one another, often corkscrewing or interconnecting. The genesis of urethral diverticula is unclear but may involve local infection or inflammation leading to obstruction of the glandular neck. The gland may then fill with mucus or purulence and is termed a *diverticulum*. If the diverticulum becomes patent again, the sac may fill with urine during voiding and empty as postmicturition incontinence. Urethral diverticula should only be excised if they are shown to be the source of recurrent cystitis or urethral symptoms, dyspareunia, or pain.

Complications of Diverticulum Excision

Excision of a urethral diverticulum (or diverticula) should consider whether the mass connects with the proximal or distal urethra. Very distal diverticula may be treated with marsupialization at the external urethral meatus (Spence procedure). Distal and midurethral diverticula should be excised completely, including the neck of the gland as it enters the urethral lumen. Diverticula of the proximal urethra are fortunately less common, and the investigation should consider the possibility of a bladder diverticulum. After excision of the sac, the urethral smooth and striated muscle should then be closed in nonoverlapping layers of fine delayed-absorbable suture. I have not found it useful to drain the bladder per urethra after such repairs.

Failure to heal properly may lead to a urethrovaginal fistula. These are diagnosed by an examination that demonstrates a defect in the urethra communicating with the vagina, by triple swab test, or by urethroscopy. Repair of a urethrovaginal fistula is more complicated than a Latzko repair of a supratrigonal post-hysterectomy fistula. The innervation of the urethra may be disturbed by an extensive dissection, leading to urinary incontinence due to an intrinsic sphincter deficiency. However, the fistulous tract must be excised and the defect closed with mobilized layers of periurethral fascia under no tension. A bulbocavernosus fat graft should be considered. Finally, the best chance for correction is with the initial attempt; therefore, the most experienced surgeon in the repair of urethrovaginal fistula should perform the operation.

Urethral Trauma

Urethral trauma uncommonly occurs with incorrect passage of a cystoscope per urethra.

The defect should be considered as for the excision of a large diverticulum and closed in multiple, nonoverlapping layers of fine delayed-absorbable suture, often over a urethral catheter.

USEFUL TECHNIQUES

Some techniques may be used in a number of situations and may avoid injury or complications to the lower urinary tract associated with gynecologic surgery.

Intentional Cystotomy at Bladder Dome

This technique should be used when there is extensive scarring or distorted anatomy in the space of Retzius. The Foley balloon is grasped through the intact bladder and pulled up to the bladder dome (most cephalad position). Either cautery or scalpel is used to make a small *vertical* incision in the bladder wall and through to the lumen. Care should be taken through this final layer to not burst the balloon: a fine mosquito clamp can be used to penetrate the bladder mucosa, or the balloon can be gently retracted at this point. The incision is vertical to permit further enlargement and visualization of the trigone and ureteral orifices, if necessary. For situations where identification of the bladder wall is important, a finger placed inside the bladder through the intentional cystotomy may be all that is required. Further dissection of the bladder away from the uterus or pubic symphysis is then facilitated, the bladder finger palpating the thickness of the bladder wall and gently retracting the wall away from the line of dissection (Fig. 8–10).

In situations where the conditions of the ureters and trigone are important, the incision may be extended from the dome down the anterior bladder wall as far as necessary to visualize the trigone. Ureteral catheters may be passed or sutures removed through the open cystotomy. The bladder wall should be closed in the usual manner and the space of Retzius drained postoperatively.

Repair of the Bladder Wall

The bladder wall should be closed in two layers: the first with continuous 3-0 chromic su-

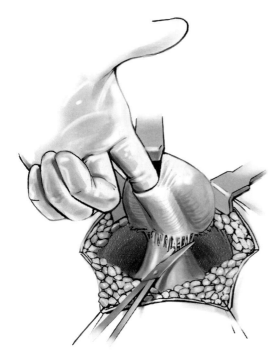

FIGURE 8–10
Intentional cystotomy at the bladder dome provides a proprioceptive guide to accurate dissection. (From Mitchell G, Walters M. Gynecologic injury to the ureters, bladder and urethra: recognition and management. In: Walters M, Karram M, eds. Clinical Urogynecology. St. Louis, Mosby–Year Book, 1993.)

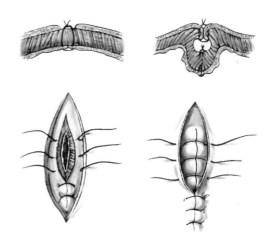

FIGURE 8–11
Double-layer closure of bladder wall abdominal or vaginal cystotomy. (From Penalver M. Urinary tract injuries. In: Hurt G, ed. Urogynecologic Surgery. Gaithersburg, MD, Aspen, 1992.)

ture (may include the mucosal epithelium), and the second with 2-0 delayed-absorbable suture reinforcing the first layer (Fig. 8–11). Two types of cystotomy should be considered. In an unintentional cystotomy, the bladder wall may be torn or weakened. These areas should be oversewn, in addition to closing the visible defect. A suprapubic catheter should be placed through a separate stab cystotomy in cases of unintentional cystotomy. In an intentional cystotomy, the defect is defined and the bladder wall otherwise uninjured. When an intentional cystotomy has been performed, a suprapubic catheter may be placed through the cystotomy without any compromise of the closure.

Retropubic Teloscopy

Timmons and Addison[14] reported the passage of a cystoscope through a stab wound in the dome of the bladder surrounded by a pursestring of suture. In this way, they were able to fill the bladder and easily visualize the ureteral orifices and trigone (Fig. 8–12). A suprapubic catheter could be placed through

the same cystotomy, and the pursestring suture used to close the defect. This is an excellent way to ensure patency of the ureters when performing abdominal surgery, especially if the patient is positioned such that there is no access to the perineum and urethra for cystoscopy per urethra. Ureteral catheters may be passed through this technique.

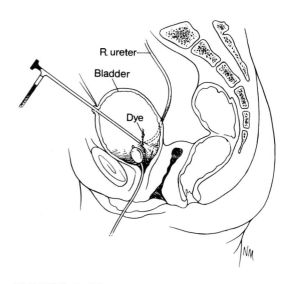

FIGURE 8–12
Suprapubic teloscopy uses a 30-degree cystoscope passed through a chromic pursestring suture in the bladder dome to view dye egress from the ureteral orifices. (From Timmons C, Addison A. Suprapubic teloscopy: extraperitoneal intraoperative technique to demonstrate ureteral patency. Obstet Gynecol 1990;75:137.)

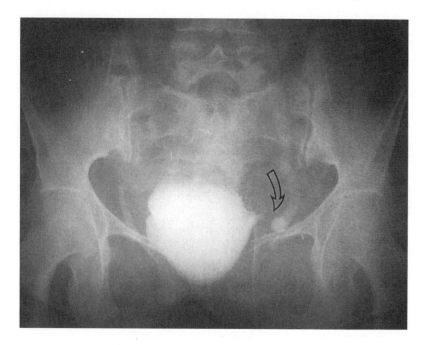

FIGURE 8-13
IVP demonstrating left ureteric obstruction after paravaginal repair. The defect is seen at the arrow, while the patent right ureter has filled the bladder. (From Wall L, Norton P, DeLancey J. Practical Urogynecology. Baltimore, Williams & Wilkins, 1993.)

Cystoscopic Ureteral Catheterization

This is a relative simple procedure to perform; nevertheless, it has only limited use in gynecologic surgery. The catheter or stent may be a 5F whistle-tip or pediatric feeding tube. The catheter is passed through the cystoscope port until its tip is visible just beyond the tip of the scope and inserted into the ureteral orifice by directing the 30-degree scope (and so the catheter) toward its lumen. The catheter is then gently threaded through the outside port, taking care to keep the catheter sterile as it is passed into the scope. Once both catheters are passed, they will continue to drain some of the urine from the ureters out their distal end. Therefore, the ends of the ureteral catheters must be drained in some manner; I prefer to make a small slit in the Foley catheter and insert the ureteral catheters into this slit for continuous drainage.

It has been suggested that the ureters be catheterized for a case in which difficult anatomy is anticipated. This is in error, because catheterization will not prevent ureteral damage, may not always identify the injury, and may cause transient edema and atony of the ureters. Once an injury is suspected, catheterization is indicated.

Intraperitoneal Ureteral Catheterization

If a ureteral defect has been recognized, a catheter should be passed in both the distal and proximal portions of the ureter to assess patency. The defect may be closed over the catheter in some cases. Consultation with a urologist or gynecologic oncologist is important in such cases.

TESTS OF THE LOWER URINARY TRACT

These tests are performed to assess the anatomy and function of the lower urinary tract in relation to gynecologic surgery.

Triple Sponge or Tampon Test

This is a clinical test in the evaluation of suspected fistula, whether vesicovaginal, ureterovaginal, or urethrovaginal. Even if a definite defect can be seen, the investigator must determine the source of leakage and whether two or more defects exist. The woman is asked to take 200 mg of phenazopyridine 3 hours before the test. The bladder is emptied and filled with 250 mL of sterile water or saline with 2 to 3 mL of indigo carmine added. If blue dye is seen in the vagina at this time, a vesicovaginal fistula may be diagnosed. The defect is often more subtle, and the test is continued: three folded gauze sponges or cup-shaped tampons are placed in tandem in the vagina, representing the apex, midvagina, and distal vagina. The woman is then asked to ambulate for 20 minutes, with activities such as bending over or standing from a chair. Ureteral urine is colored orange, and bladder sources of urine are blue. Apical orange staining is seen with ureterovaginal fistula, while apical or mid-vaginal blue staining is seen with vesicovaginal fistula. Blue staining of the distal sponge may represent a urethrovaginal fistula but is more likely to be seen with severe incontinence per urethra that has been taken up from the perineum.

Intravenous Pyelogram and Voiding Cystourethrogram

These radiologic tests are widely available and may help in the assessment of ureteric reflux, stricture, dilation, or defect (Fig. 8–13). They may also demonstrate renal anomalies or damage, duplicated ureters, bladder diverticula, and, occasionally, fistula. Duplication of the ureter is seen in approximately 0.5% of the female population. Piscatelli and colleagues[15] found that for benign gynecologic surgery, pre-

operative intravenous pyelography was useful only in cases of adnexal mass larger than 4 cm and uterine enlargement greater than the size of a 12-week gestation or for known müllerian/renal anomalies. There was no benefit in cases of endometriosis, infection, pelvic organ prolapse, or previous gynecologic surgery.

Urodynamic Testing

Urodynamic tests are available in most metropolitan areas. Preoperatively, urodynamic testing is indicated for incontinence that has multiple or obscure etiologies, has failed previous surgery, is associated with voiding dysfunction, or has significant coexisting conditions such as pelvic organ prolapse or neurologic disease. Voiding studies may help to identify patients at risk for postoperative voiding with low detrusor voiding pressures, low flow rates, low isometric detrusor contraction (stop test), and the presence of straining. Postoperatively,

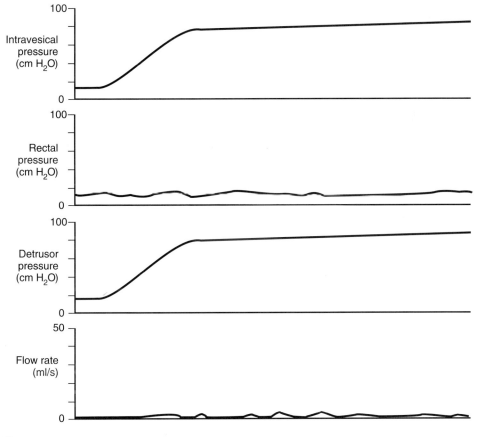

FIGURE 8–14
Obstructed voiding after bladder neck surgery. The detrusor voiding pressure is high (80 cm H_2O), while there is minimal flow. (From Wall L, Norton P, DeLancey J. Practical Urogynecology. Baltimore, Williams & Wilkins, 1993.)

urodynamic testing can be used to diagnose detrusor instability as a cause of postoperative urinary incontinence. Voiding dysfunction may be isolated as a problem of inadequate urethral relaxation (treated with muscle relaxants or self-limited), bladder atony or inadequate detrusor contraction (poorly treated with parasympathetic agonists such as bethanechol), or lack of coordination between detrusor contraction and urethral relaxation (detrusor sphincter dyssynergia). Patients with voiding difficulties associated with anti-incontinence procedures may be evaluated for obstructed voiding. In these cases, the relative obstruction of the surgical procedure prevents voiding, and very high pressures must be generated by the detrusor muscle to overcome the urethral obstruction (Fig. 8–14). Such intravesical pressure puts the upper tracts at risk for cortical necrosis due to pressure. Although these patients can be successfully managed by clean, intermittent self-catheterization, a takedown of the anti-incontinence procedure should be considered in very symptomatic patients or in patients with persistent high intravesical pressures.

Drainage

If bladder drainage is required for longer periods of time, a suprapubic catheter is more comfortable and less likely to lead to infection. If the urine is bloody, narrow suprapubic catheters such as a Bonnano may become blocked. In such cases, larger catheters such as a Foley or Malecot-type should be used. If a defect in the bladder or ureter has been repaired, external drainage should be used to prevent collection of urine in the intraperitoneal or retroperitoneal spaces.

CONCLUSION

Prevention of lower urinary tract injuries must be a priority for surgeons in the female pelvis. Preoperative radiologic studies and ureteric catheterization are less important than careful, thoughtful surgical technique and attention to anatomy. A high degree of suspicion must be maintained, and liberal use of cystoscopy, intentional cystotomy, retrograde teloscopy, and intraoperative ureteric catheterization will identify injuries if they occur. Postoperative discovery of these injuries is regrettable. Finally, few gynecologic surgeons have had sufficient experience in ureteral injury to deal with these complications, and consultation is to be encouraged.

REFERENCES

1. Gosling J, Harris P, Humpherson J, et al. Atlas of Human Anatomy. Philadelphia, JB Lippincott, 1985, p 59.
2. Wheelock J, Krebs H, Hurt W. Sparing and repairing the bladder during gynecologic surgery. Contemp Obstet Gynecol 1984;23:155–159.
3. Kuskarelis D, Sakkas J, Aravantinos D. Urinary tract injuries in gynecologic and obstetrical procedures. Int Surg 1975;60:40.
4. Peterson H, Hulka J, Phillips J. American Association of Gynecologic Laparoscopists' 1988 membership survey on operative laparoscopy. J Reprod Med 1990; 35:587–589.
5. Corriere J, Sandler C. Management of the ruptured bladder: seven years of experiences with 111 cases. J Trauma 1986;26:830.
6. Ward J, Nay H. Immediate and delayed urologic complications associated with abdominoperineal resection. Am J Surg 1972;123:642.
7. Thompson J. Operative injuries to the urinary tract. In: Nichols D, ed. Reoperative Gynecologic Surgery. St. Louis, CV Mosby, 1991, pp 163–209.
8. Blandy J, Badenoch D, Fowler C, et al. Early repair of iatrogenic injury to the ureter or bladder after gynecological surgery. J Urol 1991;146:761–765.
9. Halloway HJ. Injury to the urinary tract as a complication of gynecologic surgery. Am J Obstet Gynecol 1950;60:30–40.
10. Mann WJ, Arato M, Patsner B, et al. Ureteral injuries in an obsterics and gynecology training program: etiology and management. Obstet Gynecol 1988;72:82–85.
11. Pettit P, Petrou S. The value of cystoscopy in major vaginal surgery. Obstet Gynecol 1994;84:318–320.
12. Sandoz I, Paul D, MacFarlane C. Complications with transuretero-ureterostomy. J Urol 1977;117:39–42.
13. Lapides J, Tank E. Urinary complications following abdominal perineal resection. Cancer 1971;28:230–233.
14. Timmons M, Addison W. Suprapubic teloscopy: extraperitoneal intraoperative technique to demonstrate ureteral patency. Obstet Gynecol 1990;75:137–139.
15. Piscatelli J, Simel D, Addison A. Who should have intravenous pyelograms before hysterectomy for benign disease? Obstet Gynecol 1987;69:541–545.

9

John R. Potts III

Upper Abdominal Complications

Upper abdominal disorders are of importance to the gynecologic surgeon because of the threat they can pose in the preoperative or postoperative period and because when faced with the unexpected finding of an upper abdominal pathologic process the gynecologic surgeon must know how to respond. By virtue of being detectable to the surgeon's hand or eye, unexpected intraoperative findings represent gross anatomic abnormalities. As such, their incidence should be limited by careful preoperative evaluation. Still, even with modern imaging techniques there are several reasons why unexpected operative findings do arise. Some conditions are truly asymptomatic. The symptoms associated with other conditions are so minimal that the patient does not believe that they warrant mention or the surgeon does not believe that they warrant full evaluation. In either case, such conditions would only be detected incidentally by laboratory studies, imaging studies, or exploration at laparotomy. Although less likely with upper than lower abdominal conditions, it is possible that symptoms ascribed to a known gynecologic problem are, in fact, due to another abdominal process. Furthermore, the current economic pressures in medicine call for directed (cost effective) evaluation of complaints, fewer and briefer patient–physician interactions, and same-day operative procedures, each of which decreases one's ability to detect and pursue conditions other than the patient's chief complaint. For all of these reasons, and no less because it is simply good medical practice to do so, unexpected intraoperative findings should be actively sought.

Important in doing so is the routine performance of abdominal exploration at operation. Habitual performance of exploration allows the surgeon to be familiar with normal anatomy so that a disorder is recognized. It is best to explore at the outset of the operation. Doing so routinely ensures that this important duty is not lost in the denouement of accomplishing the planned procedure. Also, unexpected findings may well alter the priority of the proposed task. In open gynecologic procedures, exploration is usually performed almost entirely manually. Laparoscopy offers a superb opportunity to visually explore the upper abdomen, but tactile investigation of suspected pathology is markedly diminished. The key to the reliable performance of a complete examination is a standardized, systematic approach. Perhaps the simplest way of doing so is from the top down. In this approach, the diaphragm is first examined. The gastrointestinal tract is then evaluated beginning with the esophagogastric junction, followed by the stomach, the duodenum, the small intestine and its mesentery, the appendix, and, finally, the colon and its mesentery. The liver, pancreas, gallbladder, and spleen are then explored in a standardized order.

Assuming no major preexistent adhesive disease is present, such a search can almost always be completed through a low transverse or midline incision. Much of the examination is performed manually with the organs in situ, but most of the small bowel can be examined visually through a lower abdominal incision. During laparoscopic surgery, a 30-degree angled scope is useful for visual exploration of the upper abdomen. The patient must be briefly brought to a steep reverse Trendelenburg position to visualize the upper abdominal organs. This being done, the exploration can follow virtually the same order as that in which the manual exploration is performed. One exception may be that the small intestine (and to some extent the colon) can gravitate to the inferior reaches of the abdomen, making evaluation difficult while the patient remains in the reverse Trendelenburg position. In laparoscopic surgery, therefore, these organs might be evaluated first while the patient is in a Trendelenburg position. The other exception is that, barring the presence of a large mass, the pancreas cannot be assessed well through the scope without deliberate maneuvers to enter the lesser sac. In addition to visual assessment, the use of the laparoscope offers a superb opportunity to photograph any pathologic processes found. Whether static or video images are made, it is important to provide useful landmarks in those images.

Adhesive disease may hamper exploration whether performed laparoscopically or openly. If there are but a few filmy adhesions, they should be taken down and the exploration pursued. More extensive adhesions may be difficult to take down without substantially increasing the elapsed time and the risk of the procedure. These factors must be weighed against the likelihood of finding a pathologic process in the upper abdomen and a decision made as to whether complete exploration should be pursued.

Abnormal conditions detected on exploration may pose logical, ethical, and legal problems. All unanticipated findings require complete descriptive documentation (including photographs, if possible). To address some of the logical, ethical, and legal problems associated with unanticipated findings, the following questions must be answered:

Does the newly discovered lesion pose a threat to the patient in the postoperative period?

Does this condition require biopsy in addition to descriptive documentation?

Does this condition require definitive therapy?

If definitive therapy is appropriate, can it be performed in the same operation as the planned procedure?

If so, what is the best technical approach?

Which lesion takes priority if both procedures cannot be performed in the same sitting?

The surgeon's best preparation for an appropriate response to an unanticipated finding on exploration is a working knowledge of the pathology and natural history of potential pathologic findings as well as of their surgical management. Against that information, the surgeon can weigh the reason for the planned operation and the patient's condition. The ability and confidence of the surgeon in dealing with conditions outside the scope of his or her usual practice and one's access to surgical consultants with greater expertise relevant to the unanticipated lesion impact heavily in deciding on the appropriate response to a given situation. The ready availability of a reliable pathologist is clearly crucial as well. Finally, it is important that the surgeon has developed a rapport with the patient and the family and that he or she has explained preoperatively that exploration would be performed. It is also important to inform available family members during the operation of the unanticipated finding and to invite their thoughts regarding treatment of the lesion.

The aims of this chapter are to address the more common pathologic conditions of upper abdominal organs that can be incidentally discovered at the time of laparotomy as well as those that pose a threat to the patient in the perioperative period. The natural history of each is briefly reviewed, and, when appropriate, the operative approach is described. In doing so, an effort has been made to emphasize the relative incidence of each condition in women when it is known to occur with greater or lesser frequency on the basis of gender.

DIAPHRAGM

The diaphragm is a musculotendinous dome-shaped structure that separates the abdominal and thoracic cavities. It is attached posteriorly to the lumbar vertebrae, laterally to the costal arches, and anteriorly to the sternum. Three foramina exist in the diaphragm that allow passage of normal anatomic structures. Most posteriorly, the aortic hiatus contains the aorta, the azygos veins, and the thoracic duct. Anterior to the aortic hiatus is the esophageal hiatus (which also contains the vagus nerves) and to the right and somewhat anterior to that pass the vena cava and associated phrenic nerve branches. The blood supply to the diaphragm arises from the aorta, the costal arteries, and the internal mammary arteries.

Hernias

Two principal types of congenital hernias of the diaphragm are described. Children with the posterolateral hernia of Bochdalek rarely survive infancy without repair. On the other hand, hernias through the foramen of Morgagni are seldom discovered before middle age. These hernias are located anteriorly and result from failure of fusion of the sternal and costal portions of the diaphragm. They usually contain the liver but can also contain the stomach, small bowel, or transverse colon. Morgagni hernias can be incidentally found at operation and should be repaired when noted by either primary closure or the application of permanent surgical mesh.

There are also two principal types of acquired diaphragmatic hernias: traumatic and paraesophageal. *Traumatic hernias* can result from either penetrating or blunt trauma. They can occur in any portion of the diaphragm but are more common on the left. Abdominal viscera may immediately herniate through the defects or may do so slowly over months or even years. Visceral pain or obstruction may develop, or the hernia may remain asymptomatic only to be discovered on exploration of the abdomen. When noted, these injuries should be repaired because the risk of strangulation is substantial.[1] *Paraesophageal hernias* (type II hiatal hernias), occur through the esophageal hiatus, usually to the left and anterior to the esophagus. Unlike a sliding (type I) hiatal hernia, a paraesophageal hernia is a true herniation into a peritoneal sac in the mediastinum. In a pure type II hiatal hernia, the gastroesophageal junction is anchored below the diaphragm by the phrenoesophageal ligament and the herniated stomach lies alongside. Many paraesophageal hernias remain completely asymptomatic. When symptoms do arise from these hernias, they may be limited to those of esophageal reflux and their significance may be overlooked. Thus, these unusual hernias can be incidentally encountered on exploration of the abdomen. The natural history of para-esophageal hernias is one of enlargement. In addition to the stomach, organs that can become involved in these hernias include the spleen, the omentum, the colon, the small bowel, and the pancreas. Untreated paraeso-phageal hernias are prone to the development of life-threatening complications, including volvulus, strangulation, ulceration with bleeding or perforation, and acute gastric dilation with pulmonary compromise.[2] To avoid these catastrophic complications, it is generally recommended that a paraesophageal hernia be repaired when the diagnosis is made. The principles of repair include reduction of the contents of the sac, complete excision of the sac, and closure of the diaphragmatic defect. An antireflux procedure is frequently performed as an adjunct to the repair. The term *eventration* simply refers to a thinned and floppy portion of the diaphragm that bulges into the thoracic cavity. This is not a true herniation but can be electively repaired by plication when it results in pulmonary compromise.

Tumors

Primary tumors of the diaphragm are not common but can be completely asymptomatic and therefore encountered incidentally. *Lipomas* are probably the most common benign tumors of the diaphragm. *Fibromas, mesotheliomas, angiofibromas,* and *neurogenic tumors* have also been reported. In addition, congenital cysts of the diaphragm occur. Malignant primary tumors are somewhat more common than benign tumors,[3] and most of these are *fibrosarcomas* or *neurofibrosarcomas.* Simple removal is indicated for the benign tumors, and wide excision is used for the malignant varieties. Metastatic lesions to the diaphragm can arise from adjacent or remote abdominal organs.

THE STOMACH

Shaped like a wineskin, the stomach lies obliquely in the upper abdomen in continuity with the esophagus superiorly and the duodenum distally. It resides posterior and inferior to the liver, medial to the spleen, and anterior to the pancreas. For obvious reasons, the inner (right) margin of the stomach is described as the lesser curvature and the outer (left) as the greater curvature. The lesser curvature is suspended by the hepatogastric ligament (the lesser omentum) and from the greater curva-ture hangs the gastrocolic ligament (the greater omentum). The blood supply of the stomach is exceptionally rich. Entering the lesser curvature are the left gastric artery, which arises from the celiac axis, and the right gastric artery, which arises from the common hepatic artery. The greater curvature is supplied by the gastroepiploic artery, arising on the right from the the gastroduodenal artery and on the left from the splenic artery. The short gastric vessels contribute blood flow to the superior portion of the greater curvature. Three areas of the stomach are classically used for gross description. The fundus is that portion of the stomach to the left of and superior to the esophagogastric junction. The body of the stomach is that portion between the fundus and an imaginary line running between the incisura angularis (a visible indentation of the lesser curvature about 6 cm proximal to the pylorus) and a point on the greater curvature about midway between the inferiormost short gastric vessel and the pylorus. The distal portion is called the antrum. Its distal extent is described by the pylorus, a thick muscular ring usually marked externally by a transverse vein. Problems of the stomach that require surgical intervention are almost entirely limited to peptic ulcer disease and neoplasms.

Peptic Ulcer Disease and its Complications

Although the incidence of peptic ulcer disease has remained static or decreased somewhat in recent decades, the frequency of surgical intervention for complications of peptic ulcer disease has diminished dramatically due to the availability of antisecretory agents. For the same reasons, it is now distinctly unlikely that the gynecologist will incidentally encounter grossly identifiable peptic ulcer disease at operation. On careful palpation one may occasionally encounter a small mass representing the inflammation and scarring surrounding a chronic peptic ulcer but such ulceration is usually symptomatic. Operative intervention for such a mass is unnecessary because of the very high likelihood of successful medical management. On an extremely rare occasion, one may encounter a peptic ulcer presenting as lower abdominal pain due to dependent accumulation of gastric contents after perforation. Such a perforation should be securely closed. It may also be appropriate to proceed with a formal peptic ulcer operation, but a full discussion of the indications and technique of doing so is beyond the scope of this chapter.

Tumors

Benign tumors represent a very small proportion of all gastric neoplasms. The majority of these are either mucosal polyps or leiomyomas. *Mucosal polyps* tend to occur in older individuals, are usually located in the body or the fundus, and can be associated with pain or bleeding due to ulceration. Excision is warranted if they are symptomatic or greater than 2 cm. *Leiomyomas* are smooth muscle tumors of the gastric wall. They can grow to a size appreciable even on physical examination and can also be associated with bleeding or pain due to ulceration. Leiomyomas should be excised with a 2-cm margin.

Primary lymphoma of the stomach is unusual. These tumors are usually large enough to be appreciated on abdominal exploration but are rarely asymptomatic. Pain, anorexia, early satiety, nausea, and vomiting are common in these patients, and many present with constitutional symptoms of lymphoma. Stage I and stage II gastric lymphoma can be cured by surgical resection. If resection is not chosen, the mass should at least be sampled and the status of the regional and the periaortic nodes documented. By far the most common neoplasm of the stomach is *adenocarcinoma.* Early gastric carcinoma is usually asymptomatic, but a carcinoma large enough to be appreciated on exploration is probably already incurable. Despite the dismal prognosis, resection is usually recommended to avoid bleeding and obstruction. As with lymphoma, if resection is not chosen the mass should be sampled and the nodal status carefully documented as a guide for future therapy. Of note to the gynecologist is that an advanced gastric carcinoma can be associated with a Krukenberg tumor.

LIVER

The liver is the largest solid organ in the body. Located in the upper abdomen, it is nestled between the diaphragm superiorly and posteriorly and the gastrointestinal tract medially and inferiorly. The liver is suspended by several peritoneal reflections that are (anatomically incorrectly) referred to as ligaments. The falciform ligament extends to the anterior abdominal wall and incorporates the usually obliterated left umbilical vein. Continuous

with this are the anterior and posterior right and left coronary ligaments that suspend the liver from the diaphragm. Laterally the coronary ligaments form the triangular ligaments. A fibrous sheath (Glisson's capsule) invests the liver. This highly vascular organ is supplied by the proper hepatic artery (arising from the celiac axis) in about half of the population. The origin and course of the right and left hepatic arteries, though, are highly variable. The right hepatic artery often arises from the superior mesenteric artery, and the left hepatic artery not infrequently arises from the left gastric artery. The portal vein, which supplies some 70% of blood flow to the liver, enters the liver just posterior and to the right of the hepatic artery. The venous drainage of the liver is through the hepatic veins that empty into the inferior vena cava. There are three principal veins: the right, the middle, and the left. In addition, there are a number of smaller veins emptying directly into the vena cava from the caudate lobe. The right and left hepatic lobes are delineated by an invisible plane that passes from the inferior vena cava to the gallbladder fossa and through which runs the middle hepatic vein. The most useful definition of hepatic segmental anatomy is one in which the boundaries of the segments are described by the passage of the hepatic veins in the vertical plane and the portal veins in the horizontal. Thus, the right lobe and left lobes are each divided into four segments centered around the principal vein draining that lobe.[4]

General Consideration and Biopsy Technique

Most liver masses can be detected by bimanual palpation. The number, size, and location of masses in relation to major vessels should be noted because this information is crucial in determining whether to resect a lesion and how to do so. Ultrasonography is useful in these determinations. Samples need not be taken from masses previously documented to be benign and should not be taken from vascular lesions, simple liver cysts, and echinococcal cysts. Previously undocumented solid liver masses should all be sampled, as should the previously undocumented cirrhotic liver. Small superficial lesions can undergo excisional biopsy that becomes both diagnostic and therapeutic. Incisional biopsy should be used for larger superficial masses. For deeper lesions and for suspected cirrhosis, core needle biopsy is appropriate.

Liver biopsy, even in the presence of cirrhosis, is easily done and should not be associated with excessive blood loss or other complication. At laparotomy, a core biopsy is most easily taken from an anterior, inferior edge of either lobe at a point that can be easily compressed by the surgeon's fingers until cautery has controlled any resulting bleeding. At laparoscopy, biopsy can be performed by introducing the needle directly through the skin at a point overlying the liver. By necessity, the needle must be introduced into the anterior surface of the organ. The acquisition of the specimen and the application of cautery to the bleeding point can then be guided through the laparoscope. Wedge biopsy samples are obtained by placing two large absorbable sutures in a mattress fashion such that the deepest points of the two are adjacent and their most superficial points are separated by 4 to 6 cm. After the "wedge" is excised from the area described by the sutures, cautery is applied to specific bleeding points and the uncut ends of the sutures are tied together to approximate the cut surfaces.

Cirrhosis and Portal Hypertension

Cirrhosis is the end result of chronic hepatocellular injury, whether that injury be toxic, viral, cholestatic, autoimmune, or metabolic. With a history of any such insult, one may suspect the presence of liver disease. Examination may reveal splenomegaly, spider angiomas, caput medusa, palmar erythema, or ascites. Laboratory studies may demonstrate abnormalities in the liver enzyme, bilirubin, albumin, or coagulation values. However, preoperative evidence of cirrhosis is not always available. Cirrhosis is clinically diagnosed at operation by the presence of a firm, nodular liver. Corroborative evidence includes the presence of splenomegaly, dilated visceral veins, and ascites. Because of its many implications in the acute and longitudinal care of the patient, it is important to document the presence of cirrhosis. Although the experienced eye or hand can diagnose cirrhosis with great certainty, this is best done by liver biopsy. Having documented its presence, nothing further need be or should be done incidentally with respect to cirrhosis or portal hypertension. However, the surgeon should be prepared for a more difficult postoperative course than might otherwise have been anticipated. Even with minor abdominal procedures, cirrhotic patients are at risk for the development of postoperative ascites and its associated fluid and electrolyte problems. In addition, patients with cirrhosis are at much greater risk for the development of coagulopathy, postoperative bleeding, infection, and wound healing problems than the general population.

Liver Abscess

Because they are rare and are usually symptomatic,[5] it would be quite unusual for the gynecologist to encounter an unsuspected liver abscess. Liver abscesses can be associated with fever, right upper quadrant pain, malaise, nausea, vomiting, or weight loss. Laboratory studies usually reveal leukocytosis, anemia, hypoalbuminemia, and an elevation in the serum alkaline phosphatase level. *Pyogenic abscesses* are usually solitary and average about 5 cm. Most are polymicrobial, and broad-spectrum antibiosis is indicated. Drainage is usually necessary and can be performed percutaneously or at operation. Most patients who have *amebic abscesses* have traveled or lived outside the United States. Serologic testing is the best method for differentiating amebic from pyogenic abscesses. The primary treatment for amebic abscess is metronidazole, but drainage is occasionally necessary.

Hepatic Cysts

Solitary hepatic cysts are unusual, but they do occur three times more commonly in females.[6] Most are small and do not require therapy. Rarely, a larger hepatic cyst may be an incidental finding. Uncomplicated cysts can simply be unroofed or, if conveniently possible, filled by a tongue of omentum. Cysts that communicate with the biliary tree should be internally drained into a Roux-en-Y jejunal limb. *Adult polycystic liver disease* is usually symptomatic on the basis of mass effect. However, it is possible to encounter the disease incidentally. Surgical treatment is directed toward reduction of the mass effect by draining as many cysts as possible. This condition is benign, but when associated with polycystic kidney disease the patient's prognosis is dependent on the latter. Echinococcal cysts are rarely seen in patients from the United States. Usually solitary, they can remain asymptomatic for years so that even large echinococcal cysts can be incidentally found. Treatment is primarily surgical, but antihelmintics should be given before operation. Extreme care must be taken to prevent spillage of viable scoleces. The cyst should be aspirated and then infused with a scolecidal agent before being excised.

Vascular Tumors

Cavernous hemangioma is the most common benign liver tumor. Often discovered incidentally, these lesions are much more common in females than males.[7] When located on the liver surface, they are usually deep red and very soft. The natural history of the tumor is benign. Tumors smaller than 4 cm in diameter should be left alone because they rarely enlarge or become symptomatic. Indications for resection include a rapidly growing mass, symptoms (fever or pain) that are attributable to the tumor, diagnostic uncertainty, congestive heart failure, and rupture of the tumor with intra-abdominal bleeding. There are reports of cavernous hemangiomas enlarging during pregnancy. However, this is unusual, and current or future pregnancy is not an indication for resection.[8]

Primary Benign Hepatic Tumors

Focal nodular hyperplasia may represent focal cirrhosis, hamartomatous malformation, or local injury to liver tissue.[7] These lesions are usually asymptomatic and incidentally found. Most are solitary, lobulated lesions that are well demarcated and measure less than 5 cm. When found at operation, they should be sampled to confirm the diagnosis. Because their natural history is benign, they should otherwise be left alone. Excision is reasonable if it can be performed as a simple wedge.

Hepatocellular adenoma is an unusual tumor that generally affects young women.[7] There is good evidence that links hepatic adenomas to oral contraceptive use.[9] When found, these lesions are usually greater than 5 cm in diameter and are symptomatic. These tumors are hypervascular with sharp margins. They are usually located in the right lobe and are multifocal in about 30% of cases. Because of the risk of complications (rupture with bleeding or malignant transformation), resection of these "benign" tumors should be undertaken when the risk is acceptably low. Lesions that are not resected should be closely observed.

Primary Hepatic Malignant Tumors

Hepatocellular carcinomas usually occur against a background of cirrhosis. They often remain asymptomatic until they reach substantial size so that it is possible to incidentally encounter them at operation. These tumors appear as soft masses without central umbilication, often with areas of bleeding and necrosis, and may be surrounded by satellite lesions. Core needle biopsy can be safely done to confirm the diagnosis. When found in the noncirrhotic patient, or in a particularly accessible location in the cirrhotic patient, they should be resected with a 2-cm tumor-free margin, provided the patient is a suitable surgical candidate.[10]

Metastatic Liver Tumors

Hepatic metastases from extrahepatic tumors are common. Because therapy and prognosis demand a precise diagnosis, a tissue biopsy is essential. All patients with suspected hepatic metastases should be sampled. When the patient does not have a known primary tumor site, an extensive search of the abdomen and retroperitoneum should be performed. The colon, rectum, pancreas, and stomach are the most common primary tumor sites that metastasize to the liver.

Most authors agree that metastatic colorectal carcinoma limited to the liver and located in accessible locations should be resected because such treatment appears to improve 5-year survival. Conversely, resection of hepatic metastases from tumors in other organs is rarely indicated. The principles established for elective hepatic resection for colorectal metastasis should be observed when performing incidental resections.[11] All tumor tissue should be encompassed by the liver resection. Portal or celiac nodal involvement is considered a contraindication to liver resection because of the almost universal failure of combined hepatic and nodal resections. The tumor should not be violated during resection, and margins of resection should be at least 1 cm. Wedge resection is just as efficacious as formal resection and spares more normal parenchyma. Age, gender, tumor size, and tumor site (left lobe, right lobe, or both) do not appear to affect prognosis in patients who undergo resection of colorectal metastases. The effect on 5-year survival of the number of resected metastases remains a topic of debate. The status of the remaining liver is clearly of importance in as much as cirrhotics are at much greater risk for bleeding and other complications, including liver failure. When nonresectable metastatic disease in the liver is encountered, placement of an arterial catheter should be considered for delivery of postoperative chemotherapy.

GALLBLADDER AND BILIARY TREE

The right and left hepatic ducts unite into the common duct either just within or just outside liver substance in the hilum. The duct is known as the common hepatic duct above its union with the cystic duct; below that point it is the common bile duct. Distally, the common duct courses behind the first portion of the duodenum, through the head of the pancreas, and into the medial wall of the second portion of the duodenum. There it is enveloped by a complex and delicate regulatory muscular sleeve—the sphincter of Oddi. Superior to the duodenum, the hepatic artery lies to the left of the bile duct and the portal vein behind it. The gallbladder is a pear-shaped vesicle suspended by the visceral peritoneum of the liver. Its function is to store and concentrate bile until it is needed in the digestive process. At its proximal end, the gallbladder narrows into an infundibulum before joining a 2- to 4-cm cystic duct that connects it to the common duct. The cystic artery supplies the gallbladder and usually arises from the right hepatic artery. The latter generally passes behind the common hepatic duct. The surgeon must be aware, however, that the anatomy in this area is highly variable and is often the cause of surgical misadventure.

The Gallbladder

CARCINOMA

There are about 6000 cases of carcinoma of the gallbladder per year in the United States.[12] The prognosis of this disease is dismal. If a tumor in the gallbladder is grossly visible or palpable, the fate of the patient is probably already sealed. The so-called porcelain gallbladder (one with a rim of calcium visible on plain film) is strongly associated with gallbladder cancer and is an indication for cholecystectomy.

CHOLELITHIASIS

Some 20 million Americans have gallstone disease, and women are afflicted about three times more commonly than men. Complications that can occur as a result of cholelithiasis include choledocholithiasis (with or without obstructive jaundice and with or without cholangitis), biliary pancreatitis, and, less frequently, gallstone ileus. By far the most common complication of cholelithiasis, however, is acute cholecystitis in which the neck of the gallbladder becomes obstructed by one of the stones. This complication results in pain that is unrelenting until the stone becomes dislodged or until cholecystectomy. These complications are much more likely to develop in patients who are symptomatic, are older, and have nonfunctioning gallbladders on oral cholecystography. Because the risk of elective cholecystectomy is low, it is almost always the recommended treatment for symptomatic cholelithiasis.[13] In a woman with documented and symptomatic gallstones deemed fit to undergo a gynecologic operation, it is quite reasonable to perform *en passant* cholecystectomy.[14]

In 50% to 85% of patients with gallstones there are no symptoms or the symptoms are so mild and nonspecific that they have never been fully evaluated. Given the number of persons with gallstones, the preponderance of women in that group, and the high percentage who are "asymptomatic," gallstones could reasonably be expected to represent one of the more common incidental findings during abdominal exploration. Furthermore, it is possible for an "asymptomatic" woman to have stones discovered on an ultrasonogram done in preparation for a gynecologic operation. Available data on the natural history of asymptomatic gallstones are imperfect,[13] but they seem to indicate that the risk of developing serious complications is fairly low. Whether that risk is outweighed by the risk of *en passant* cholecystectomy is not truly known, but most authors believe that, in a patient who is fit on the conclusion of the primary operation, incidental cholecystectomy is a reasonable procedure. The case for *en passant* cholecystectomy in the asymptomatic patient is strengthened if she is young (therefore both better able to tolerate the additional operating time now and at greater cumulative risk for the development of symptoms or complications in the future), if the primary operation was for benign disease, or if the gallbladder is shrunken or thickened, indicative of chronic cholecystitis. Also, the case for proceeding with incidental cholecystectomy is strengthened if the primary procedure is performed through laparoscopy or through a midline incision extending into the upper abdomen.

The Bile Duct

Surgical diseases of the bile duct include stones, benign strictures, primary tumors, and congenital abnormalities. It is unlikely that *choledocholithiasis* or a *benign stricture* not previously diagnosed would be detected with even the most deliberate abdominal exploration. *Cholangiocarcinoma* is uncommon (3000 cases per year in the United States).[12] It can occur anywhere in the biliary tree but most commonly arises superior to the cystic duct. These tumors progress insidiously, and it is conceivable that one could be incidentally found as a sclerotic tubular mass in the porta. Faced with such a finding, the surgeon should simply document the size and location of the mass, the status of the liver (particularly of the hilum), and the status of regional lymph nodes. If an adjacent node seem suspicious, biopsy would be both safe and appropriate. *Choledochal cysts* are rare congenital abnormalities. They are usually detected in childhood, but perhaps 20% are initially found in adults.[15] They range in size from 2 to 20 cm and can have a fusiform or a saccular configuration. On the rare occasions when they are found incidentally, they should merely be documented because the treatment of these lesions is far too complicated to be performed as a secondary procedure.

THE PANCREAS

The pancreas is a complex organ of great consequence in both endocrine and digestive physiology. Because of its retroperitoneal position, both benign and malignant diseases of the pancreas can proceed to advanced states with little or no evidence from the history or physical examination. The pancreas lies obliquely in the upper abdomen from the C-loop of the duodenum to the hilum of the spleen. Anteriorly lies the stomach, the first portion of the duodenum, and the lesser omentum. Posteriorly (from right to left) lie the right renal vein, the inferior vena cava, the aorta, the superior mesenteric vessels, the left adrenal gland, and the left kidney. To the left of the aorta, the splenic artery lies superior to the pancreas throughout its course and the splenic vein is intimately associated with the posterior and superior aspect of the gland. For descriptive purposes the pancreas is divided into four regions. The head is that portion between the C-loop of the duodenum and the superior mesenteric vessels. The neck overlies those vessels. The body lies to the left and (with no distinguishing landmark between the two) the tail abuts the hilum of the spleen. In the adult, the pancreas is from 10 to 20 cm in length, 3 to 6

cm in superior to inferior dimension, and 1 to 2.5 cm from anterior to posterior. It normally weighs 70 to 100 g. As with so many other organs in the upper abdomen, the pancreas has a very rich and redundant blood supply. The head shares its supply with the C-loop of the duodenum in the form of four pancreaticoduodenal vessels arising from the gastroduodenal and superior mesenteric arteries. The body and tail are supplied by the splenic artery. The veins parallel the arteries, and all empty into the portal system. Most surgical diseases of the pancreas are of an inflammatory or neoplastic nature.

Pancreatitis

Acute pancreatitis is characterized by inflammation of the gland that resolves without residual fibrosis and with no detectable loss of parenchymal mass or function.[16] Gallstones and alcohol abuse account for probably 70% of acute pancreatitis, but there are a host of other etiologic agents. Certain drugs, including thiazide diuretics, furosemide, azathioprine, estrogens, corticosteroids, and tetracycline, have been implicated in acute pancreatitis. Trauma, operations, viral infections, lipid abnormalities, ductal obstruction, and hyperparathyroidism occasionally cause pancreatitis. No specific cause is found for the disease in 15% to 25% of cases. Upper abdominal pain is almost always present in acute pancreatitis. Other findings include nausea, vomiting, ileus, and elevated serum levels of amylase and lipase. There are no symptoms, physical findings, or laboratory or routine radiologic tests that are diagnostic of the disease. Acute pancreatitis thus remains a clinical diagnosis.

Some 95% of acute pancreatitis attacks are self-limited. In such cases, the patient requires only bowel rest, intravenous hydration, and analgesia. The reason that acute pancreatitis is of such great importance to surgeons and physicians is because of the 5% of individuals who develop severe pancreatitis. Early in its course, the major complications that can be associated with severe acute pancreatitis are volume depletion, hyperglycemia, electrolyte abnormalities, and failure of remote vital organs. Exploration of the abdomen is contraindicated in the presence of acute pancreatitis except as necessary to treat a specific surgical complication. However, occasionally one is faced with the operative finding of acute pancreatitis either incidentally or when operating for diagnosis in the acute abdomen. In such settings, acute pancreatitis may be manifest simply by edema or minor fat opsonification in the pancreatic bed. In more severe cases, one may find visible hemorrhage in the pancreas with or without extension to adjacent areas. Should these findings be encountered, it is best to leave the area undisturbed because any manipulation only enhances the risk of secondary infection. Surgical complications of acute pancreatitis include pancreatic pseudocyst, pancreatic ascites, hemorrhage, fistulas, and pancreatic abscess.

Pancreatic pseudocysts result from ductal disruption with leakage of pancreatic enzymes. These lesions are not true cysts and are simply contained by adjacent structures. Most are located in the lesser omentum, but they can extend to any location in the abdomen, including the pelvis. Acute pancreatic pseudocysts need not be drained because most spontaneously resolve.[17]

Pancreatic ascites results when a disruption in the pancreatic ductal system is not walled off by surrounding organs. It can be readily identified by its extremely high amylase concentration. Pancreatic ascites can often be managed medically.

Chronic pancreatitis generally results from alcohol abuse. Unusual causes include familial pancreatitis, lipid abnormalities, ductal obstruction, and nutritional deficiencies. Chronic pancreatitis is defined by permanent scarring and loss of exocrine parenchyma. Pain is experienced by 95% of patients. At least a third have associated exocrine insufficiency (steatorrhea), endocrine insufficiency (diabetes), or both. Serum amylase and lipase levels in these patients are frequently normal and are of little help in diagnosis. Calcifications seen in the pancreatic parenchyma on a radiograph are diagnostic but are present in a minority of patients. Most patients with chronic pancreatitis experience substantial weight loss. Uncomplicated chronic pancreatitis is represented on exploration by the finding of a very firm, often shrunken and ropy, pancreas gland. Biopsy of such a gland is warranted only when a discrete mass is palpated. Pseudocysts and pancreatic ascites are potential complications of chronic pancreatitis.

Tumors

Owing to the dual functions of the pancreas, this gland is subject to a variety of neoplasms: benign and malignant, cystic and solid, endo-crine and exocrine, functional and nonfunctional.

ENDOCRINE TUMORS

Endocrine cells in the pancreas are thought to originate from the neural crest and such amine precursor uptake and decarboxylation (APUD) cells are pleuripotential. Grossly and by standard histologic techniques, all of these tumors have a similar appearance. The clinical history, serum assays, and special histologic techniques are necessary to differentiate the cells producing the predominant hormone. Diagnosis of malignancy of these tumors is not based on their histologic appearance but by spread to regional lymph nodes, the liver, or other more distant sites. Endocrine tumors of the pancreas are rare. Typical clinical syndromes have been described for each of several tumor types.[18] Benign pancreatic endocrine tumors are small and are unlikely to be incidentally encountered. It is much more likely that an endocrine tumor discovered at operation will be malignant. The majority of glucagonomas, somatostatinomas, and VIPomas are malignant at the time of diagnosis as are one half of gastrinomas and 15% of insulinomas. Most nonfunctional islet cell tumors of the pancreas are also malignant. Treatment for benign endocrine tumors of the pancreas is complete excision. Most malignant endocrine tumors should be debulked as thoroughly as possible. Chemotherapy and endocrine therapy are thought to be beneficial.

CYSTIC EXOCRINE TUMORS

Although cystic neoplasms are usually symptomatic, it is possible that smaller tumors could be incidentally encountered. About 90% of all cystic lesions of the pancreas are simple pseudocysts, but the possible neoplastic nature of a cystic lesion must be born in mind.[19] *Serous cystadenomas* are usually well-circumscribed lesions containing multiple small cysts that on cut section have the appearance of a sponge. They are thought to have no malignant potential but should be completely excised if possible. *Mucinous cystadenomas* have a predilection for women of middle age or older. They, too, are well circumscribed but can be unilocular or multilocular. They are filled with mucus and have a smooth lining, often with papillary projections. These tumors have definite malignant potential and should be completely excised. *Cystadenocarcinomas* are thought to arise uniformly from mucinous cystadenomas. These are large tumors (therefore unlikely to be incidentally encountered), and some 25% are metastatic at diagnosis. They, too, should be completely excised if possible. Of interest to the gynecologist (because it almost exclusively occurs in young women) is an unusual tumor known as solid-and-papillary neoplasm of the pancreas. These tumors are usually large and contain areas of hemorrhage. Resection is often curative.

SOLID EXOCRINE TUMORS

Ductal adenocarcinoma comprises the preponderance of all pancreatic tumors. These tumors can occur anywhere in the gland but are predominantly located in the head. They tend to arise in older individuals, blacks more commonly than whites, urban populations more commonly than rural populations, and men more commonly than women. These are particularly virulent tumors. Most occur in areas other than the head of the pancreas and are unresectable at the time of diagnosis. Even with primary tumors located in the head of the pancreas and less than 2 cm, the vast majority of patients have nodal metastases at the time of diagnosis. When the diagnosis is suspected, it should be confirmed by core needle biopsy or fine-needle aspiration cytology and a thorough search made for nodal or hepatic metastases. Five-year survival after pancreaticoduodenectomy for ductal adenocarcinoma has been reported to be as high as 25%,[20] but most centers still report long-term survival rates of less than 10%. For these reasons, patients are very carefully chosen for resection.

Acinar cell carcinoma is much less common than ductal adenocarcinoma. An interesting feature of this tumor is that many of the patients have elevated serum levels of lipase and many have fat necrosis in remote and unusual sites. Almost all of these patients are elderly and have distant metastases at the time of diagnosis. The prognosis is even more dismal than that seen in ductal adenocarcinoma.

APPROACH TO PANCREATIC TUMORS

Faced with a mass in the pancreas, one should first determine whether it is cystic or solid. This can be done by palpation, intraoperative ultrasonography, or needle aspiration. If the mass is cystic and there is history of pancreatitis, it is probably a pseudocyst. Aspiration with chemical and cytologic analysis of the fluid is safe and should be performed. The site of aspiration should be carefully oversewn with figure-of-eight sutures to prevent leakage of cyst contents into the peritoneal cavity. A cystic mass in the pancreas should be carefully documented as to size and location in addition to the status of the regional lymph nodes. Follow-up is critical to determine resolution or growth because surgical intervention might be necessary given the latter. If the presence of a cystic neoplasm is determined by cytology, resection is necessary and should be considered at the time of diagnosis. Needle aspiration cytology, core needle biopsy, or both should also be performed if a solid mass is encountered. The size and location of the mass should once again be documented along with nodal status to guide future therapy.

SPLEEN

The spleen is located in the left upper quadrant of the abdomen between the stomach, the diaphragm, the splenic flexure of the colon, and the kidney. It is dark purple and shaped somewhat like a coffee bean. The normal spleen is about 12 cm in greatest dimension and weighs 100 to 150 g. It is suspended from the diaphragm by the phrenicolienal ligament and from the kidney by the lienorenal ligament and is attached to the colon by the lienocolic ligament. The gastrolienal ligament is also supportive and is traversed by the short gastric vessels. The spleen is covered by peritoneum and a fibroelastic capsule. The principal blood supply to this highly vascular organ is the splenic artery arising from the celiac axis and traversing along or within the superior aspect of the pancreas until dividing into six or more hilar segmental branches. The splenic vein is analogous to the artery through most of its course but joins the superior mesenteric vein to form the portal vein.

Splenic Injury

In the course of an operation it is possible for a splenic injury to result from retraction or, less commonly, from errant dissection. For the most part, these are relatively minor capsular tears or superficial parenchymal injuries that should be readily reparable. A grade I injury consists of a nonexpanding subcapsular hematoma involving less than 10% of the surface area of the organ or a nonbleeding capsular tear associated with a laceration of the splenic parenchyma less than 1 cm in depth.[21] A grade II injury consists of a nonexpanding subcapsular hematoma that encompasses less than 50% of the surface area of the spleen, a nonexpanding intraparenchymal hematoma less than 2 cm in diameter, or a capsular tear with active bleeding. This is probably the most common type of intraoperative splenic injury. Grade III injuries are defined by the presence of a subcapsular hematoma that covers more than 50% of the surface area of the spleen or is expanding; a ruptured subcapsular hematoma with active bleeding; an intraparenchymal hematoma that is greater than 2 cm in diameter or expanding; or a parenchymal laceration that is greater than 3 cm in depth or involves trabecular vessels. A grade III injury would be an unusual intraoperative event. Grade IV and V injuries should not occur as operative complications.

The key to assessment and treatment of any splenic injury is mobilization of the spleen into the wound. In doing so, an adequate abdominal wall incision is necessary. Two other simple maneuvers can make operations on the spleen much less tedious. One is to roll the table 15 to 20 degrees toward the operating surgeon (who should now be on the patient's right side). The second is to place folded linen under the patient's left flank to further elevate the splenic bed. The phrenicolienal, lienorenal, and lienocolic ligaments must be divided. The latter is vascular and requires clamping and tying. If a hilar injury is noted or suspected, the short gastric vessels must also be clamped and divided to allow visualization of that area. If examination of the injury reveals formed clot with no oozing, nothing further need be done except for the surgeon to remember to reassess the area before closure. If there is any bleeding, clot must be thoroughly removed to visualize the underlying injury. This can be accomplished by irrigation or by gently lifting the clot away with forceps. Repair of the spleen (splenorraphy) can be a time-consuming process. Therefore, splenectomy should be considered in a patient who has a short life expectancy on the basis of operative findings or preoperatively documented disease, a patient who has already sustained a prolonged operative procedure against a background of significant comorbid conditions, or a patient with other contraindication to further prolongation of operation such as hypothermia, coagulopathy, or hemorrhagic shock. It is desirable to salvage the spleen whenever the condition of the organ and the patient allow. In addition to its hematologic functions, which include the culling of senescent or otherwise defective cellular elements of the blood, the spleen has several important immunologic functions. It is an important source of IgM, opsonins, and ele-

ments in the alternate complement pathway. In addition, the spleen plays a vital role in the removal of bloodborne antigens. Absence of the latter function appears to be the primary cause of the increased susceptibility of the splenectomized patient to septic phenomena. In trauma patients who have undergone splenectomy, the risk of septicemia has been estimated to be approximately 140 times that of the general population.[22] For the remainder of life, the splenectomized patient is at risk for overwhelming postsplenectomy infection. Most of these infections have occurred in children and young adults, but mature adults are susceptible as well. The mortality with this syndrome can be as high as 80%.[23]

Techniques of Splenorrhaphy

Grade I splenic injuries rarely require intervention. Most grade II injuries can be managed using simple, readily available means that should be applied in a stepwise fashion. Tamponade with a gauze sponge or with available tissue (omentum or subcutaneous fat) for a few minutes is often successful in controlling bleeding from a superficial laceration.[21] If this fails, electrocautery can be applied to specific bleeding points. If these basic maneuvers fail, commercial hemostatic agents can be applied (absorbable purified bovine collagen, oxidized regenerated cellulose, or topical thrombin). More extensive splenic injuries require more surgical intervention, and it may be advisable for an individual experienced in the techniques of splenorrhaphy to be consulted intraoperatively. In the presence of a grade III injury, blood clot and devitalized tissue should be removed and expanding subcapsular hematomas should be opened to search for a source of parenchymal hemorrhage. Lacerations should be approximated to their full depth by placement of sutures through the capsule well away from the laceration. Horizontal mattress sutures with pledgets under the exposed portions of the sutures are often useful in such injuries.

In any attempt at splenorrhaphy, the condition of the patient vis-à-vis the degree of success in achieving hemostasis must be continually reassessed. Deterioration of the patient's hemodynamic status, the necessity for excessive blood transfusions, and prolonged failure to achieve hemostasis are indications to proceed with splenectomy. Whether splenorrhaphy or splenectomy is ultimately performed, the area should be once again checked for hemostasis before closure is undertaken. Drains should not be routinely placed.

Splenic Artery Aneurysm

Splenic artery aneurysms are unusual, but they occur twice as commonly in women as in men. In the elderly they appear to be of atherosclerotic origin. In women of child-bearing age the aneurysms are thought to be congenital, with the hormonal milieu influencing their enlargement and potential for rupture. These lesions can also result from local inflammation such as pancreatitis. In most patients, the aneurysms are located near the splenic hilum. They can be completely asymptomatic and therefore found incidentally. Alternatively, they can be diagnosed by a calcific rim on plain radiographs or by the presence of a bruit. Symptoms of left upper quadrant pain, nausea, and vomiting are ominous in that they suggest impending rupture. Approximately 20% of reported ruptures of splenic artery aneurysms have occurred during pregnancy.[24] Therefore, sudden hypotension and the presence of blood in the abdominal cavity during pregnancy should alert one to assess the splenic artery. Incidentally detected splenic artery aneurysms in the elderly can probably safely be left alone. In younger patients, aneurysmectomy is probably advisable to prevent rupture, particularly in women of child-bearing age. Arteriographic embolization may be a suitable alternative to aneurysmectomy.

Splenic Cysts

Splenic cysts are unusual.[25] Trauma is probably the most common etiology. Congenital, dermoid, epidermoid, and endothelial cysts of the spleen have been reported, and pancreatic pseudocysts can also present in the spleen. Operation is necessary only if such cysts persist, enlarge, or become symptomatic. Parasitic cysts of the spleen are almost always echinococcal. Such cysts may be asymptomatic and detected by the presence of splenomegaly, eosinophilia, or calcification on radiographs. Serology is confirmatory. Operation should be considered only if the cavity is persistent or symptomatic after medical treatment. The cyst should not be entered before killing the parasites to avoid precipitating an anaphylactic reaction.

Primary Tumors of the Spleen

NONLYMPHOID

Nonlymphoid tumors of the spleen are unusual.[26] They include *hemangiomas, lymphangiomas,* and *hamartomas.* These benign tumors are rarely significant, but splenectomy may be necessary. Splenectomy is both diagnostic and therapeutic for the extremely rare *angiosarcoma.*

LYMPHOID

The spleen is the largest single lymphoid organ in the body. As such, it is subject to involvement by many systemic lymphoid malignancies. Although they are much more common than primary nonlymphoid tumors of the spleen, it is unlikely that lymphoid tumors involving the spleen will be primarily encountered by the gynecologist except in the setting of previously undiagnosed splenomegaly. Furthermore, most lymphoid malignancies involving the spleen are less common in women than in men. There is a role for splenectomy in some cases of Hodgkin's lymphoma, hairy cell leukemia, chronic myelogenous leukemia, and chronic lymphocytic leukemia. In non-Hodgkin's lymphoma, splenectomy is indicated only for local symptoms.

Metastatic Tumors

The spleen is a relatively common target of metastasis from remote tumors, but this is of little clinical significance.

Abscesses of the Spleen

Splenic abscesses can result from hematogenous spread, direct extension from other organs, or secondarily in a splenic hematoma.[27] Although involvement of the spleen per se may be occult, these patients are almost always symptomatic from the septic process.

Ectopic Spleen, Accessory Spleen, and Splenosis

Ectopic ("wandering") spleens are often more common in women than in men. In addition, the ectopic spleen is often found in the lower abdomen or pelvis, where it can present as a pelvic mass by virtue of a long vascular pedicle. The ectopic spleen is at risk of torsion so splenopexy or splenectomy should be considered when this condition is identified. *Accessory spleens* are common. They tend to occur near the hilum of the spleen and the tail of the pancreas. *Splenosis* refers to the implantation and growth of spleen fragments after trauma. More commonly found in the left upper quadrant, such implants can occur anywhere in the abdomen. Accessory spleens and splenosis are of no significance except in patients with certain hematologic disorders. Biopsy is not advocated because of the risk of bleeding.

Hypersplenism

Hypersplenism is not a disease but a syndrome consisting of splenomegaly, decreased cellular blood elements, and secondary bone marrow hyperplasia. *Primary hypersplenism* is more common in women than in men but is still quite rare. Splenectomy is therapeutic but should be done only after a thorough search for a primary etiology. Hypersplenism is usually *secondary* to other identifiable conditions including portal hypertension, chronic inflammatory diseases, infections, and metabolic abnormalities. Disparate in origin and in mechanism, these processes have in common the increased sequestration of cellular blood elements in the spleen. Splenectomy is contraindicated in those cases secondary to generalized portal hypertension.[28] Splenectomy is the treatment of choice in splenic vein thrombosis. In secondary hypersplenism due to other causes, splenectomy may also be indicated for severe manifestations of the syndrome.

REFERENCES

1. Smithers BM, O'Loughlin B, Strong RW. Diagnosis of ruptured diaphragm following blunt trauma: results from 85 cases. Aust NZ J Surg 1991;61:737.
2. Skinner DB, Belsey RHR. Surgical management of esophageal reflux and hiatus hernia. J Thorac Cardiovasc Surg 1967;54:33.
3. Anderson LS, Forrest JV. Tumors of the diaphragm. Roentgenol Radium Ther Nucl Med 1973;119:259.
4. Couinaud C. Les enveloppes vasculobiliaires du foie ou capsule de Glisson: leur intérêt dans la chirugie vesiculaire, les resections hepatiques et l'abord du hile du foie. Lyon Chir 1954;49:589.
5. Frey CF, Zht Y, Xuzuki M, et al. Liver abscesses. Surg Clin North Am 1989;69:259.
6. Doty JR, Tompkins RK. Management of cystic disease of the liver. Surg Clin North Am 1989;69:285.
7. Nichols FC III, van Heerden JA, Weiland LH. Benign liver tumors. Surg Clin North Am 1989;69:297.
8. Schwartz SI, Husser WC. Cavernous hemangioma of the liver: a single institution report of 16 resections. Ann Surg 1987;205:456.
9. Kerlin P, Davis GL, McGill DB, et al. Hepatic adenoma and focal nodular hyperplasia: clinical, pathologic, and radiologic features. Gastroenterology 1983;84:994.
10. Cady B. Liver tumors. In: Cameron JL, ed. Current Surgical Therapy, 3rd ed. Toronto, BC Decker, 1989, p 212.
11. Hughes K, Scheele H, Sugarbaker PH. Surgery for colorectal cancer metastatic to the liver: optimizing the results of treatment. Surg Clin North Am 1989;69:339.
12. Pitt HA, Dooley WC, Yeo CJ, et al. Malignancies of the biliary tree. Curr Probl Surg 1995;32:1.
13. Potts JR III. What are the indications for cholecystectomy? Cleve Clin J Med 1990;57:40.
14. Stevens ML, Hubert BC, Wenzel FJ. Combined gynecologic surgical procedures and cholecystectomy. Am J Obstet Gynecol 1984;149:350.
15. Lipsett PA, Pitt HA, Colombani PM, et al. Choledochal cyst disease: a changing pattern of presentation. Ann Surg 1994;220:644.
16. Potts JR III. Acute pancreatitis. Surg Clin North Am 1988;68:281.
17. Yeo CJ, Bastidas JA, Lynch-Nyhan A, et al. The natural history of pancreatic pseudocysts documented by computed tomography. Surg Gynecol Obstet 1990;170:411.
18. Mozell E, Stenzel P, Woltering EA, et al. Functional endocrine tumors of the pancreas: clinical presentation, diagnosis, and treatment. Curr Probl Surg 1990;27:301.
19. Yang EY, Joehl RJ, Talamonti MS. Cystic neoplasms of the pancreas. J Am Coll Surg 1994;179:747.
20. Cameron JL, Pitt HA, Yeo CJ, et al. One hundred and forty-five consecutive pancreaticoduodenectomies without mortality. Ann Surg 1993;217:430.
21. Shackford SR, Molin M. Management of splenic injuries. Surg Clin North Am 1990;70:595.
22. Green JB, Shackford SR, Sise MJ, et al. Late septic complications in adults following splenectomy for trauma: a prospective analysis of 1444 patients. J Trauma 1986;26:999.
23. Scully RE, Mark EJ, McNeely BU. Case records of the Massachusetts General Hospital (20-1983). N Engl J Med 1983;308:1212.
24. Caillouett JC, Merchant EB. Ruptured splenic artery aneurysm in pregnancy—twelfth reported case with maternal and fetal survival. Am J Obstet Gynecol 1993;168:1810.
25. Moir C, et al. Splenic cysts: aspiration, sclerosis, or resection. J Pediatr Surg 1989;24:646.
26. Hahn PF, et al. MR imaging of focal splenic tumors. AJR 1988;150:823.
27. Paris S, Weiss SM, Ayers WH Jr, et al. Splenic abscess. Am Surg 1994;60:358.
28. El-Khishen MA, Henderson JM, Millikan WJ Jr, et al. Splenectomy is contraindicated for thrombocytopenia secondary to portal hypertension. Surg Gynecol Obstet 1985;160:233.

10

Robert L. Coleman

CHAPTER

The Retroperitoneal Mass

Occasionally, the gynecologic surgeon is confronted, sometimes unexpectedly, by a mass or disease process arising primarily from or located within the retroperitoneum. Statistically, the majority of these disease processes are neoplastic, and their operative management has proved to be challenging and memorable for many surgeons. Precise knowledge of the natural history and a clear understanding of the surgical goals are paramount to the successful management of these clinical problems. The objective of this chapter is to review the critical anatomy of the retroperitoneum, to present an exhaustive differential diagnosis, and to discuss perioperative management for various primary retroperitoneal disease processes.

ANATOMY AND SURGICAL EXPOSURE

The retroperitoneum is generally defined by its boundaries and represents both a potential and an actual space. Anatomically, the retroperitoneum is limited cephalad by the diaphragm and caudad by the levator ani muscles. The anterior margin is the parietal peritoneum, and, posteriorly, the retroperitoneal space is bounded by the quadratus lumborum and psoas muscles and the vertebral column. The quadratus lumborum and the tendinous sections of the transversus abdominis muscles demarcate the anatomic lateral borders. The retroperitoneum includes tissues derived embryologically from the ectoderm, mesoderm, endoderm, and embryonal remnants (Table 10–1). These tissues occupy the actual space of the retroperitoneum. The retroperitoneal space consists of loose areolar tissue and blood ves-

TABLE 10–1
Tissues Located Within the Retroperitoneal Space

Adrenal glands
Kidneys
Ureters
Bladder
Lumbar sympathetic chain
Splenic artery and vein
Renal artery and vein
Abdominal aorta
Inferior vena cava
Common, external, and internal iliac arteries and veins
Pancreas
Duodenum
Mesentery of the large and small intestine

sels and, generally, is easily displaced from underlying tissues.

Surgically, the peritoneum can be easily dissected with few exceptions. Posteriorly, dissection is limited by the major tributaries of the abdominal aorta. Cephalad, the peritoneum is fused to the undersurface of the diaphragm. Under the rectus muscles, the peritoneum is differentially attached to the anterior abdominal wall. Below the semicircular line the peritoneum is easily dissected free from the rectus adventitia. However, above the semicircular line, the peritoneum is densely attached and access to the subrectus plane can only be reached by incising the lateral margin of the fused internal oblique–transversalis fascial attachments.

Access to the retroperitoneum is important not only for resection purposes but also for exposure of tissues to be salvaged during intraperitoneal and extraperitoneal operations. Entering the retroperitoneal space can be easily gained through strategically planned incisions (Fig. 10–1). For access to the lateral and dependent pelvis, an incision of the peritoneum over the external iliac artery between the round ligament and ovarian vessel pedicle is made. Gentle blunt medial dissection easily exposes the upper retroperitoneal structures with attendant lymphatics and nerve tissues. Through this technique, visualization of the pelvic ureter and main branches of the internal iliac vasculature is accomplished. Identification of these structures is important to the successful resection of lateral retroperitoneal pelvic masses. Exposure to the lateral retroperitoneum of the abdomen or the midline retroperitoneum over the great vessels is accomplished either by continuing the lateral pelvic peritoneal separation (along the line of Toldt) or by division of the peritoneum at the root of the small bowel mesentery immediately over the abdominal aorta (Fig. 10–2). With reflection of the duodenum cephalad (best accomplished by transection of the peritoneal attachment to the ligament of Treitz), exposure to the renal vessels, superior mesenteric artery, and celiac axis is made. This is a common method of access to the high common iliac and para-aortic lymphatics.

PATHOLOGY AND NATURAL HISTORY

Development of a precise diagnosis and an effective management strategy for a retroperitoneal mass depends on an exhaustive consideration of its potential causes. Development of

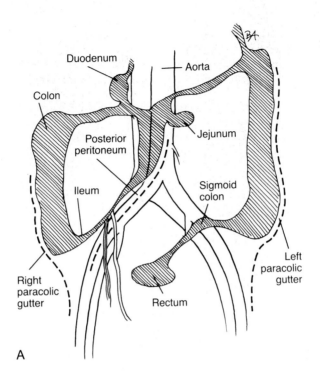

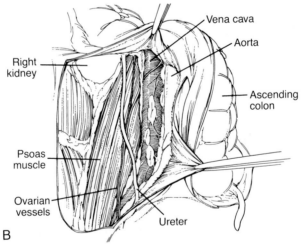

FIGURE 10-1

A, Retroperitoneal exposure of the vena cava and abdominal aorta can be obtained by vertically incising the peritoneum of the right and left paracolic gutter as outlined by the lateral markings. This is most easily accomplished by caudally extending the incisions made in the pelvic peritoneum created at the time of hysterectomy and pelvic node sampling. Medial mobilization of the large bowel and its mesentery provides access to the vena cava or aorta. An alternative approach is to open the posterior peritoneum along the anterior surface of the common iliac artery and lower aorta as indicated by the middle line. Dissection to the level of the arterial wall permits lateral mobilization of the more superficial structures and provides access to both the right and left para-aortic nodal chains. *B*, The cecum and ascending colon have been retracted medially to expose the vena cava. The ovarian vessels and right ureter are identified lying on the surface of the psoas muscle and can be protected with a large curved retractor. The duodenum is identified and mobilized superiorly. (From Gershenson DM, DeCherney AH, Curry SL. Operative Gynecology. Philadelphia, WB Saunders, 1993, p 384.)

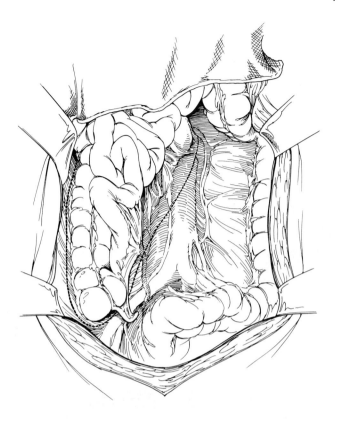

FIGURE 10–2
An incision for mobilization of the right colon to adequately expose the high para-aortic nodes in patients in whom they are palpable or when nodes in the area of the renal vessels should be removed, as in some patients with ovarian carcinoma. This is also a useful incision in the obese patient, in whom exposure is limited. The incision may be utilized on the left to expose the left para-aortic nodes, depending on the operator's preference. (From Gershenson DM, DeCherney AH, Curry SL. Operative Gynecology. Philadelphia, WB Saunders, 1993, p 144.)

a differential diagnosis takes into consideration the primary tissues and organs contained in the retroperitoneum (Table 10–2). These lesions are rare, accounting for 0.07% to 0.2% of all neoplasms reported annually in the United States.[1] Tumors arising primarily from the retroperitoneum have been classified histologically by their cell type and are derived from either mesodermal tissues (75%), nerve tissues (24%), or embryologic remnants (1%).[2] The re-

TABLE 10–2
Benign and Malignant Retroperitoneal Tumors by Tissue Source

Source	Benign Tumors	Malignant Tumors
Adipocyte	Lipoma	Liposarcoma
Fibroblast	Fibroma	Fibrosarcoma
Myocyte smooth	Leiomyoma	Leiomyosarcoma
Myocyte striated	Rhabdomyoma	Rhabdomyosarcoma
Endothelium	Hemangioma	Malignant hemangiopericytoma
Mesothelium	Adenomatoid tumor	Malignant mesothelioma
Neurocyte	Neurilemoma	Malignant schwannoma
Nerve ganglion	Ganglioneuroma	Neuroblastoma
Glandular formation	Adenoma (fibroma)	Carcinoma
Embryonal remnants	Nephrogenic cysts	Urogenital ridge tumor
Lymph nodes	Lymphangioma	Lymphoma (lymphosarcoma)

Adapted from Adams JT. Abdominal wall, omentum, mesentery and retroperitoneum. In: Schwartz SJ, Shires GT, Spencer FC, eds. Principles of Surgery. New York, McGraw-Hill, 1994.

ported incidence of malignancy is varied but ranges from 60% to 85%.[1–5] The natural history of these lesions varies according to the histologic cell type. For example, lymphomatous lesions frequently have distant tissue involvement at the time of initial diagnosis. However, retroperitoneal tumors arising from the other tissues of the mesoderm are locally aggressive, with metastatic lesions representing a late effect. Overall, the reported frequency of distant metastatic disease ranges from 5% to 43% but is most frequently reported around 20% at diagnosis.[1, 6, 7] Even in the absence of metastatic disease, complete surgical excision rates are modest (20%–40%), owing to the invasiveness of these tumors into adjacent vital structures.

Consideration must also be given to traumatic and space-occupying lesions that may result from an underlying disease or recent manipulation. In contradistinction to neoplasms, hematomas, lymphoceles, and abscesses are much more common conditions that occupy the retroperitoneal space and can present as primary retroperitoneal masses. In general, identification of these processes can be reliably made by radiographic evaluation.

ETIOLOGY AND PATHOGENESIS

Biologic study of soft tissue tumors arising in the retroperitoneum have suggested that genetic alteration of cell regulatory genes such as the *p53* tumor suppressor gene and mutation of mesenchymal stem cells are central to the development of these lesions.[8–13] The exact pathogenesis as to how these events occur is largely unknown. Study of hereditary cancer syndromes in which soft tissue sarcomas are manifest, such as the Li-Fraumeni syndrome and familial retinoblastoma, has demonstrated that inherited germline mutations of these genes are predictors of phenotypic expression.[10] In addition, exposure to environmental toxins (e.g., asbestos), chemical agents, carcinogenic drugs (e.g., xylene, alkylating chemotherapeutic agents), chronic immunosuppression, and ionizing radiation has been linked to occurrence of these rare lesions. Although malignant degeneration of benign lesions rarely occurs, sudden changes in size should raise clinical suspicion and warrant further evaluation.[11] Careful consideration of these factors helps narrow the differential diagnosis and direct an appropriate and cost-effective evaluation of the patient.

PRESENTATION

Retroperitoneal masses, whether arising from the pelvis or abdomen, have no classic symptomatology. This is largely due to the relative vastness of the potential space and the abdominal cavity "hiding" these lesions until they obtain considerable size. Of those patients diagnosed with primary retroperitoneal lesions, as many as 20% are completely asymptomatic. An equal number of patients present with abdominal fullness as a solitary complaint. The majority, however, present with multiple complaints resulting from compression and obstruction of neighboring organs and structures. Most often, symptoms are related to location and size and, to some extent, histology of the disease process. Malignant conditions of the sacral area commonly induce pain relative to sacral and lower lumbar nerve roots and muscles. Motor dysfunction of the gluteal, hamstring, and gastrocnemius muscles may be evident. Disease involving the lateral retroperitoneum of the abdomen commonly causes back or flank pain. Centrally located retroperitoneal masses can produce symptoms of gastric outlet obstruction or ileus as an initial complaint. Benign and traumatic processes can similarly produce pain, fever, and malaise, but the lack of bone or muscle invasion may alter the degree of motor dysfunction seen as a whole. Symptoms generally are nonacute and can be traced for several months before presentation. In one series of malignant retroperitoneal masses, 50% of the patients identified reported symptoms between 2 and 6 months, with nearly another third reporting symptoms up to 1 year before diagnosis.[14]

DIAGNOSIS

The advent of computed tomography (CT), magnetic resonance imaging (MRI), and ultrasonography has made precise localization and diagnosis of retroperitoneal masses far less difficult. The great advantage of these studies is not only their ability to evaluate local invasion and extension of the primary lesion but also their ability to evaluate the relationship of the lesion to other organs. The importance of accurate preoperative evaluation cannot be overstated, especially for masses situated near the great vessels. Most patients found with abdominopelvic masses on physical examination not believed to be from the adnexa will undergo either ultrasonography or CT. Contours of the mass to the bony pelvis and adjacent organs as well as the size, shape, and consistency of the

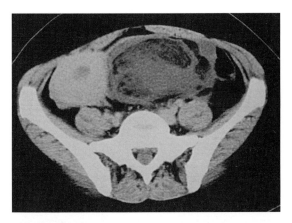

FIGURE 10–3
Retroperitoneal liposarcoma presenting as a pelvic mass of the broad ligament. The margins of resection were limited by invasion into the adventitia of the common, external, and internal iliac vessels and the inferior pole of the left kidney.

mass can be exploited with the CT scan (Fig. 10–3). In addition, these studies become extremely important in identifying early residual or recurrent disease. In one series of 44 cases, CT proved to identify the retroperitoneal mass in all cases, correctly characterize the lesion in 43 cases, and delineate the origin in 41 cases.[15] However, determination of resectability and malignancy potential has been less rewarding. In the study of Pistolesti and coworkers,[15] prediction of successful resection was confirmed in 60% of the cases and local invasiveness was reported in 57%. MRI has improved the prediction of local invasion, but improvement in the prediction of a successful resection has not been altered. Refinements in both CT and MRI continue to be made, and reliance on them for accurate pretreatment planning will likely increase as well.

Although a vast amount of information can be gained anatomically from CT and MRI, information regarding functional characteristics of a tumor are obtained by alternate sources. Because many of the tumors identified in Table 10–2 have the potential for prolific vascularity or vascular invasion, angiography and venography can be extremely helpful in the pretreatment planning. Certain lesions, such as the leiomyosarcoma, can present as an intravascular mass of the retroperitoneum where venography of the vena cava can give important preoperative information. The posterolateral abdominal retroperitoneum is supplied in large part by the lumbar arteries, and deviation of the aorta or stretching or displacement of these vascular pedicles can also aid in treatment planning.

Radiographic surveys of the intestine are commonly ordered in these patients primarily to rule out more common neoplasms primary to these organs. In one series, results of 86% of barium enemas and 75% of upper gastrointestinal series were abnormal; however, the findings were nonspecific and generally represented displacement of the soft tissue and intestines.[14] Intravenous pyelography is another commonly obtained test in this group of patients and has the ability to outline the course of the ureter and to visualize local invasion of the kidney or bladder. Abdominal and pelvic ultrasonography is often used in conjunction for lesions occupying the renal fat. The addition of Doppler flow analysis can provide information regarding the flow of blood or fluid in an identified mass. There is a great temptation to obtain multiple radiographic studies. This is not cost effective and adds little to the formulation of a plan of management. In most cases, initial CT evaluation can direct further studies.

Fine needle aspiration (FNA) for the establishment of a diagnosis may be considered in cases where the information will potentially alter the management strategy. A common example of this is among tumors arising from the hematopoietic system. Several studies have addressed the diagnostic accuracy of FNA and have compared its use to core needle biopsies in patients with soft tissue masses.[15a, 15b] These studies have shown the information obtained to be favorable and reliable. Theoretical concern for tract implantation (as in sarcomas) requires that the diagnostic pathway be excised with a surgical margin when operative intervention is warranted. The technique is largely practiced for retroperitoneal masses with the aid of CT or ultrasound. A 22-gauge needle is commonly used and provides adequate cytologic material for study. Other biologic parameters, such as flow cytometry and receptor data, can be obtained with some of these specimens.[15a] When evaluation of a cystic, complex, or air containing mass such as a lymphocele, hematoma, or abscess is performed, a drain can be placed in the area at question for therapy.

TREATMENT

Surgical Considerations

Treatment planning encompasses consideration of the differential diagnosis, review of the physical and radiographic findings, histopathology if obtained, and proper patient preparation. In cases in which lymphoma is considered preoperatively, fine needle aspiration may alleviate unnecessary surgical procedures. All patients undergoing surgical exploration should undergo mechanical bowel preparation combined with orally administered antibiotics. It is common practice to provide systemic antibiotics and antithromboembolic measures perioperatively. Appropriate blood products should be available. The principal surgeon should be skilled in retroperitoneal dissection with appropriate consultation of supporting services should vascular, renal, or radiotherapeutic procedures be needed.

Surgical exposure is generally best through a transperitoneal, midline approach, although one must be prepared to use alternate incisions such as a thoracoabdominal or abdominoinguinal incision to best approach the lesion in question. An exception to this axiom would be a low presacral mass, which may be best approached through a Kraske position. In all cases, en bloc resection should be the goal even if this incorporates adjacent viscera. Bryant and colleagues[14] reported that all nine patients in their series undergoing complete tumor excision required removal of at least one adjacent organ. In cases in which subtotal tumor resection is accomplished, it is unclear that tumor "debulking" can improve survival. However, it is clear that cytoreduction may improve symptomatology when derived from structural compression. Patients with subtotal resections may undergo intraoperative radiation therapy and should have the residual tumor margins marked with surgical clips for future treatment planning.

On occasion, the surgeon may be confronted with the unexpected intraoperative finding of a retroperitoneal mass when the patient was explored for what was thought to be a pelvic mass arising from the female reproductive tract.

Therapeutic Considerations

Although overall survival among patients with nonlymphomatous primary retroperitoneal neoplasms is dependent, in part, on histology, grade, and stage, the degree of resection and the amount of residual disease appear to be the most important predictors of long-term treatment success. This is fundamentally supported by the lack of benefit offered from adjuvant chemotherapy and radiation therapy. Thus, primary complete surgical resection has been the primary therapeutic goal for more than 50 years. Differential survival has been demonstrated among patients whose tumors

have been resected completely. Serio and colleagues[7] reported an overall 5-year survival of 46% and 10-year survival in 38% among 35 patients with primary malignant retroperitoneal tumor. Of these 35 patients, 23 (65%) underwent complete resection with a 5-year survival of 65% compared with 12 who underwent biopsy or partial resection with a median survival of 6 months. The survival curves are demonstrated by resection outcome in Figure 10–4. Similar survival data have been presented by others.[6, 16, 17] However, recurrence among those patients undergoing complete resection continues to taint long-term survival results. In the series reported by Serio and colleagues,[7] recurrence was identified locally in 35% and distantly in 23%. Cody and coworkers[6] reported that whereas 40% of their completely resected patients were alive at 5 years, only 22% were disease free. Similarly, McGrath and colleagues reported a 70% 5-year survival among 18 completely resected patients but only a 50% 5-year disease-free survival; at 10 years of follow-up this difference was 56% and 10%, respectively.[16] In addition, these series failed to demonstrate an improvement on these statistics with any adjuvant therapy.

In view of the importance of aggressive surgical resection, appropriate consultation should be sought when the diagnosis of a retroperitoneal mass is made. The margins of the neoplasm should be marked with surgical clips to direct postoperative radiation therapy fields if this treatment is recommended.

Adjuvant Therapy: Radiation Therapy and Chemotherapy

Despite the lack of randomized trials employing prospective treatment protocols, many investigators have sought to elucidate the role of adjuvant therapy to the primary surgical effort. Much of the clinical acumen regarding chemotherapeutic and radiotherapeutic response of soft tissue neoplasms comes from data produced by treatment of lesions located in the extremities. In these trials, inoperable lesions have been made operable, local recurrence was decreased, and limb-sparing outcomes were achieved (often with lower morbidity) with the use of preoperative radiation therapy. Unfortunately, tissue tolerance of the abdominal viscera is lower than that of the extremities (which are usually much smaller in size), thus limiting extrapolation of these treatment results to those neoplasms arising in the retroperitoneum. For example, many peri-

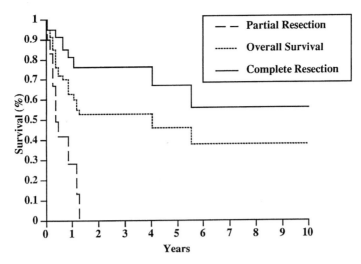

FIGURE 10–4
Log-rank survival curves among 36 patients undergoing resection for primary retroperitoneal soft tissue sarcomas. A significant improvement in survival was seen only if the neoplasm was completely resected. Overall survival was significantly influenced by the proportion of patients able to undergo a complete excision; however, few were disease free. (Adapted from Serio G, Tenchini P, Nifosi F, Iacono C. Surgical strategy in primary retroperitoneal tumours. Br J Surg 1989; 76:385.)

operative (limb-preserving) radiation protocols will plan to deliver between 6000 and 6500 cGy to the tumor bed. Therefore, radiation therapy among patients with primary retroperitoneal tumors is delivered in an adjunctive role to attempt decrease in local recurrence. Several nonrandomized trials have incorporated adjuvant radiation therapy in their treatment protocols.[6, 16–19] From these it is difficult to discern whether radiation therapy (either intraoperative or postoperative) added any survival or disease-free benefit. Table 10–3 summarizes the results of two of these trials. In a trial assessing the benefit of radiation therapy, four patients who were deemed unresectable at first exploration underwent complete resection after a course of preoperative radiation therapy.[20] This group appeared to have an improved survival once undergoing a complete resection compared with those unable to undergo this degree of resection. Morbidity was modest. Catton and coworkers[17] reviewed the Princess Margaret Hospital experience of 104 patients with

retroperitoneal soft tissue sarcomas managed with radiation and surgery. Of the 45 patients undergoing complete resection, 36 received adjuvant radiation therapy (40 Gy). In comparison to the 9 patients receiving no additional therapy after complete resection, there was no difference in survival or relapse-free survival. There was a trend in delaying local-regional recurrence among those irradiated and a significant decrease of "in-field" recurrences among this group, but this benefit failed to translate into prolonged disease-specific survival. These investigators concluded that because local control was the only factor independently predicting survival, further efforts should be directed toward preoperative irradiation. Trials evaluating this approach are underway. In addition, treatment protocols evaluating intraoperative radiation therapy have demonstrated an ability to provide excellent local control (70% in one series) with acceptable toxicity.[21, 22] Long-term evaluation has yet to confirm the efficacy of this approach. Fur-

TABLE 10–3
Studies Evaluating Benefit of Adjuvant Radiation Therapy to Primary Surgical Resection

Author	Surgical Survival (n)	Surgical + Radiation Therapy Survival (n)	P
McGrath (incomplete)	6 months (11)	15 months (18)	NS
McGrath (complete)	9.66 years (12)	5 years (6)	NS

NS, not significant.

thermore, it is usually the bias of individual institutions to treat with adjuvant radiation therapy cases in which incomplete resection was performed, surgical margins were positive or inevaluable, or lesions were of high-grade or large size (i.e., >100 mm). Lesions of more favorable prognosis and histology probably benefit little from additional therapy.

The role of chemotherapy for retroperitoneal malignancies has undergone somewhat more scrupulous analysis. This has resulted from anticipated extrapolation of prospective trials performed in soft tissue sarcomas of the extremity. Whereas overall survival statistics tend to be worse with nonextremity soft tissue neoplasms, chemosensitivity is more uniform between sites. Clinical trials have evaluated the role of chemotherapy in completely resected tumors, in advanced or recurrent disease, in low-grade neoplasms, and in drug combinations with or without irradiation. Randomized trials of patients with primary retroperitoneal neoplasms are lacking, but preliminary information suggests that little additional benefit is gained in the adjuvant setting. Glenn and coworkers[18] randomized 15 patients with primary retroperitoneal sarcomas to doxorubicin and cyclophosphamide versus no therapy. There was one disease-related death in the no-treatment arm and four disease-related deaths in the chemotherapy arm. Although obviously of little power, results from this trial failed to demonstrate a benefit to therapy. Most of the additional information regarding adjuvant therapy among completely resected cases of primary retroperitoneal soft tissue sarcoma comes from unifactorial and multifactorial analysis of prognostic factors in nonrandomized clinical series.[7, 14, 16–18, 23–27] Almost uniformly, the administration of cytotoxic chemotherapy is excluded from the statistical model when survival and disease-free survival are considered. In contrast, data from larger prospective, randomized trials of soft tissue extremity sarcomas have suggested a potential benefit in both disease-free and overall survival with adjuvant chemotherapy. Meta-analysis of data obtained from 11 randomized trials by Zalupski and associates[28] demonstrated a highly significant disease-free survival (68% vs. 53%) and overall survival (81% vs. 71%) for patients treated with adjuvant therapy. The much higher survival figures represent the better overall prognosis of sarcomas arising in the extremity and probable nonapplicability to primary retroperitoneal soft tissue sarcomas. The obvious exception is among lymphomas where chemosensitivity provides a dramatic response.

Therapy for Advanced or Recurrent Disease

Although chemotherapy administration has not been proven as an adjuvant modality for sarcomas, responses have been achieved in advanced or recurrent disease. To date, many agents have been evaluated alone and in combination for advanced disease. A listing of these is presented in Table 10–4. Overall response rates range from 10% to 30%. The most active agents appear to be ifosfamide and doxorubicin. Randomized trials of the combination of these agents versus use of either drug alone have demonstrated superiority in the former. In two multi-institutional cooperative group studies, the combination of doxorubicin (with or without dacarbazine) and ifosfamide was superior in overall response rate to doxorubicin alone.[29, 30] However, responses were short-lived and median survival times were similar in the two treatment arms. One European Organization for Research in Cancer Therapy study failed to demonstrate any difference in response rate among 549 patients randomized to doxorubicin; doxorubicin plus ifosfamide; or doxorubicin plus cyclophosphamide, dacarbazine, and vincristine.[31] Although dose-intensity trials are suggesting a linear response effect with doxorubicin and alkylator therapy, clinical benefit with the addition of the various cytokines (e.g., granulocyte colony-stimulating factor, granulocyte-macrophage colony-stimulating factor, PIXY-321) has yet to be determined.

TABLE 10–4
Response Rates Achieved in Soft Tissue Sarcomas From Clinical Trials of Single Agent Chemotherapeutics

Agent	Response Rate (%)
Ifosfamide	30
Doxorubicin	26
Methotrexate	13–21
Dacarbazine	16
Vincristine	12
Cisplatin	12
Cyclophosphamide	8
Etoposide	8
Bleomycin	6

CONCLUSIONS

Primary retroperitoneal masses should be viewed as potentially malignant processes. Precise knowledge of the lesion, its extent, and a prospective treatment plan should be obtained before surgical exploration. Through conscientious use of appropriate radiographic studies reasonably accurate determinations of resectability can be made, greatly helping preoperative treatment planning. Complete resection with a margin of normal tissue is the preferred and only proven modality of therapy. Many of these lesions will present with a pseudocapsule, and enucleation should be avoided if possible in establishing surgical margins. In those cases not completely resectable, available evidence supports surgical debulking, knowing that adjuvant therapy plays little role in the long-term therapy plan. Patients with a suspicion of lymphoma should undergo needle biopsy in an effort to avoid unnecessary laparotomy. Patients with advanced or unresectable recurrent disease should be offered chemotherapy because short-term responses are obtainable with a combination protocol involving doxorubicin and ifosfamide with or without dacarbazine or vincristine. Adjuvant radiation therapy for completely resected disease may be of benefit locally, especially if given as an intraoperative boost, but appears, at this time, to have little effect on long-term disease-specific and overall survival. Clearly, prospective randomized treatment protocols as well as delineation of the natural history of these tumors will be tantamount to any additional progression in clinical knowledge. Currently, soft tissue sarcoma tissue banks and national tumor registries are being developed that should provide clinical investigators with the resources to progress in the understanding of these rare but lethal tumors.

REFERENCES

1. Pack GT, Tabah EJ. Primary retroperitoneal tumours: a study of 120 cases. Surg Gynecol Obstet 1954;99:209.
2. Acherman LV. Tumors of the retroperitoneal mesentery and peritoneum. In: Lund HZ, ed. Atlas of Tumor Pathology, section II, fasicle 23-24. Washington, DC, Armed Forces Institute of Pathology, 1954, p 136.
3. Braasch JW, Mon AB. Primary retroperitoneal tumors. Surg Clin North Am 1967;47:663.
4. Jacobsen S, Juul-Jorgensen S. Primary retroperitoneal tumors. Acta Chir Scand 1974;140:498.
5. Moore S, Aldrete J. Primary retroperitoneal sarcomas: the role of surgical treatment. Am J Surg 1981;142:358.
6. Cody HS, Turnbull AD, Fortner JG, Hajdu SI. The continuing challenge of retroperitoneal sarcomas. Cancer 1981;47:2147.
7. Serio G, Tenchini P, Nifosi F, Iacono C. Surgical strategy in primary retroperitoneal tumours. Br J Surg 1989;76:385.
8. Seale KS, L Dange TA, Monson D, Hackbarth DA. Soft-tissue tumors of the foot and ankle. Foot Ankle Int 1988;9:19.
9. Salloum E, Slamant F, Caillaud JM, et al. Diagnostic and therapeutic problems of soft tissue tumors other than rhabdomyosarcoma in infants under 1 year of age: a clinicopathological study of 34 cases treated at the Institut Gustave Roussy. Med Pediatr Oncol 1990;18:37.
10. Wunder JS, Czitrom AA, Kandel R, Andrulis IL. Analysis of alterations in the retinoblastoma gene and tumor grade in bone and soft-tissue sarcomas. J Natl Cancer Inst 1991;83:194.
11. Dei Tos AP, Doglioni C, Laurino L, et al. p53 protein expression in non-neoplastic lesions and benign and malignant neoplasms of soft tissue. Histopathology 1993;22:45.
12. Kawai A, Noguchi M, Beppu Y, et al. Nuclear immunoreaction of p53 protein in soft tissue sarcomas: a possible prognostic factor. Cancer 1994;73:2499.
13. Fanburg JC, Rosenberg AE. Pathology of soft tissue sarcomas. Cancer Control 1994;1:581.
14. Bryant RL, Stevenson DR, Hunton DW, et al. Primary malignant retroperitoneal tumors: current management. Am J Surg 1982;144:644.
15. Pistolesi GF, Procacci C, Caudana R, et al. CT criteria of the differential diagnosis in primary retroperitoneal masses. Eur J Radiol 1984;4:127.
15a. Willem H, Akerman M, Carlen B. Fine needle aspiration (FNA) in the diagnosis of soft tissue tumours; a review of 22 years experience. Cytopathology 1995;6:236.
15b. Barth R, Merino M, Solomon D, et al. A prospective study of the value of core needle biopsy and fine needle aspiration in the diagnosis of soft tissue masses. Surgery 1992;112:536.
16. McGrath PC, Neifeld JP, Lawrence W Jr, et al. Improved survival following complete excision of retroperitoneal sarcomas. Ann Surg 1984;200:200.
17. Catton CN, O'Sullivan B, Kotwall C, et al. Outcome and prognosis in retroperitoneal soft tissue sarcoma. Int J Radiat Oncol Biol Phys 1994;29:1005.
18. Glenn J, Sindclar WF, Kinsella T, et al. Results of multimodality therapy of resectable soft-tissue sarcomas of the retroperitoneum. Surgery 1985;97:316.
19. van Doorn RC, Ballee MP, Hart AA, et al. Resectable retroperitoneal soft tissue sarcomas, the effect of extent of resection and postoperative radiation therapy on local tumor control. Cancer 1994;73:637.
20. Wang YN, Zhu WQ, Shen ZZ, et al. Treatment of locally recurrent soft tissue sarcomas of the retroperitoneum: report of 30 cases. J Surg Oncol 1994;56:213.
21. Gunderson LL, Nagorney DM, McIlrath DC, et al. External beam and intraoperative electron irradiation for locally advanced soft tissue sarcomas. Int J Radiat Oncol Biol Phys 1993;25:647.
22. Willett CG, Suit HD, Tepper JE, et al. Intraoperative electron beam radiation therapy for retroperitoneal soft tissue sarcoma. Cancer 1991;68:278.
23. Shiloni E, Szold A, White DE, Freund HR. High-grade retroperitoneal sarcomas: role of an aggressive palliative approach. J Surg Oncol 1993;53:197.
24. Bevilacqua RG, Togatko A, Hajdu SE, Brennan MF. Prognostic factors in primary retroperitoneal soft-tissue sarcomas. Arch Surg 1991;126:328.
25. Storm FK, Mahvi DM. Diagnosis and management of

retroperitoneal soft-tissue sarcoma. Ann Surg 1991;214:2.

26. Gottlieb JA, Baker LH, Quagliana JM, et al. Chemotherapy of sarcomas with a combination of adriamycin and dimethyl triazeno imidazole carboxamide. Cancer 1972;30:1632.

27. McGrath PC. Retroperitoneal sarcomas. Semin Surg Oncol 1994;10:364.

28. Zalupski M, Ryan J, Hussein M. Defining the role of adjuvant chemotherapy for patients with soft-tissue sarcoma of the extremities. In: Salmon SE, ed. Adjuvant Therapy of Cancer VII. Philadelphia, JB Lippincott, 1993, p 385.

29. Antman K, Crowley J, Balcerzak SP, et al. An intergroup phase III randomized study of doxorubicin and dacarbazine with or without ifosfamide and mesna in advanced soft tissue and bone sarcomas. J Clin Oncol 1993;11:1276.

30. Edmonson JH, Ryan LM, Blum RH, et al. Randomized comparison of doxorubicin alone versus ifosfamide plus doxorubicin or mitomycin, doxorubicin, and cisplatin against advanced soft tissue sarcomas. J Clin Oncol 1993;11:1269.

31. Santoro A, Rouesse J, Steward W. A randomized EORTC study in advanced soft tissue sarcomas: ADM vs ADM + IFOS vs CYVADIC. Proc Am Soc Clin Oncol 1990;9:309. (abstract).

11

John M. Malone, Jr.

CHAPTER

Wound Closure

Incisional closure is an often overlooked part of the operative procedure and is frequently relegated to the most junior person present. A secure closure is of utmost importance. Attention to detail and technique can measurably reduce the incidence of dehiscence, evisceration, and herniation. The intelligent use of available suture material and proper closure technique can go a long way toward reducing these problems.

In this chapter the focus is on wound healing, suture material, and surgical technique as they pertain to the closure of a surgical defect. The recognition and management of wound complications are discussed in Chapter 15.

WOUND HEALING

Secure healing depends on the approximation of tissue, the maintenance of blood supply, and the avoidance of infection. If this is successfully accomplished, neovascularization and fibroblast proliferation will commence and complete the process. Wound healing starts at the time of tissue approximation and continues until the scar has matured. This process can be considered as four separate yet overlapping parts: (1) inflammation, (2) epithelialization, (3) fibroplasia, and (4) maturation. At the time of tissue injury, an inflammatory process begins and vascular constriction results in blood clot formation, which is followed by leukocyte migration and margination.[1] The initial cellular response includes the phagocytization and digestion of bacteria, foreign debris, and necrotic tissue. In the absence of infection, this process is completed within 3 days. At the same time, epithelialization results in the development of a thin covering of epithelial cells that act as a barrier against bacteria and foreign material.[2] Within 48 hours, the approximated wound surfaces are completely epithelialized.

Fibroblasts follow the leukocytes into the wound and within 3 to 5 days start to lay down a collagen matrix that ultimately becomes the scar.[3] Over the subsequent weeks the collagen matrix becomes more organized and the scar matures. By the third week a wound has achieved 20% of its "pre-wound" strength. Complete maturation occurs after 8 to 9 weeks and the wound regains 60% of its pre-wound strength.

A number of conditions can impede the healing process and contribute to fascial disruption (Table 11–1). Fascial disruption leading to either dehiscence, evisceration, or herniation occurs in 1% to 3% of all major abdominal sur-

TABLE 11–1
Conditions That May Affect Wound Healing

Length of operation
Obesity
Diabetes
Infection
History of prior wound problems
History of prior radiation or chemotherapy
Malnutrition
Current malignancy
Liver dysfunction
Kidney disease
Poor surgical technique

gery. Numerous factors, some inherent to the patient and others within the purview of the surgeon, contribute to fascial separation.[4] By attention to detail, the surgeon can minimize these wound complications.

The suture material used at the time of fascial closure is important. The surgeon needs to choose one that maintains its tensile strength and causes minimal tissue reaction.[5] When tissue is approximated there must be sufficient tension to keep the tissue edges together. However, excess tension at the fascial edge can lead to ischemia and pressure necrosis of the wound, which is believed to be the primary cause of wound dehiscence.[6] The suture material should have sufficient intrinsic strength to hold the tissue edges together long enough for the body's own reparative processes to accomplish their tasks. This is a delicate balance.

SUTURE MATERIAL

When choosing suture material the surgeon must consider tensile strength, functional life expectancy, and tissue reactivity. The ideal suture material must be strong enough to hold the wound together yet absorbable and associated with minimal tissue reaction. The surgeon needs to remember that any type of suture is a foreign body that is capable of causing tissue reaction. As a rule of thumb, the smallest and least reactive material capable of accomplishing the task at hand should be used.

Suture material may be characterized in several ways. Suture tensile strength refers to the amount of force needed to pull apart a strand of suture. This is a function of density of the material, molecular cohesiveness, and the diameter of the strand.[7, 8] Suture material is also characterized as either absorbable or nonabsorbable (Table 11–2). Absorbable sutures tend to cause more tissue reaction then the nonab-

TABLE 11–2
Suture Material

Absorbable

  Natural
    Plain gut
    Chromic gut
  Synthetic
    Polyglycolic acid (Dexon)
    Polyglactin 910 (Vicryl)
    Polydioxanone (PDS)
    Polyglyconate (Maxon)

Nonabsorbable

  Silk
  Cotton
  Polypropylene (Prolene)
  Braided synthetics (Tevdek, Mersilene, Dacron)
  Stainless steel wire
  Nylon

sorbable materials. On the other hand, they are less likely to cause irritation and inflammation. Absorbable suture materials can be divided into naturally occurring and synthetic materials.

Both plain gut and treated (chromic) gut are naturally occurring materials.[9] Derived from either subserosa of sheep intestine or the serosa of beef intestine, plain "gut" is exposed to formaldehyde to increase its tensile strength. Treated gut is produced by treating plain gut material with chromium salts, which further increases tensile strength and durability. Both plain and treated gut are well known for their handling and knot-holding characteristics. Disadvantages include an intense inflammatory reaction and a short half-life.

The synthetic absorbable suture materials include polyglycolic acid (Dexon),[10] polyglactin 910 (Vicryl), polydioxanone (PDS), and polyglyconate (Maxon).[11] The synthetic absorbable sutures come as both braided and monofilament strands. On the whole these materials are stronger with greater tensile strengths and have less local inflammatory response than "gut" suture. The braided synthetics offer ease of handling and knot tying. The monofilament synthetics are harder to handle and tie but maintain their tensile strength longer than the braided materials.

The nonabsorbable sutures offer the advantage of long half-lives, but they can cause significant local irritation that can persist indefinitely. The nonabsorbable materials also come as either monofilament or braided. Braided suture is associated with an increased risk of wound infection.

Nonabsorbable suture materials are derived

from natural or synthetic materials. The naturally occurring materials, such as cotton and silk, are easy to handle and tie but they also induce an intense inflammatory reaction that can weaken the incision. Steel wire is considered a natural material; it is strong and it will maintain its tensile strength indefinitely. However, wire is very difficult to work with, and its sharp ends can be dangerous, cutting the surgeon or the patient. The nonabsorbable synthetic materials include nylon, Dacron, Tevdek, and Prolene. These materials can be either single stranded or braided. With the exception of Prolene, all of these may induce a marked inflammatory response.

Ultimately the suture chosen is predicated on the preference of the surgeon. Factors that influence the surgeon's selection include familiarity with the material, the surgical objectives at hand, and whether there are extenuating circumstances, such as infection, the need for irradiation or chemotherapy, malnutrition, and obesity.

OBJECTIVES OF WOUND CLOSURE

The objectives at the time of wound closure are to approximate the tissue edges with sufficient tension to keep the edges together yet with adequate laxity to avoid tissue ischemia. Tissue ischemia increases the risk of infection and subsequent wound breakdown.

Approximation of the wound can be done in either a layered fashion or by mass closure. Many standard closure techniques have been described.[12] The method chosen depends on the type of incision, surgeon preference, and factors unique to each patient. Most surgeons will become familiar with and use only a couple of different techniques.

CLOSURE OF A TRANSVERSE INCISION

Transverse incisions are frequently used in gynecology for purposes of exposure and cosmesis. Although some surgeons traditionally reapproximate the peritoneum, the necessity of this step may be questioned. Because reperitonealization is completed within 24 hours, there seems to be little advantage in surgically reapproximating it and there may be a disadvantage in terms of adhesion formation. Recent evidence attributes a higher adhesion rate to those women who have had a peritoneal closure.[13] On the other hand, Tulandi and associates[14] reported on a group of patients who subsequent to their laparotomy underwent a laparoscopic procedure. In this report there was no increase in adhesion formation in patients who had undergone peritoneal closure.

If the rectus muscle has been detached from the pubic bone (Cherney incision), it should be reattached. If the muscle has been cut (Maylard incision), some surgeons advocate that the muscle edges be approximated. Other surgeons suggest this is unnecessary because a strong, fibrous bridge occurs as a consequence of normal healing with no adverse effect on abdominal wall function. Following attention to the rectus muscle, the overlying fascia is then reapproximated with a delayed absorption synthetic material. The fascia should not be approximated under tension because this causes ischemia. The subcutaneous fat is then vigorously irrigated, and the overlying skin is reapproximated.

CLOSURE OF A VERTICAL INCISION

Vertical incisions are frequently used because of their versatility. They afford good exposure to the pelvis and can be easily extended if the surgery requires exposure in the mid and upper abdomen. Vertical incisions may be closed using variations of layered or en bloc closures. A layered closure involves separate approximation of the peritoneum, fascia, subcutaneous tissue, and skin. Although a layered closure is satisfactory for uncomplicated situations, an en bloc closure is generally preferred because it is less likely to result in short-term or long-term complications.

The Smead-Jones internal retention suture is an interrupted, en bloc wound closure that is considered the gold standard to which other closures are compared. It is associated with a very low dehiscence and hernia rate.

The Smead-Jones technique[15] is a far-far near-near stitch that is placed through the fascia, rectus muscle, and peritoneum. If placed properly, it is in essence a vertical mattress or internal retention suture. To place these stitches a large needle is used. Bucknell[1] compared a layered closure versus a Smead-Jones closure and found that the latter was associated with fewer hernias and dehiscences. Banarjee and Chatterjee[16] compared conventional closure versus a single-layer closure and found that the single-layer closure had a significantly lower

incidence of burst abdomens. Cameron and coworkers[17] compared the use of absorbable polydioxanone versus nonabsorbable polypropylene for mass wound closure. They found that wound dehiscence and infection were lower in the polydioxanone group, and at 1 year the rate of incisional hernia was similar between the two groups.

Many surgeons now use a running en bloc closure rather than the Smead-Jones closure for vertical incisions, even in patients at increased risk of wound complications. Sutton and Morgan[18] compared the Smead-Jones closure against a running en bloc closure. A looped suture was started at either end of the incision, and full-thickness bites were placed no greater than 2 cm apart and at least 2 cm lateral to the cut fascial edges. In the midline the suture ends were tied together, so that the knot was inverted under the fascia. In this study, operating time and expense incurred were less in the group in whom closure was done with a running looped suture. The patients whose incisions were closed en bloc had a slightly higher incidence of herniation and dehiscence than the Smead-Jones group, but the difference was not statistically significant. The authors concluded that a running closure was acceptable, less costly, and expeditious.

Wissing and associates[19] compared four techniques of fascial closure in patients with midline incisions. Compared were interrupted closure with polyglactin, continuous polyglactin closure, continuous polydioxanone-S closure, and continuous nylon closure. The frequency of hernias detected at 1 year was similar (10%–20%). However, those patients closed with continuous nylon had much higher rates of pain and suture sinuses. As a rule of thumb nonabsorbable sutures should be avoided when possible because of potential problems with ongoing tissue reaction and the development of draining sinuses. Separate closure of the subcutaneous fat is not necessary.[20]

When there is evidence of a wound infection, it is best not to close the skin at the time of initial surgery because of the risk of a wound infection. Rather, the skin edges and the subcutaneous tissue should be left open. A delayed primary closure can be performed 3 to 5 days later or the incision can be allowed to heal by secondary intention.

The use of incisional drains is controversial. Drainage of the subcutaneous adipose tissue can be done to decrease fluid collections and seromas. If used, these drains are best brought out through a separate cutaneous stab wound.

In the circumstances of excessive contamination, prior dehiscence, or large patient size, the surgeon may elect to place retention sutures. These are mass sutures placed through the entire abdominal wall in addition to the regular fascial sutures. These retention sutures can be closed either at the time of surgery or later if there is no sign of infection.

CONCLUSION

Incisional closure is an art that is frequently overlooked. Careful attention to detail reduces the risk of complication and increases the chances of a successful closure.

REFERENCES

1. Bucknell TE. Wound healing in abdominal operations. Surg Annu 1985;17:1–22.
2. Odland G, Ross R. Human wound repair: I. Epidermal regeneration. J Cell Biol 1968;39:135.
3. Howes EL, Harvey SC, Hewitt WJ. Rate of fibroplasia and initiation in the healing of cutaneous wounds in different species of animals. Arch Surg 1939;38:934.
4. Poole GV. Mechanical factors in abdominal wound closure: The prevention of fascial dehiscence. Surgery 1985;97:631–640.
5. Hugh TB. Abdominal wound dehiscence. Aust NZ J Surg 1990;60:53–55.
6. Bartlett LC. Pressure necrosis is the primary cause of wound dehiscence. Can J Surg 1985;28:27–30.
7. Fraunhofer JAV, Storey RS, Stone IK, Masterson BJ. Tensile strength of suture materials. J Biomed 1985;19:595–600.
8. Fraunhoffer JAV, Storery RJ, Masterson BJ. Tensile properties of suture materials. Biomaterials 1988;9:324–327.
9. Stone IK, Fraunhoffer JAV, Masterson BJ. A comparative study of suture materials: chromic gut and chromic gut treated with glycerin. Am J Obstet Gynecol 1985;151:1087–1093.
10. Katz AR, Mukherjee D, Kaganov AL, Gordon S. New synthetic monofilament absorbable suture made from polytrimethylene carbonate. Surg Gynecol Obstet 1985;161:213–222.
11. Metz SA, Chegini N, Masterson BJ. In vivo and in vitro degradation of monofilament absorbable sutures, PDS, and Maxon. Biomaterials 1990;11:41–45.
12. Ellis H, Bucknell TE, Cox PJ. Abdominal incisions and their closure. Curr Probl Surg 1985;4:1–51.
13. Hugh TB, Nankivell C, Meagher AP, Li B. Is closure of the peritoneal layer necessary in the repair of midline surgical abdominal wounds? World J Surg 1990;14:231–234.
14. Tulandi T, Hum HS, Gelfand IV. Closure of laparotomy incisions with or without peritoneal suturing and second-look laparoscopy. Am J Obstet Gynecol 1988;158:536–537.
15. Jones TE, Newell ET, Brubaker RE. The use of alloy steel wire for the closure of abdominal wounds. Surg Gynecol Obstet 1941;72:1056.
16. Banarjee P, Chatterjee A. Critical evaluation of conventional abdominal closure with single-layer closure in adult and elderly. J Indian Med Assoc 1989;87:277–278.
17. Cameron AEP, Parker CJ, Field ES, et al. A randomized comparison of polydioxanone (PDS) and polypropylene (Prolene) for abdominal wound closure. Ann R Coll Surg Engl 1987;69:113–115.
18. Sutton G, Morgan S. Abdominal wound closure using a running looped monofilament polybutester suture: comparison to Smead-Jones closure in historic controls. Obstet Gynecol 1992;80:650–654.
19. Wissing J, Van Vroonhoven JMV, et al. Fascia closure after midline laparotomy: results of a randomized trial. Br J Surg 1987;74:738–741.
20. Hussain SA. Closure of subcutaneous fat: a prospective randomized trial. Br J Surg 1990;77:107.

12

Vicki V. Baker

Principles of Postoperative Care

The period of postoperative care begins when the patient enters the recovery room and continues until she has recovered from the surgical procedure. Even with the most meticulous perioperative care, complications can and do occur. It has been estimated that approximately 10% of all surgical patients will experience a perioperative complication of varying clinical significance.[1] With respect to gynecologic surgery, complications are reported to occur in 10% to 60% of cases. The incidence varies not only with the age of the patient, the presence of comorbid illnesses, and the type of procedure but also with the definitions used to define complications.

At the outset, it is acknowledged that there are several ways to manage the same clinical situation. However, diligence and attention to detail are universally applicable principles of management that are the cornerstone of good perioperative care regardless of the specific therapy that is implemented. The goal of this chapter is to review the basic principles of postoperative care. Antibiotic therapy, deep venous thrombosis prophylaxis, detection of pulmonary thromboembolism, and administration of blood products are discussed in separate chapters. The reader is also referred to general medical textbooks for detailed information concerning the management of specific medical complications that may occur in the postoperative period.

MEDICAL RECORD DOCUMENTATION

After the surgical procedure is completed, a detailed operative note should be written. Although the format varies from institution to institution, the procedure performed, the specimens removed, the blood loss, and the intraoperative findings should always be noted (Table 12–1). A formal operative note should be dictated within 24 hours of the procedure.

Postoperative orders should be finalized in the recovery room after the patient's status has been carefully assessed. Individualized orders, reflecting the fact that each patient and her operation are unique, are the rule. A systematic, organized approach to postoperative care is encouraged. This minimizes the likelihood of overlooking important details of management and facilitates the organized communication of information to the nursing staff. The major issues that should be addressed in the postoperative orders are listed in Table 12–2. Orders should be frequently reviewed

TABLE 12–1
Components of the Operative Note

Date of surgery
Preoperative diagnosis
Postoperative diagnosis
Procedure(s) performed
Attending surgeon
Assistants
Anesthesia
Estimated blood loss
Fluids administered
Specimens submitted for pathologic analysis
Cultures
Drains
Complications
Intraoperative findings

and rewritten as the patient's condition changes.

Postoperative patients should be seen daily and a progress note written. Patients with complications or serious comorbid illnesses should be seen more often, as necessitated by their conditions, and notes written more frequently. The progress note should accurately reflect the patient's condition. Any abnormal test results should be specifically addressed and a plan of management outlined in the medical record. Any procedures performed on the patient, such as insertion or removal of a central venous line, removal of a pack or drain, or blood transfusion, should be clearly documented in the medical record.

TABLE 12–2
Postoperative Orders

Diagnosis
Procedure performed
Condition
Known medical illnesses
Frequency and type of monitoring
   Vital signs, urine output, body weight, pulse oximetry, telemetry, fingerstick glucose
Diet
Intravenous fluids
Medications
   Pain, antibiotics, preoperative medications
Activity
Deep venous thrombosis prophylaxis (if applicable)
Respiratory care
Instructions regarding management of dressings, lines, packs
Laboratory tests
   Blood work, chest radiograph, electrocardiogram
Physician notification parameters
   Temperature, respiratory rate, urine output, blood pressure, acute bleeding, change in mental status, inadequate pain relief

FLUID AND ELECTROLYTE THERAPY

Postoperative fluid administration is based on estimated blood loss, the patient's urine output, and her vital signs. Individualized decisions regarding intravenous fluid therapy should be formulated in the context of the patient's general condition and the risks and benefits assessed. A standard "cookbook" approach for every patient should be avoided.

Twenty-four-hour maintenance fluid requirements include 1 L of 0.25% normal saline or lactated Ringer's solution to provide for renal solute excretion in addition to 600 to 900 mL of dextrose 5% in water to replace insensible losses. Increased fluid requirements occur with long cases, extensive gastrointestinal losses, and third space losses. Specific body fluid losses should be replaced with an intravenous fluid that approximates the composition of the losses (Table 12–3).

Daily measurements of body weight and careful monitoring of input and output point to fluid imbalances. Although patients are in a catabolic state postoperatively, it is not unusual for the patient to gain weight during the first 24 to 48 hours after surgery followed by a return to baseline. These fluctuations in weight are associated with a phase of water and sodium retention followed by a brisk diuresis that reflects the endocrinologic responses to the stress of surgery.[2] The administration of intravenous fluids should be carefully monitored to avoid progressive postoperative weight gain and peripheral edema. The adverse effects of systemic fluid overload include decreased chest wall compliance, decreased tissue oxygenation, impaired wound healing, and ileus.[3–5]

Oliguria

In general, urine output greater than 1 mL/kg/h is considered adequate in the postoperative patient. Oliguria is defined as urine output

TABLE 12–3
Replacement Fluids for Body Fluids

Gastric drainage	0.5% normal saline
Proximal small bowel	Lactated Ringers'
Distal small bowel	Lactated Ringers'
Isotonic urine	Lactated Ringers' or normal saline
Diarrhea	0.5% normal saline

TABLE 12–4
Causes of Postoperative Oliguria

Prerenal Oliguria

Intravascular volume depletion
Hypoperfusion (secondary to congestive heart failure)
Increased reabsorption of sodium and water secondary to increased aldosterone and vasopressin

Renal Oliguria

Acute tubular necrosis
Renal artery thrombosis
Hypoperfusion
Nephrotoxicity

Postrenal Oliguria

Foley catheter occlusion
Bilateral ureteral obstruction
Urinary retention

less than 0.5 mL/kg/h rather than the more commonly used definition of urine output less than 30 mL/h. Whenever oliguria occurs, the patient should be promptly evaluated. Oliguria may be divided into prerenal, renal, and postrenal etiologies (Table 12–4). After the patient has been examined, a number of tests may be obtained to aid in the determination of the cause of decreased urine output (Table 12–5). The value of these tests is limited in the patient who has received diuretics, is malnourished, has chronic renal disease, or has suffered gastrointestinal bleeding.

In the postoperative gynecology patient with normal renal function, oliguria most commonly reflects intravascular volume depletion. The rapid infusion of 250 mL of normal saline or lactated Ringer's solution generally results in a prompt increase in urine production and concomitantly establishes the diagnosis of volume depletion. Empiric diuretic therapy in the postoperative oliguric patient is not appropriate. However, diuretic therapy is appropriate in the patient who has normal intravas-

TABLE 12–5
Evaluation of Postoperative Oliguria After the Exclusion of Postrenal Causes

Test	Normal	Prerenal	Renal
Urine specific gravity	Variable	>1.020	1.010
Osmolality (urine)	Variable	>500	<350
BUN/creatinine	Variable	20:1	10:1
Fractional excretion of sodium		<1	>3
Urine sodium	Variable	<20	>30
Urine BUN/blood BUN		>8	<3

BUN, blood urea nitrogen.

cular volume and decreased output secondary to increased antidiuretic hormone levels or in a hypertensive patient who is "diuretic dependent."

An oliguric patient who has limited cardiopulmonary reserve may not tolerate a fluid bolus. In addition, this patient often has other pathophysiologic derangements in addition to volume depletion. In this situation, central hemodynamic monitoring may be helpful. One must keep in mind that although central venous pressure measurements reflect intravascular volume status in a healthy patient, these measurements are of limited value in the patient with heart or lung disease. In addition, central venous pressure measurements are only as good as the personnel observing them. Invasive hemodynamic monitoring using a Swan-Ganz catheter permits the acquisition of data that cannot be obtained by other means.[5] However, use of the Swan-Ganz catheter is associated with a number of serious complications, including catheter breakage with right-sided heart embolization, infection, arrhythmia, and rupture of the pulmonary artery. Because of these potentially life-threatening complications, careful consideration should be given to the use of this monitoring tool.

Patients with gastrointestinal obstruction and women who have undergone cytoreductive surgery for ovarian cancer often exhibit oliguria secondary to third space fluid shifts that cause intravascular volume depletion. Normal saline is the fluid of choice for initial volume resuscitation in these patients. It is also appropriate to use this fluid in the patient with moderate hyponatremia (sodium level of 118 to 132 mEq/L), and when blood must be given through the same line. However, the prolonged administration of normal saline in large volumes and its use in the patient sensitive to sodium loads (e.g., congestive heart failure, significant hypertension) should be avoided because of the fluid and electrolyte abnormalities that may occur. Lactated Ringer's solution results in fluid and electrolyte abnormalities less commonly, but it is not an appropriate fluid when glucose is needed, when more free water and less sodium is required, or when blood must be transfused through the same line. Other intravenous fluids provide larger amounts of free water than normal saline or lactated Ringer's and may exacerbate peripheral edema (Table 12–6).

Because of the potential problems associated with all crystalloid solutions when administered in large volumes, some clinicians advocate the use of colloids in patients with intra-

TABLE 12–6
Expansion of the Three Compartments That Can be Achieved with Different Intravenous Fluids

Fluid	Intravascular Volume (mL)	Interstitial Volume (mL)	Intracellular Volume (mL)
Lactated Ringers'	175	825	0
Normal saline	250	750	0
0.5% normal saline	165	500	333
5% saline	987	2962	−2950
5% albumin	1000	0	0
Dextran	790	210	0
Hetastarch	710	290	0

vascular volume depletion secondary to third space fluid losses. The appropriateness of colloids versus crystalloids as a means to expand the intravascular volume is an ongoing debate that has spanned the past 15 years. Colloids are more efficient volume expanders than crystalloids because they remain in the intracellular space for longer periods of time. In general, two to four times the volume of crystalloid as 5% albumin or 6% Hetastarch is required to achieve the same physiologic endpoints.[6]

Commonly used colloids include Hetastarch and Dextran. Hetastarch consists of modified amylopectin, which is a branched glucose polymer that is cleared by the kidneys and reticuloendothelial system. Dextrans are colloid suspensions of glucose polymers of various sizes. In terms of volume expansion, 6% Dextran 70 is equivalent to 6% Hetastarch. Although colloids rapidly restore the intravascular volume, side effects include hypersensitivity reactions and possible platelet aggregation dysfunction.

One of the complications of intravascular volume depletion is acute tubular necrosis (ATN). Other predisposing factors to the development of ATN include renal ischemia, exposure to nephrotoxins including aminoglycosides and intravenous contrast media, advanced age, chronic renal failure, congestive heart failure, diabetes, and prolonged intraoperative hypotension. ATN is a serious condition. Typically, the 40% to 90% mortality associated with this condition occurs in the surgical setting.[7, 8] The mortality is influenced by the number of other failed organ systems, ranging from 10% in cases of isolated renal failure to 60% when a second system fails to 90% when three systems fail.[9, 10]

Dopamine is occasionally administered at a

starting dose of 3 µg/kg/min in an effort to maintain renal perfusion and decrease the incidence of ATN in patients who are thought to be at increased risk. Investigations of the efficacy of prophylactic dopamine in general surgical patients have yielded conflicting results. The role of prophylactic dopamine in gynecology patients, particularly those who undergo extended surgical procedures for cancer, has not been critically evaluated.

The diagnosis of ATN is based on increasing serum creatinine values. The quantity of urine output separates ATN into two categories: non-oliguric (>400 mL/d) versus oliguric (<400 mL/d). After the diagnosis of ATN, management strategies include volume expansion, support of blood pressure, and avoidance of electrolyte abnormalities. After establishing a normal intravascular volume, furosemide may be administered in an effort in increase urine output. Oliguric ATN is typically associated with a prolonged course that may be complicated by metabolic acidosis, hyperkalemia, hyponatremia, and hypocalcemia. Diuretic therapy may convert oliguric ATN into nonoliguric ATN, which simplifies fluid and electrolyte management and may improve long-term prognosis. Indications for dialysis include hyperkalemia, acidosis, or volume overload that cannot be controlled medically.

Electrolytes

Serum electrolytes do not need to be routinely monitored in the postoperative patient. Patients with normal renal function preoperatively rarely exhibit clinically significant electrolyte alterations postoperatively. Exceptions are made for certain patients with medical conditions such as cardiac disease in whom electrolyte fluctuations may potentiate adverse drug reactions. As an example, patients requiring digitalis are at increased risk of toxicity in the presence of hypokalemia.

Hyponatremia

Mild hyponatremia is a common observation in the postoperative patient. The stress-induced release of antidiuretic hormone and aldosterone results in decreased free water clearance with retention of water relative to sodium. Other causes of postoperative hyponatremia include inappropriate intravenous fluid administration, gastrointestinal losses, third space fluid losses, congestive heart failure, potassium

depletion, and diuretic therapy. The serum sodium value does not reflect the patient's intravascular volume status. The hyponatremic patient may be hypovolemic, isovolemic, or hypervolemic.

In general, mild hyponatremia is a self-limited condition and will correct spontaneously as the stress-induced endocrinologic alterations secondary to surgery resolve. Serum sodium values less than 130 mEq/L are treated by restricting free water. The administration of hypertonic saline solutions is potentially hazardous and is rarely necessary in the postoperative gynecology patient.

Hypokalemia

Hypokalemia commonly occurs in the postoperative patient. Causes include beta-agonist therapy, alkalemia, acute glucose loads, anabolic conditions, diarrhea, aminoglycoside therapy, prolonged therapy with certain penicillins, reduced potassium intake, magnesium deficiency, and renal losses.

Symptomatic hypokalemia generally occurs at serum levels less than 2.5 mEq/L. The consequences of hypokalemia may include weakness, ileus, orthostatic hypotension, worsening of hypertension, and arrhythmias.

As a general guideline, each 0.75-mEq/L decrease in serum potassium reflects a total body deficit of 100 mEq. When potassium supplementation is indicated, 10 to 20 mEq of potassium chloride can be placed in 50 to 100 mL of normal saline and infused over a minimum of 1 hour. To minimize the pain caused by the peripheral intravenous administration of potassium chloride, the addition of 0.5 mL of 1% lidocaine is helpful. This will decrease the pain of the potassium chloride infusion but will not prevent venous sclerosis.

CARDIOVASCULAR MANAGEMENT

During and immediately after surgery, the cardiovascular system is significantly stressed as a consequence of the surgical procedure as well as by hypothermia, pain, and intravascular volume fluxes. Age-related changes in ejection fraction, myocardial compliance, and inotropic responsiveness to catecholamines may limit the patient's ability to respond to these stresses.

Hypothermia after surgery is a fairly common occurrence, particularly in elderly patients.[11] Hypothermia is defined as a core temperature less than 35°C. Most patients become somewhat hypothermic during surgery. Contributing factors include removal of clothing, cool ambient room temperature, and loss of body heat from the incision. The most important cause is inhibition of central thermoregulatory vasoconstriction by the anesthetic.

The physiologic consequences of hypothermia correlate with the core body temperature. Core body temperatures less than 33°C are associated with vasoconstriction, a decrease in intravascular volume, arrhythmias, decreased oxygen availability at the tissue level, bronchospasm, hyperglycemia, and impaired renal function. Recovery from hypothermia results in shivering, which may increase oxygen consumption beyond that of thyroid storm or febrile episodes. Elderly patients may have inadequate cardiovascular reserves to meet these physiologic demands. Suggested measures to minimize intraoperative hypothermia include extensive draping of the patient, the use of warmed anesthetic gases, the administration of prewarmed fluids, and peritoneal irrigation with warm fluids. In addition to the use of radiant lamps, supplemental oxygen and warmed intravenous fluids should be given to the hypothermic patient while in the recovery room. The hypothalamic shivering response can be blocked pharmacologically using meperidine, chlorpromazine, or morphine.

Hypothermia can cause hypertension during the immediate postoperative period, but a number of other causes should be considered (Table 12–7). Systolic pressures greater than 180 mm Hg, diastolic pressures greater than 120 mm Hg, or an increase in either parameter greater than 20 mm Hg as compared with the preoperative values requires treatment. Several pharmacologic agents can be used to control hypertension in the postoperative patient (Table 12–8). Excessive reductions in blood pressure should be avoided, particularly in elderly patients and hypertensive patients because of the risk of myocardial ischemia, infarction, and stroke. The goal of therapy is to reduce the elevated blood pressure to the patient's baseline rather than to achieve a normotensive value.

TABLE 12–7
Causes of Postoperative Hypertension

Pain	Hypoxemia
Anxiety	Hypercarbia
Fluid overload	Hypothermia
Bladder distention	

TABLE 12–8
Management of Postoperative Hypertension

Drug	Dosage
Nitroprusside	0.5–1.0 µg/kg/min to a maximum dose of 15 µg/min. Cyanide toxicity is a potential problem with long-term use.
Nitroglycerin	10–20 µg/min initially. Increase by 5–10 µg/min every 5 minutes until the desired pressure is achieved.
Hydralazine	5 mg IV q 20 minutes
Propranolol	1 mg IV q 5 minutes to a maximum dose of 7 mg every 4 hours. Avoid using in patients with depressed cardiovascular function.
Labetalol	20 mg IV
Nifedipine	10 mg sublingually

Hypotension may result from narcotics and other medications, but intravascular volume depletion must always be considered in the differential diagnosis. The surgeon must exclude inadequately replaced intraoperative blood loss, continued bleeding postoperatively, third space losses, cardiogenic shock, and sepsis. Transfusion remains the most effective way to treat hypotension secondary to acute anemia.

Tachycardia is common in the postoperative patient, particularly in the first 12 to 24 hours. Tachycardia in the postoperative patient may be the result of congestive heart failure, infection, infarction, hypoxemia, pain acidosis, hypokalemia, or anemia. It is important to establish the specific cause because this directs the selection of therapy. Generally, supraventricular tachycardia spontaneously resolves and does not require treatment in the absence of decreased cardiac output or evidence of myocardial ischemia.

The risk of myocardial infarction is increased in the postoperative patient, particularly in the elderly and in those with pre-existing cardiac disease. The first 3 days after surgery are the greatest period of risk for myocardial infarction.[12] Continuous electrocardiogram monitoring and serial cardiac enzymes should be obtained in patients with coronary artery disease who exhibit any alteration in cardiac function or who complain of symptoms suggestive of myocardial ischemia. Because patients with coronary artery disease are more susceptible to myocardial ischemia, factors that may compromise oxygen delivery, such as anemia, hypotension, tachycardia, hypoxia, fluid overload, and inadequately controlled pain, should be avoided. Daily electrocardiograms are recommended for diabetic patients because they are at increased risk of silent infarction.

Congestive Heart Failure

The hypertensive patient with concentric left ventricular hypertrophy is sensitive to fluid boluses and may develop congestive heart failure with limited fluid infusions. In the elderly patient, congestive heart failure secondary to volume overload may appear on postoperative day 2 or 3 as extracellular fluids are mobilized and returned to the intravascular space.

PULMONARY CARE

Pulmonary function is adversely affected by inhalational anesthetics, and postoperative hypoxemia is the rule rather than the exception. Generally, the decrease in PaO_2 postoperatively is well tolerated unless the patient's preoperative PaO_2 was marginal. Supplemental oxygen should be given as necessary to maintain a PaO_2 of 60 to 70 mm Hg. Arterial oxygen pressures greater than 60 to 70 mm Hg are of little physiologic benefit by virtue of the shape of the oxyhemoglobin dissociation curve. In addition, the prolonged administration of inspired oxygen concentrations greater than 50% is potentially harmful because it may cause absorption atelectasis.

Basilar atelectasis is the most common pulmonary complication that occurs in the postoperative patient. It results from the gradual and progressive collapse of alveoli secondary to altered patterns of ventilation. Clinically, atelectasis is associated with a decrease in total lung capacity, functional residual capacity, residual volume, and lung compliance. These postoperative changes are most apparent on the second or third day after surgery. Atelectasis generally resolves by the fifth to the seventh day after surgery.

A key goal for postoperative pulmonary management is to minimize atelectasis by restoring functional residual lung capacity to the preoperative level as quickly as possible. Incentive spirometry has been demonstrated superior to intermittent positive-pressure breathing or vigorous exhalational therapy in the prevention of atelectasis.[13, 14] When indicated, bronchodilators such as inhaled beta-adrenergic agonists should also be used. Aminophylline has a very limited role in the management of postoperative pulmonary problems. Aminophylline infusions are not as efficacious as beta-

adrenergic agonists in the treatment of acute exacerbations of chronic obstructive pulmonary disease or asthma.[15, 16] In addition, the therapeutic index for aminophylline is narrow.

Other measures that may decrease the incidence of postoperative pulmonary complications include early ambulation and positioning of the patient in the modified semi-Fowler position. Adequate pain control is also important in that it permits the patient to make deep inspiratory efforts. Epidural analgesia is superior to narcotic analgesics as a means of providing adequate pain control after pelvic and abdominal surgery without suppressing respiratory rate.[17–19]

POSTOPERATIVE NUTRITION

The caloric requirements of the postoperative patient are influenced by the extent of the surgical procedure, the patient's preoperative nutritional condition, and the postoperative course. Nutritional requirements, reflecting metabolic demands, usually peak 5 to 10 days after surgery and then return to normal in the absence of complications such as fever and infection.

In general, the small bowel exhibits return of normal peristaltic activity within hours of lower abdominal surgery. The stomach does not resume its normal activity for approximately 24 hours, and many patients will not tolerate enteral feeding until the first postoperative day. The colon does not regain its normal function for approximately 72 hours after surgery. Patients with a history of constipation or laxative abuse typically require longer periods of time to regain baseline bowel function. In addition to interindividual variation, resumption of preoperative bowel function is also influenced by the extent of surgery and the occurrence of postoperative complications. The administration of medications such as metoclopropamide does not facilitate gastric emptying in the immediate postoperative period. Similarly, stimulants of colonic function are rarely helpful before the third postoperative day.

To maintain nitrogen balance and meet the increased metabolic demands of a surgical procedure, supplemental nutrition may be required if the patient is unable to consume adequate calories for a prolonged period of time. As a general rule, the gastrointestinal tract should be used whenever possible rather than resorting to parenteral alimentation. Failure to use the gastrointestinal tract results in villous atrophy, diminished gastrointestinal enzyme

TABLE 12–9
Indications for Enteral and Parenteral Nutrition Relevant to Gynecologic Surgery

	Enteral Nutrition	Parenteral Nutrition
Routine	Inadequate oral intake for >5 days	Patients who have lost >10% of usual body weight; catabolic patient in whom gastrointestinal tract cannot be used for 5–7 days
Usually Helpful		After major surgery if patient cannot eat for 5–7 days; enterocutaneous fistula
Limited Value	Immediate postoperative period, acute enteritis	Immediate postoperative period
Contraindicated	Obstruction, ileus, severe diarrhea	Patient who can tolerate enteral feeding; period of anticipated nutritional support <5 days

Data from American Society for Parenteral and Enteral Nutrition Board of Directors. Guidelines for the use of total parenteral nutrition in the hospitalized adult patient. JPEN 1986;10:441; and guidelines for the use of enteral nutrition in the adult patient. JPEN 1987;11:435.

activity, and decreased hepatobiliary and pancreatic secretions. Indications for enteral and parenteral nutrition have been proposed by the American Society for Parenteral and Enteral Nutrition (Table 12–9).

PAIN RELIEF

Adequate pain relief is an important component of postoperative care. Postoperative pain that is inadequately controlled may result in hypertension, tachycardia, postoperative ileus, impaired respiratory effort, and delayed ambulation.[20, 21]

The two primary modalities for pain control after major gynecologic surgery are epidural analgesia and patient-controlled analgesia. Each modality is associated with potential advantages and disadvantages (Table 12–10). Both modalities provide good pain relief after

surgery, and the superiority of one over the other has not been established.

Factors that influence the selection of epidural versus patient-controlled analgesia include patient preference, body habitus, pulmonary status, nursing support, availability of infusion pumps, and cost considerations.

FEBRILE MORBIDITY

Febrile morbidity is very common after gynecologic surgery, occurring in approximately 31% of abdominal hysterectomies and 38% of vaginal hysterectomies.[22] Febrile morbidity is defined as a temperature greater than 38°C on two separate occasions after the first 24 hours after surgery. Fever after surgery is a common occurrence and does not invariably reflect infection and the need for antibiotic therapy.[23, 24] There is an unfortunate tendency to order a

TABLE 12–10
Advantages and Disadvantages of Epidural Analgesia and Patient-Controlled Analgesia

	Epidural	Patient-Controlled
Advantages	Immediate pain relief	Requires no special nursing or anesthesia support postoperatively
	May improve colon motility	Gives the patient "personal control" over administration of pain medication
	May improve postoperative pulmonary function after lower abdominal and pelvic surgery	
	Less sedating than patient-controlled analgesia	
Disadvantages	Requires a skilled anesthesiologist for correct placement	Patient may experience pain in the recovery room until an adequate serum level of medication is achieved
	May interfere with ambulation	
	May delay removal of Foley catheter	

battery of tests in the febrile postoperative patient. These tests are often unnecessary, unduly expensive, and infrequently diagnostic. A specific cause is identified in less than 20% of patients who have fever during the first 24 hours after surgery.

The first step in the management of the febrile postoperative patient is examination of the patient. Subsequent laboratory tests should be selected prudently, recognizing their potential limitations. As an example, a complete blood cell count during the first 24 to 48 hours after surgery invariably reveals an elevated white blood cell count. A radiograph of the chest is unlikely to show anything in the absence of findings on physical examination, although a notable exception may be the febrile, neutropenic patient. Although antibiotics are not invariably required when the postoperative patient exhibits an elevated temperature, interventions to decrease the fever should be implemented. A febrile response causes increased metabolic demands, increased cardiac output, and patient discomfort.

The more common causes of postoperative fever are relatively limited and may be considered in two broad categories: infectious and noninfectious (Table 12–11). The most common infectious cause of postoperative fever is a urinary tract infection. The distal urethra is typically colonized, and catheterization significantly increases the risk of a clinically significant urinary tract infection. The most common causes of noninfectious postoperative fever are atelectasis and tissue trauma.[25]

CRITERIA FOR DISCHARGE FROM THE HOSPITAL

Discharge criteria after surgical procedures are changing, primarily motivated by the need to reduce health care costs. Many of the services previously provided by the hospital are now

TABLE 12–11
Causes of Postoperative Fever

Noninfectious	Infectious
Tissue trauma	Pelvic cellulitis
Atelectasis	Abscess at operative site
Drug reaction	Pneumonia
Phlebitis (nonseptic)	Wound infection
Halothane hepatitis (rare)	Urinary tract infection
Dehydration	Septic phlebitis
Blood transfusion	

TABLE 12–12
Components of the Discharge Summary

Patient name
Admission date
Discharge date
Diagnosis
Procedures / operations
Discharge medications
Allergies

Condition of patient at time of discharge (as compared with condition on admission)

Reason for admission

Brief history and physical examination (address all significant and abnormal findings and pertinent negative findings)

Hospital course
  Diagnosis
  Procedures / operations
  Significant events
  Pertinent clinical findings and laboratory results
  Response to treatments
  Any complications
Discharge instructions
  Medications
  Diet
  Physical activity
  Follow-up care

available on an outpatient basis. In general, the patient should be afebrile and tolerating oral feedings prior to discharge.

At the time of discharge, the patient should be given a prescription for pain medication. Postoperative instructions should be reviewed with the patient, and this should be documented in the medical record. Arrangements for follow-up should be made, and the patient should be given instructions concerning whom to call in the event of problems or questions after discharge from the hospital. Any test results that are not available should be noted in the discharge note with a comment concerning how these test results will be followed up and acted upon.

A discharge summary, following a standard format (Table 12–12), which notes the key events that transpired during the hospitalization, should be dictated in a timely fashion.

REFERENCES

1. Cohen MM, Duncan PG, Pope WDB, Wolkerstein C. A survey of 112,000 anesthetics at one teaching hospital (1975–1983). Can Anesth Soc J 1986;33:22.
2. Thoren L. Metabolic response to surgery. In: Lloyd M, Hughes TA, eds. Surgery Annals. New York, Appleton-Century-Crofts, 1975, p 53.
3. Heughan C, Niinikoski J, Hunt TK. Effect of excessive

infusion of saline on tissue oxygen transport. Surg Gynecol Obstet 1972;135:257.

4. Falk JL. Fluid administration and colloid-crystalloid controversy: new thoughts on an old debate. Crit Care Med 1991;19:451.

5. Stole JE, Bender JS. Use of the pulmonary artery catheter to reduce operative complications. Surg Clin North Am 1993;73:253–264.

6. Rackow EC, Falk JL, Fein IA, et al. Fluid resuscitation in circulatory shock: a comparison of the cardiorespiratory effects of albumin, hetastarch, and saline solutions in patients with hypovolemic and septic shock. Crit Care Med 1983;11:839.

7. Turney JH, Marshall DH, Brownjohn AM, et al. The evolution of acute renal failure, 1956–1988. Q J Med 1990;74:83–104.

8. Cameron JS. Acute renal failure in the intensive care unit today. Intensive Care Med 1986;12:64–70.

9. Cioffi WG, Ashikaga T, Gamelli RL. Probability of surviving postoperative acute renal failure. Ann Surg 1984;200:205–211.

10. Smithies MN, Cameron JS. Can we predict outcome in acute renal failure? Nephron 1989;51:297–300.

11. Collins K, Dore C, Exton-Smith AN, et al. Accidental hypothermia and impaired temperature regulation homeostasis in the elderly. BMJ 1977;1:353.

12. Stern P, Tinker JH, Tarban S. Myocardial reinfarction after anesthesia and surgery. JAMA 1978;239:2566.

13. Bartlett RH, Bazzaniga AB, Geraghty TR. Respiratory maneuvers to prevent postoperative pulmonary complications. JAMA 1973;224:1017.

14. Dohi S, Gold MI. Comparison of two methods of postoperative respiratory care. Chest 1978;73:592.

15. Fanta CH, Rossing TH, McFadden ER. Emergency room treatment of asthma. Am J Med 1982;72:416.

16. Siegel D, Sheppard D, Gelf A, et al. Aminophylline increases the toxicity but not the efficacy of an inhaled beta-adrenergic agonist in the treatment of acute exacerbations of asthma. Am Rev Respir Dis 1985;132:282.

17. Spence AA, Smith G. Postoperative analgesia and lung function: a comparison of morphine with extradural block. Br J Anaesth 1971;43:144.

18. Modig J. Lumbar epidural nerve blockade versus parenteral analgesics. Acta Anaesthesiol Scand (Suppl) 1978;70:30.

19. Cushieri RJ, Moran CG, Howie JC, et al. Postoperative pain and pulmonary complications: a comparison of three analgesic regimens. Br J Surg 1985;72:495.

20. Benedetti C, Bonica JJ, Bellucci G. Pathophysiology and therapy of postoperative pain: a review. Adv Pain Res Ther 1984;7:373–407.

21. Bonica JJ. Pathophysiology of pain. Hosp Pract 1978;13:4–14.

22. Ledger WJ, Child MA. The hospital care of patients undergoing hysterectomy: an analysis of 12,026 patients from the Professional Activity Study. Am J Obstet Gynecol 1973;117:423.

23. Galicier C, Richet H. A prospective study of postoperative fever in a general surgery department. Infect Control 1985;6:487.

24. Drago JJ, Jacobs AM, Oloff LM. Elevated temperature in the postoperative patient. J Foot Surg 1982;21:269.

25. Watters JM, Redmond ML, Desai D, March RJ. Effects of age and body composition on the metabolic responses to elective colon resection. Ann Surg 1990;212:89–96.

26. American Society for Parenteral and Enteral Nutrition Board of Directors. Guidelines for the use of total parenteral nutrition in the hospitalized adult patient. JPEN 1986;10:441.

27. American Society for Parenteral and Enteral Nutrition Board of Directors. Guidelines for the use of enteral nutrition in the adult patient. JPEN 1987;11:435.

13

Manuel Penalver
Heather Lafferty

CHAPTER

Postoperative Genitourinary Tract Complications

GENITOURINARY INJURY

The anatomic proximity of the genital and urinary systems requires that the gynecologic surgeon have a thorough understanding of the anatomic relationship between these systems. The best measure against prevention of iatrogenic injury to the urinary system is a thorough understanding of the surgical planes that exist between these closely positioned organs. Familiarity with the normal anatomy as well as the occasionally encountered anomalies will help prevent iatrogenic injury to the ureter and bladder during gynecologic surgery.

Wheelock and colleagues reported bladder injuries in 1.8% of abdominal hysterectomies and 0.4% of vaginal hysterectomies.[1] Predisposing factors to bladder injury include pelvic inflammatory disease, endometriosis, cesarean section, and anatomic distortion by tumors (e.g., fibroids, adnexal masses). Bladder injuries may occur during opening of the peritoneal cavity, while dissecting the vesicovaginal space during hysterectomy, and at the time of closure of the vaginal cuff. While opening the peritoneum, attention must be given to the bladder, especially in cases of previous abdominal surgery, because the bladder may be adherent to the anterior abdominal wall. To avoid bladder injury, while dissecting the bladder from the anterior surface of the uterus, sharp dissection with scissors should be used and the surgical plane of the vesicovaginal space entered. Bleeding while dissecting in this plane indicates a warning of close proximity to the bladder or to the uterus. To avoid bladder injury at the time of vaginal cuff closure the bladder should be dissected free for a distance of at least 0.5 cm from the area where the vaginal closure will be performed. This careful dissection of the bladder from the cervix and vagina should be done whether a suture or a staple closure of the vagina will be performed.

If bladder injury is not obvious during surgery but is suspected, the bladder can be filled with methylene blue or sterile milk through the Foley catheter. Sterile milk is preferable because it does not stain the tissues. As an alternative, indigo carmine can be injected intravenously. Once the injured bladder has been noted, its relationship to the ureteral orifices must be determined. If the bladder injury is in close proximity or includes the ureteral orifices, a ureteral reimplantation should be done to avoid ureteral stricture. The use of ureteral catheters may obviate the need for a reimplantation of the ureter. Bladder injuries should be repaired in two layers with running absorbable

sutures. The first layer should incorporate the entire thickness of the bladder wall, and the second layer should include the seromuscular layer to invert the first layer. A suprapubic or urethral bladder catheter should be used to drain the bladder for 7 to 10 days after the repair. Radiographic tests to illustrate healing of the bladder after repair are not necessary after a simple two-layer repair of a fundal injury; however, this should be done in all injuries that are in close proximity to the ureteral orifices in the posterior bladder wall. A drain should be left in the space of Retzius for retroperitoneal bladder injuries in case of extravasation of urine.

Ureteral injury has been reported to occur in 0.5% to 2.5% of gynecologic malignancies.[2] In a major teaching hospital, Mann and colleagues documented ureteral injury in 0.5% of major gynecologic cases.[3] Before the management of ureteral injury is discussed, the anatomy, embryology, nerve supply, and preoperative evaluation are reviewed.

Anatomy

The ureters are bilateral, tubular urinary conduits (25 to 30 cm in length) that connect the kidneys to the urinary bladder. The ureters have an abdominal and a pelvic course, and throughout the abdominal course they travel anterior to the psoas muscle. At the level of the bifurcation of the common iliac artery the ureters enter the pelvis and have a pelvic course from the pelvic brim to the ureteral orifices in the bladder. Throughout the course of the ureters, they obtain blood supply from the renal arteries, abdominal aorta, and ovarian, uterine, internal iliac, and the vesical arteries. Microscopically, three layers of the ureters have been identified (the inner layer, which is transitional epithelium; the middle layer, which is circular and longitudinal smooth muscles, and the outer-layer adventitial sheath). In cases in which the ureter has to be dissected, it is important to maintain the integrity of the adventitial layer because it is in this layer that the blood supply of the ureter travels. When a periaortic lymphadenectomy is done, the location of the ureters and of their lower abdominal course is identified and throughout their pelvic course the gynecologist should be aware of the proximity of the ureters to the level of the dissection. The ureters course posterior to the uterine artery at the level of the parametrium and then continue their course into the bladder. Within the parametrium the ureters are approximately 1.5 cm lateral to the cervix and in close proximity to the lateral vaginal fornices. When the ureters enter the bladder, their lumina expand as their muscle fibers mingle with those of the bladder. The two ureteral orifices and the internal urethral meatus form the trigone of the bladder.

Embryology

The ureters are outgrowths of the mesonephric ducts. The ureteric buds give rise to the ureters, the renal pelvis, and the kidney's collecting tubules. As the ureters elongate, the kidneys migrate in a cephalad direction to end up in the abdominal retroperitoneal location. As the kidney migrates cephalad, this movement can be obstructed by the bifurcation of the common iliac artery, resulting in a pelvic kidney, or it can be arrested by the inferior mesenteric artery, resulting in a horseshoe kidney. The most common congenital anomaly of the ureter is the double ureter, occurring in 0.5% of the population and is the result of the splitting of the ureteric bud. The splitting can be complete or incomplete, with the incomplete form being the most common. The incomplete splitting of the ureteric bud gives rise to a partially duplicated (i.e., double) ureter.

Nerve Supply

The ureters, like the bladder, are profusely innervated with nerve fibers of the autonomic nervous system. Their nerve supply originates from both abdominal and pelvic sources (mesenteric and pelvic plexus). The efferent and afferent nerve supply to the bladder and ureters travels in the connective tissue ligaments of the pelvis (cardinal and uterosacral). In performing radical pelvic surgery a more extensive dissection to the nerve supply to the bladder occurs. Bladder and ureteral stasis are more common in radical than in simple abdominal hysterectomy. Also, the bladder should be kept catheterized for a longer time in radical pelvic surgery because of the more extensive denervation of the structures. The nerve supply to the ureter travels in the outer adventitial sheet. This outer layer also contains the blood supply, and careful dissection of the ureter must maintain the integrity of this layer.

Preoperative Evaluation

Methods of preoperative evaluation that have been documented include intravenous urogra-

phy and preoperative stenting of the ureters. Although both of these methods have been used widely in gynecologic surgery, the most important step in trying to avoid ureteral injury is intraoperative identification of the ureters by retroperitoneal dissection. The retroperitoneal space is opened by incising the broad ligament, and on the medial leaf of the broad ligament the ureters are identified. This should be done at the start of the pelvic dissection when the operative field is hemostatic because most studies have documented that the most common cause of ureteral injury is that, in an attempt to provide hemostasis, a suture ligature or a transection of the ureter occurs. Early localization of the ureter intraoperatively can help avoid this complication during the operation when trying to achieve hemostasis.

Symmonds has stated that the most important means of preventing ureter injury is to identify the ureters at the time of surgery and to demonstrate their pelvic course and to keep them out of harm's way.[4] Preoperative intravenous urography should be done in adnexal masses, endometriosis, and tubo-ovarian abscess disease and as part of staging of gynecologic cancers. Preoperative routine intravenous urography in all pelvic surgery should not be advocated because this is not cost effective. Piscatelli and coworkers performed intravenous urography routinely on patients to undergo gynecologic surgery.[5] They found that the only significant factors associated with abnormal findings on intravenous urography were a uterine size greater than 12 cm or an adnexal cyst greater than 4 cm.

Management of Injury

Optimally, genitourinary injuries are recognized intraoperatively because the management is easier if appropriately done at the time of surgery. Intraoperatively, leakage of urine as well as obvious recognition of ureteral or bladder injury can occur. The three most common locations of ureteral injury are at the pelvic brim, close to the infundibulopelvic ligament, in the cardinal ligament where the uterine artery crosses the ureter, and at the cervicovaginal junction. Intraoperatively, minor injuries such as superficial ureteral trauma or a superficial crush injury of the ureter can be treated by simply removing the clamp and placing ureteral stents. The stents should be left in place for approximately 10 days to minimize the likelihood of stricture formation.

When a significant injury to the ureter is

identified, the most important determining factor in the management of the injury is the location of the injury. For injuries of the ureter cephalad to the pelvic brim, a direct end-to-end anastomosis (ureteroureterostomy) is performed with good results. To perform an adequate ureteroureterostomy, careful mobilization of the ureter should be done to avoid tension on the anastomosis. A ureteral stent should be inserted and left in place for approximately 10 days along with a perianastomotic drain. The perianastomotic drain should not be removed until an intravenous urogram has shown an intact anastomosis at approximately 10 days postoperatively. If there is leakage of the anastomosis, the perianastomotic drain can drain the extravasated urine. A spatulation of both ends of the ureters is performed to increase the circumference of the anastomotic site and to prevent stricture. Carlton and colleagues have reported excellent results in 84% of the patients who have had ureteric injury managed by ureteroureterostomies.[6] Ureteral injuries that are located above the midplane of the pelvis and involve more than 2 cm of the ureter can be treated by intraposition of a bowel segment, transureteroureterostomy, or cutaneous ureterostomy. Most surgeons are hesitant to use transureteroureterostomy because of the potential compromise of the recipient ureteral renal unit.[7]

Injuries to the ureter that occur below the pelvic brim are most commonly treated by reimplantation of the ureter into the bladder (ureteroneocystostomy). A ureteroureterostomy at this level of the pelvis is a difficult and tedious procedure because of the depth of the pelvis and because of the vascularity of the pelvis in this region. To obtain good results with ureteroneocystostomy the ureter must be mobilized to avoid undue tension. The bladder is opened at the fundus of the bladder, and a hiatus is created in the posterior wall through which the ureter is inserted into the bladder. The end of the ureter is spatulated for a distance of approximately 1.5 cm and sutured with interrupted absorbable sutures to the mucosa and submucosal layers of the bladder. A ureteral stent is inserted for 8 to 10 days and a perianastomotic drain is also used. Submucosal tunneling as described by Politano and Leadbetter[8] is performed whenever possible in an effort to prevent reflux. Landau and Lee and Symmonds[9] have reported good long-term renal and ureteral functioning on patients having direct ureteral reimplantation without subcutaneous mucosal tunneling. If there appears to be tension on a ureteral anastomosis the bladder should be extended toward the site of the anastomosis by performing a psoas hitch or a Boari flap. The Boari flap procedure is a method of extending the bladder by constructing tubes out of portions of the bladder wall. The ureter is anastomosed with the most cephalad portion of the bladder. The ureteral vascular anastomosis and extraperitoneal perianastomotic drain techniques are similar to that previously described. If a psoas hitch or Boari flap cannot be performed without tension on the suture line, downward mobilization of the ipsilateral kidney and upper aspect of the ureter can be undertaken.

Symptoms of ureteral injuries unrecognized at operation include flank pain, fever, ileus, and urinary leak or anuria. The presence of any of these symptoms should prompt suspicion of the possibility of genitourinary injury, and an intravenous pyelogram should be requested. If the intravenous pyelogram shows obstruction or hydronephrosis, this may not be the optimal time for repair because of the associated inflammation, edema, and infection. However, Hoch and colleagues reported a 93% success rate with immediate ureteral repair in 19 patients whose injuries were first recognized 1 to 24 days after surgery.[10]

The goal of intervention when postoperative obstruction is diagnosed is the relief of obstruction to avoid kidney damage. Recommended procedures include the passage of a retrograde catheter through the bladder or percutaneous nephrostomy. A retrograde catheter through the bladder should be attempted first, and if this is not successful, a percutaneous nephrostomy should be performed. If placement of the retrograde catheter is successful, it should be left in place from 14 to 21 days. After the stent is removed, a follow-up intravenous pyelogram should be performed at 4- to 6-week intervals to rule out stenosis or stricture. When percutaneous nephrostomy is necessary, definitive surgery should be delayed for 8 weeks because some injuries resolve with percutaneous nephrostomy alone. In addition, this interval of time permits much of the associated tissue edema, inflammation, and induration to subside.

VESICOVAGINAL FISTULA

Bender and Beck have reported the frequency of vesicovaginal fistula after total abdominal hysterectomy at a rate of 0.6%.[11] The frequency was 1% after vaginal hysterectomy and 1.5% after radical abdominal hysterectomy. Careful dissection of the bladder from the anterior aspect of the uterus and vagina and careful closure of the vaginal cuff are important in the prevention of a vesicovaginal fistula. Incorporation of bladder tissue in the closure of vaginal cuff whether done by suture or staple techniques can lead to vesicovaginal fistula formation. Vesicovaginal fistulas after hysterectomies usually present between 7 to 10 days from the day of surgery. The patient usually complains of urinary incontinence and leakage.

The cause of vesicovaginal fistulas is predominantly ischemia, owing to interruption of the blood supply to a segment of the bladder. Fistulas most often result from placement of sutures or clamps on a portion of the bladder. A properly repaired laceration or crushing injury to the bladder rarely results in a fistula. In diagnosing a vesicovaginal fistula, methylene blue should be instilled directly into the bladder through a urethral catheter, and if the contrast medium drains per vagina a vesicovaginal fistula is the most likely diagnosis. If this test does not demonstrate a fistula, contrast material such as indigo carmine should be injected intravenously to see if there is extravasation into the bladder. If the extravasation into the vagina occurs within 10 minutes of intravenous injection, this is suggestive of ureterovaginal fistula. If more than 10 minutes elapse, the contrast medium may be extravasating from the bladder. Most vesicovaginal fistulas occur in the posterior bladder wall above the bladder trigone near the midline. If the patient with the fistula has a diagnosis of a gynecologic malignancy, the fistula margins must be sampled to rule out tumor. Whether or not a fistula is visible by vaginal examination, cystoscopy and intravenous pyelography should always be performed to identify multiple fistulas or a more complex situation involving the ureter and the bladder.

After the diagnosis of a vesicovaginal fistula is made, the bladder should be catheterized for 6 to 8 weeks. The reason for the delay of 6 to 8 weeks is the inflammatory reaction and edema that occurs around the fistula site that complicates dissection of the fistula borders and interferes with wound healing. In addition, many small fistulas heal spontaneously. If the patient feels uncomfortable from the catheter, disposable diapers or rubber pants can be offered. If the fistula does not spontaneously close, a surgical repair should be undertaken. During the conservative management of the fistula with catheter drainage, antibiotic treatment and estrogen replacement therapy should be given to the patient when appropriate.

The decision to use a vaginal or abdominal approach for surgical repair of a vesicovaginal fistula depends on the location and size of the fistula and the surgeon's experience. The vaginal approach is preferred for simple fistulas. When more complicated fistulas are treated (post irradiation, large, multiple, or in close proximity to the ureteral orifices) a transabdominal approach is more appropriate. When a fistula repair is performed through a vaginal approach good exposure is required. A Schuchardt incision may sometimes be needed if the vaginal introitus is small. Table 13–1 summarizes success rates of several techniques. Whether an abdominal or a vaginal approach is chosen, the basic surgical technique and principles originally described by Sims should be followed.[12] There should be adequate mobilization of the bladder and vaginal walls with excision of the fistula tract. The layer of the bladder is closed with absorbable suture in an interrupted fashion. A second layer of sutures, inverting the initial layer, is performed with similar sutures in an interrupted or continuous fashion. The vaginal wall is then closed with absorbable sutures usually in an interrupted fashion. The basic surgical principle is that the bladder wall should be approximated in a tension-free manner with excellent hemostasis.

The Latzko technique has been described for fistulas high in the vaginal vault that occur most commonly after hysterectomy.[13] In this procedure a four-quadrant denudation of vaginal mucosa around the fistula tract is done. Approximately 2 cm of vaginal wall is de-

TABLE 13–1

Success Rates for Various Closure Techniques for Vesicovaginal Fistulas

Technique	No. of Patients	Successful Closure (%)
Vaginal Route		
Doderlein	29	96
Sims-Simon	157	94
Latzko	38	92
Futh-Mayo	34	76
Moir	40	70
Abdominal Route		
Omental flap	27	100
Peritoneal flap	54	91
Rotation flap of urinary bladder	56	87
Suprapubic	54	75

From Friedberg V, Altwein JE, Petri E. Vaginaler oder abdominaler Verschluss von Blassen-Scheiden-Fisteln? In: Petri E, ed. Gynekologische Urologie. Stuttgart, Georg Thieme, 1983, pp 73–85.

nuded around the fistula tract and a partial colpocleisis approximates the upper part of the anterior and posterior vaginal wall. The denuded area is then approximated in such a fashion that the initial layer is invaginated toward the bladder lumen. A second layer is used to invert the initial layer, and a third layer closes the vaginal wound.

The postoperative management of the repair of the vesicovaginal fistula should include at least 7 days of catheter drainage to prevent overdistention and disruption of the bladder sutures. Although a suprapubic catheter may be needed for complicated fistulas, a transurethral catheter can be used for simple fistulas that have been repaired. Early ambulation is allowed in patients with fistula repair. Maintenance of an adequate urine output and the prevention of urinary tract infection are important postoperative considerations. During this time antibiotics and estrogen therapy may be indicated.

URINARY TRACT ABNORMALITIES IN CANCER

Urologic injury may occur as a result of cancer therapy. It is most often associated with radical hysterectomy, pelvic exenteration, or radiation therapy. A radical hysterectomy is a resection of the uterus with a portion of the parametrium and upper vagina to obtain adequate margins. During this resection the ureter must be dissected from the parametrium and the paracolpos, and in doing so special care must be given to the adventitial layer of the ureter to avoid necrosis and possible fistula formation. The incidence of ureteral fistulas as a result of radical pelvic surgery has decreased from 20% as reported by Green and Morse to less than 1%.[14] Reasons include improved surgical technique with regard to handling of the ureter, extraperitoneal drainage, prophylactic antibiotics, better hemostasis, and continuous postoperative bladder drainage. Techniques that have been recommended to reduce the incidence of ureter fistulas include suturing the ureters to the obliterated hypogastric artery,[15] wrapping the ureter with a layer of peritoneum,[16] and using retroperitoneal suction drains.[17] The use of routine postoperative intravenous pyelography after radical hysterectomy has been challenged. Larson and coworkers, in a study of 233 patients who had undergone a radical hysterectomy, showed abnormal findings on intravenous pyelography in six patients, all of whom were symptomatic and would have required further evaluation on the basis of symptoms alone.[18]

Patients who develop a ureterovaginal fistula after radical hysterectomy most commonly complain of urinary leakage between 7 and 10 days postoperatively. These patients should not be treated surgically at this time because of the postoperative edema and inflammation. The repair should be delayed until fresh surgical margins are obtained, which usually takes 2 to 3 months. Initial management of the ureterovaginal fistula should be conservative with the placement of ureteral stents (retrograde or antegrade) or percutaneous nephrostomy drainage.

With the decrease in incidence of ureterovaginal fistulas after radical hysterectomy, the most common postoperative complication nowadays is bladder dysfunction.[19] Urodynamic studies have shown an initial hypertonic phase followed by a prolonged hypotonic period. Although most patients ultimately achieve a normal voiding pattern, intermittent self-catheterization may be necessary.

Although cystitis after radiation therapy still affects approximately one third of the patients, significant radiation injury (stricture, stenosis, fistula) has been reduced to a low incidence of 2% to 3% owing to improved radiation techniques. In the presence of a urologic abnormality after radiation therapy especially in the first 2 years after treatment, recurrent cancer must be excluded. Krebs and colleagues reported that 83% of recurrent cancer of the cervix occurs within 2 years of treatment.[20] Review of the data from M. D. Anderson Hospital from 1948 to 1964 shows a low incidence of radiation damage to the bladder.[21] Results of this study also confirm that lower urinary tract problems after radiation therapy are usually associated with recurrent cancer.

In vesicovaginal fistulas after radiation therapy, the principle of neovascularization should be used. The histologic response to radiation is endarteritis and fibrosis, which makes spontaneous healing of a fistula unlikely. When surgically treating a vesicovaginal fistula after radiation therapy a fresh blood supply should be provided to the healing tissue by using an omental flap,[22] a bulbocavernosus flap (Martius flap),[23] and, in indicated cases, a muscle flap such as the gracilis muscle.[24]

Urologic complications that occur after pelvic exenteration are usually the result of urinary diversion. These complications include hydronephrosis, anastomotic stenosis, and urinary leaks. The incidence of a urinary leak from a conduit is between 5% and 22%.[25] A conservative approach to these leaks is recommended because the mortality of an additional surgical procedure ranges from 30% to 50%.[26] When a urinary diversion has been performed, postoperative management can include periodic intravenous urography and retrograde dye studies.

Abnormal urologic findings may be the result of the extent of the cancer and not directly related to cancer therapy. Hydroureter and hydronephrosis are sometimes identified during the course of the staging workup of patients with gynecologic malignancies. In patients with locally advanced gynecologic cancers it is not unusual to find elevated blood urea nitrogen or creatinine levels, along with radiologic evidence of obstruction noted by intravenous pyelography or by computed tomography. Unless renal function is markedly compromised, there is no need to treat the hydronephrosis or hydroureter initially because the condition will be improved once the treatment for cancer is initiated. In gynecologic cancers this clinical situation is most common with cervical cancer because of its predilection for lateral spread into the parametria and obstruction of the ureters. Occasionally, patients with locally advanced cervical cancer present with anuria and uremia, and these patients can be initially treated with percutaneous nephrostomy before the onset of therapy. The management of these patients should include adequate recording of input and output because initially they will undergo postobstructive diuresis and the electrolyte levels must be carefully monitored during this period of time. Subsequently, internal ureteral stents (double-J) or other internal devices can replace the nephrostomy catheter. Dudley and coworkers reported the importance of the percutaneous nephrostomy at the M. D. Anderson Hospital.[27] Renal function was recovered in 70% of patients who had elevated creatinine values. The majority of patients with malignant obstructions received further therapy. It is unusual to find hydroureter or hydronephrosis with ovarian cancer because the spread pattern is mainly through peritoneal dissemination.

POSTOPERATIVE URINARY INCONTINENCE

Postoperative urinary incontinence is sometimes encountered after anterior vaginal wall surgery mainly for a cystocele repair and rarely after simple abdominal or vaginal hysterectomy. When a patient presents with postoperative urinary incontinence the presence of a vesicovaginal or ureterovaginal fistula should be ruled out. If the appropriate tests have been performed and there is no presence of a genitourinary fistula, then medical treatment of this condition can be entertained.

Urinary continence depends on adequate urethral pressures and the intra-abdominal location of the urethrovesical junction where the continence sphincter exists. The urethra is mainly innervated by α-adrenergic receptors of the autonomic nervous system, and good results have been obtained with α-adrenergic stimulants. Stimulation of these receptors produces a significant increase in urethral pressure. α-Adrenergic medication such as ephedrine, pseudoephedrine, and phenylpropanolamine has been used with good results. Urinary stress incontinence has been reported to be improved or cured in 80% of women who are placed on α-adrenergic medication. Potential side effects of α-adrenergic agents include hypertension and anxiety, and these agents should be used with caution in patients with hypertension or cardiovascular disease. The use of anticholinergic medication has proven efficacious in patients whose incontinence is secondary to a neurogenic unstable bladder in the postoperative period. Oxybutynin (Ditropan) can be used in this group of patients. Urethroscopy and cystoscopy are not necessary unless voiding difficulties persist for more than 2 months.

Postmenopausal women treated with oral estrogen replacement have reported improvement in urinary incontinence. Although estrogen does not increase the urethral pressure, transmission of pressure to the urethrovesical junction can be improved markedly. Thus, the effect of estrogen is to increase the efficiency of the urethral continence mechanism.

OLIGURIA IN THE POSTOPERATIVE PATIENT

Oliguria is defined as excretion of less than 400 mL/day of urine.[28] Acute renal failure is the inability of the kidney to excrete nitrogenous waste, which results in accumulation of this substance. One of the first functions lost in intrinsic renal disease is the ability to concentrate urine above plasma osmolality. To achieve a concentration of urine of 1200 mOsm/kg of water the kidneys must secrete 400 to 500 mL/24 h to clear the body of nitrogenous waste.

In the gynecologic surgical patient who presents with oliguria in the postoperative period, the differential diagnosis includes prerenal azotemia, acute tubular necrosis, and obstructive uropathy. Acute tubular necrosis can occur after ischemic injury to a kidney that may be secondary to significant intraoperative blood loss. Toxic injuries account for 11% to 25% of cases of acute tubular necrosis.[29] Most notable nephrotoxins include the aminoglycosides,[30] cisplatin,[31] and radiographic contrast medium. In patients who present with acute tubular necrosis, the urine osmolality is similar to that of the serum and the urinary sodium excretion is elevated. The urinalysis shows moderate amounts of proteinuria and the urinary sediment includes erythrocytes, leukocytes, renal tubular cells, or granular casts. Initial therapy of these patients includes consultation with a nephrologist and placement of a Swan-Ganz catheter for adequate documentation of hemodynamic volumes and pressures. Fluid balance must be monitored carefully because it is easy for these patients to be in fluid overload from renal compromise. The efficacy of diuretics to increase urinary output remains questionable but is safe therapy. Studies indicate that acute tubular necrosis may present in a nonoliguric fashion, and this condition accounts for 20% to 30% of acute renal failure. Nephrotoxic failure is more frequent in nonoliguric than in oliguric patients.

Laboratory values in obstructive uropathy are similar to those of acute tubular necrosis. However, the urinalysis is generally normal in the patient with an obstructive uropathy, unlike the patient with acute tubular necrosis. Obstructed uropathy most commonly is due to a mechanical obstruction; however, postoperative edema can also lead to this situation. Postoperative edema generally subsides by the fourth or fifth postoperative day and is of itself not a common cause of postoperative inability to void. A catheter that is silicone coated has been known to reduce mucosal edema, which allows residual edema to subside and alleviate the obstruction. The diagnosis can be made with a renal ultrasound examination; however, the ultrasound image can be normal if it is an early obstruction (less than 24 hours). Under these circumstances, the study should be repeated several hours later. The treatment of a significant mechanical obstruction requires that it should be relieved promptly, which in the majority of cases requires surgical intervention.

Relieving the obstruction may be as simple as placing a Foley catheter. Transvesical placement of ureteral stents and percutaneous nephrostomy are the procedures of choice for temporarily relieving obstruction proximal to the bladder to preserve kidney function until more definitive therapy can be undertaken. Postobstructive diuresis often follows the relief of an obstruction. The urinary potassium content is usually low, and the serum levels are high. One-half isotonic saline may be used safely to replace losses. Occasionally, postobstructive diuresis is significant and induces a severe hypovolemic state if fluid loss is not corrected rapidly. In this instance, a central venous pressure catheter may assist in monitoring volume status to allow adequate resuscitation.

Prerenal azotemia is usually secondary to intravascular volume depletion from blood loss during surgery. The diagnosis of prerenal azotemia can often be made clinically. Hypovolemic patients demonstrate tachycardia, low blood pressure, and poor skin turgor. Orthostatic blood pressure changes can be a valuable clinical sign in assessment of hypovolemia. In these patients the urine osmolality is concentrated and the urinary sodium is low. Both of these parameters are physiologic responses to volume depletions. In patients with prerenal oliguria, the urinalysis is usually normal. Other possible causes of prerenal azotemia during the postoperative period include myocardial infarction, sepsis, and congestive heart failure. The Swan-Ganz catheter is helpful in differentiating these conditions. Hypovolemia is characterized by a decrease in pulmonary artery and pulmonary capillary wedge pressure with an elevated systemic vascular resistance. Because of the increase in systemic vascular resistance the blood pressure is often normal. Other common causes of hypovolemia after extensive surgery are hemorrhage and third space fluid losses. Third space losses are most commonly seen after cancer operations owing to the more extensive nature of dissection and tissue injury. This is especially true after ultraradical operations such as pelvic exenteration owing to the large amount of raw surfaces resulting from the dissection. Third space volume loss must also be accounted for in the patient after a debulking procedure for ovarian cancer because of the possibility of rapid reaccumulation of ascitic fluid. Intraperitoneal chemotherapy such as thiotepa has been shown to be helpful in diminishing the amount of third space volume loss in patients with ovarian cancer after a debulking procedure.

Management of prerenal azotemia should consist of fluid administration and correction of the underlying cause. Treatment necessitates restoring renal profusion by establishing an adequate blood volume. Whole blood or packed red cells are appropriate for volume restoration when significant blood loss has occurred. Isotonic fluids should be used to replace the loss of electrolyte-rich fluids. The presence of prerenal azotemia as a result of either congestive heart failure or cirrhosis implies severe disease and often a poor prognosis. Maintenance of an adequate urine output and tissue perfusion are important postoperative considerations. Volume replacement should continue until a minimal of urine output of approximately 30 mL/h is achieved with a rise in the pulmonary capillary wedge pressure to within the normal range. Initial fluid expansion can be started with crystalloid solution.

INABILITY TO VOID POSTOPERATIVELY

On rare occasions, gynecologic surgical patients are unable to void postoperatively. This situation is most commonly seen after anterior vaginal surgery for cystocele or for urinary stress incontinence. A postvoid residual study should always be performed after removal of the Foley catheter after any type of anterior vaginal surgery because overdistention of the bladder must be avoided in these patients. A postvoid residual of over 150 mL is considered abnormal and the patient should be retested in 24 hours or perhaps discharged home with continuous catheter drainage. Watchful waiting is the best form of management for postoperative urinary retention. The patient can be discharged with a transurethral or a suprapubic urinary catheter and reassured that in most cases the catheter will be removed.

The autonomic innervation of the bladder is dominated by cholinergic receptors and that of the urethra by α-adrenergic receptors. For this reason, cholinergic medication and α-adrenergic blockers have been recommended in the treatment of postoperative urinary retention. Most studies have not shown cholinergic medication, such as bethanechol (Urecholine) to be efficacious; and, in fact, some studies suggest that bethanechol might inhibit effective bladder function. For this reason, the most commonly used medications are α-adrenergic blockers that decrease urethral pressure. The recommended dosage is 10 to 20 mg/d. Potential side effects include reflex tachycardia and postural hypotension. Cystoscopy, urodynamics, and urethral dilation are not necessary unless the urinary retention persists for longer than 2 months.

URINOMAS (PERITONEAL EXTRAVASATION OF URINE)

Urinomas, although sometimes seen after benign gynecologic surgery, are most common after radical pelvic surgery, particularly pelvic exenteration. Postexenterative complications involving the urinary tract are serious. Subclinical urinary leaks after urinary diversion probably occur frequently. Possible causes for most significant leaks include dehiscence of the ureteroconduit anastomosis or conduit necrosis secondary to compromised blood supply. The majority of exenterations in gynecologic surgery are done on patients previously treated with radiation. Reoperation to repair the leak is associated with significant mortality and should be undertaken only for life-threatening infection or deteriorating renal function. Conservative management of urinoma includes percutaneous drainage, and retrograde/antegrade stenting of the ureteroconduit anastomosis, which is associated with spontaneous closure in 30% of patients.[32]

BLADDER INFECTION IN THE POSTOPERATIVE PERIOD

Cystitis can sometimes be seen in the postoperative gynecologic surgical patient because of the common use of the transurethral or suprapubic catheter. The patient usually presents with dysuria, which can be accompanied by lower abdominal or low back pain and fever. The decision as to which antibiotic to use should be based on efficacy, side effects, and cost. Before the result of the urine culture and sensitivity is obtained a good initial treatment is the use of nitrofurantoin (Macrodantin), 100 mg four times daily for 10 days. This medication can be modified when the results of the culture and sensitivity are available. Nitrofurantoin achieves a high concentration in the bladder and has a low incidence of resistance. To avoid upper tract involvement, a 10-day course is recommended. Nitrofurantoin is rapidly absorbed from the gastrointestinal tract and has no systemic side effects. Elevated antibiotic concentrations are not achieved in plasma after oral therapy because the drug is rapidly eliminated. Nitrofurantoin is associated with a 2% emergence of *Escherichia coli* resistance compared to 40% with ampicillin. Ampicillin use is also commonly associated with the concomitant development of vaginal candidiasis. Use of cephalosporin is efficacious but expensive. The indications for use of a cephalosporin include allergies to penicillin or sulfonamides. Dysuria can be relieved with the use of phenazopyridine (Pyridium), 100 to 200 mg three times daily, warning the patient about the possibility of orange discoloration of the urine.

Patients who are discharged from the hospital with a transurethral catheter because of high residual volumes after gynecologic surgery should be kept on urinary suppression. Suprapubic catheters are associated with a much lower risk of urinary tract infection, and prophylactic antibiotic therapy is not routinely necessary.

REFERENCES

1. Wheelock JB, Krebs H-B, Hurt WG. Sparing and repairing the bladder during GYN surgery. Contemp Ob Gyn 1984;163:163–171.
2. Halloway HJ. Injury to the urinary tract as a complication of gynecologic surgery. Am J Obstet Gynecol 1950;60:30–40.
3. Mann WJ, Arato M, Patsner B, Stone M. Ureteral injuries in an obstetrics and gynecology training program: etiology and management. Obstet Gynecol 1988;72:82–85.
4. Symmonds RE. Ureteral injuries associated with gynecologic surgery: prevention and management. Clin Obstet Gynecol 1976;19:623–644.
5. Piscatelli JT, Simel DL, Addison WA. Who should have intravenous pyelograms before hysterectomy for benign disease? Obstet Gynecol 1987;69:541–545.
6. Carlton E Jr, Scott R Jr, Guthrie AG. The initial management of ureteral injuries: a report of 78 cases. J Urol 1971;105:335–340.
7. Sansoz IL, Paul DP, Macfarlane CA. Complications with transureteroureterostomy. J Urol 1977;117:39–42.
8. Politano VA, Leadbetter WF. An operative technique for the correction of vesicoureteral reflux. J Urol 1958;79:932–941.
9. Lee RA, Symmonds RA. Ureterovaginal fistula. Am J Obstet Gynecol 1971;109:1032–1035.
10. Hoch WM, Kursch ED, Persky L. Early aggressive management of intraoperative ureteral injuries. J Urol 1975;114:530.
11. Bender HG, Beck L. Surgery for vesicovaginal fistulas. In: Gynecologic Surgery. Oradell, NJ, Medical Economics, 1988, pp 229–239.
12. Sims JM. On the treatment of vesicovaginal fistula. Am J Med Sci 1852;23:59–82.
13. Latzko W. Postoperative vesicovaginal fistulas: genesis and therapy. Am J Surg 1942;58:211–228.
14. Green TH, Morse WJ Jr. Management of invasive cervical cancer following inadvertent simple hysterectomy. Obstet Gynecol 1969;33:763–769.
15. Green TH. Ureteral suspension for prevention of ureteral complications following radical Wertheim hysterectomy. Obstet Gynecol 1966;28:1–11.
16. Novak F. Surgical Gynecological Techniques. New York, John Wiley & Sons, 1978.
17. Baronow RC, Rutledge F. Vesicovaginal fistula, radiation in gynecologic cancer. Am J Obstet Gynecol 1971;111:85–90.
18. Larson DM, Malone JM, Copeland LJ, et al. Ureteral assessment after radical hysterectomy. Obstet Gynecol 1987;69:612–616.
19. Christ F, Wagner U, Debus G. Early bladder function disorders after Wertheim surgery: causes and therapeutic consequences. Geburtshilfe Frauenheilkd 1983;43:380–383.
20. Krebs HB, Helmkamp BF, Sevin BU, et al. Recurrent cancer of the cervix following radical hysterectomy and pelvic node dissection. Obstet Gynecol 1982;59:422–427.
21. Buchler DA, Kline JC, Peckham BM, et al. Radiation reactions in cervical cancer therapy. Am J Obstet Gynecol 1971;111:745–750.
22. Kiricuta I, Goldstein AMB. The repair of extensive vesicovaginal fistulas with pedicled omentum: a review of 23 cases. J Urol 1972;108:724–727.
23. Patil U, Waterhouse K, Laungani G. Management of 18 difficult vesicovaginal and vaginal fistulas with modified Ingelman-Sundberg and Martius operations. J Urol 1980;123:653.
24. Becker DW Jr, Massey FM, McCraw JM. Musculocutaneous flaps in reconstructive pelvic surgery. Obstet Gynecol 1979;54:178–183.
25. Morley GW, Lindenauer SM. Pelvic exenterative therapy for gynecologic malignancy: analysis of 70 cases. Cancer 1976;38:581–586.
26. Orr JW Jr, Shingleton HM, Hatch KD, et al. Urinary diversion in patients undergoing pelvic exenteration. Am J Obstet Gynecol 1982;42:883–889.
27. Dudley VJ, et al. Percutaneous nephrostomy catheter use related to gynecological malignancy. Gynecol Oncol 1986;24:273.
28. Grossman RA. Oliguria and acute renal failure. Med Clin North Am 1981;65:413.
29. Anderson RJ, Linas SL, Berns AS, et al. Nonoliguric acute renal failure. N Engl J Med 1977;296:1134.
30. Rasmussen HH, Ibels LS. Acute renal failure: multivariate analysis of causes and risk factors. Am J Med 1982;73:211.
31. Blachley JD, Hill JB. Renal and electrolyte disturbances associated with cisplatin. Ann Intern Med 1981;95:628.
32. Lichtinger M. Small bowel complications after supravesical urinary diversion in pelvic exenteration. Presented before the annual meeting of the Society of Gynecologic Oncologists, February 1985. (Abstract)

14

Daniel L. Clarke-Pearson

Venous Thromboembolic Complications

Deep venous thrombosis and pulmonary embolism are two major complications of gynecologic surgery. Pulmonary embolism accounts for 40% of all deaths that occur after gynecologic surgery[1] and is a leading cause of death in women who undergo a legally induced abortion[2] and in high-risk patients with uterine, ovarian, or cervical carcinoma.[3–5]

Most pulmonary emboli are preceded by deep venous thrombosis in the legs or pelvis. The incidence of postoperative deep venous thrombosis, when detected by iodine-125–labeled fibrinogen scanning, varies widely, based in large part on the risk factors of the particular group of gynecologic surgery patients. Deep venous thrombosis is detected in 24% to 29% of patients with benign conditions.[6,7] Patients with gynecologic malignancies have an increased risk of between 17% and 45%.[8,9] In this chapter the factors associated with an increased risk of venous thromboembolism are reviewed, the natural history, diagnosis, and treatment of deep venous thrombosis and pulmonary embolism are outlined, and strategies are emphasized to prevent the occurrence of deep venous thrombosis in high- and moderate-risk patients.

RISK FACTORS

Acquired conditions associated with venous thrombosis in medical and surgical patients have been reviewed by Goldhaber and associates.[10] Based on their review, factors important to the gynecologist include patients who are obese, are elderly, have hypercoagulable states, are pregnant, or are taking oral contraceptives.

In gynecologic surgery, two prospective studies have evaluated risk factors associated with the postoperative occurrence of ^{125}I-fibrinogen–detected deep venous thrombosis.[11,12] Clayton and associates studied 125 patients undergoing vaginal and abdominal surgery predominantly for benign gynecologic conditions.[12] Using logistic regression analysis, five factors were associated with postoperative deep venous thrombosis: (1) age, (2) varicose veins, (3) percentage overweight, (4) euglobulin lysis time, and (5) serum fibrin-related antigen. In a subsequent study, a prognostic index score, created on the basis of these five variables, was used to select high-risk patients who might most benefit from intensive perioperative thromboembolism prophylaxis.[13]

My colleagues and I have also assessed clinical factors associated with venous thromboembolic complications in 411 patients undergoing major abdominal and pelvic gynecologic surgery.[11] Risk factors associated with postoperative deep venous thrombosis identified in this study included age, nonwhite race, increasing stage of malignancy, a past history of deep venous thrombosis, lower extremity edema or venous stasis changes, varicose veins, excessive weight, and a past history of radiation therapy. Intraoperative factors associated with postoperative deep venous thrombosis included increased anesthesia time, increased blood loss, and transfusion requirements in the operating room. When all of these factors were evaluated in a stepwise logistic regression model, the type of surgical procedure, age, ankle edema, nonwhite race, varicose veins, prior radiation therapy, a past history of deep venous thrombosis, and duration of surgery were found to be the most important variables associated with postoperative thromboembolic complications. Table 14–1 shows the relative risk of these factors.

Recognition of the factors associated with venous thromboembolism in gynecologic sur-

TABLE 14–1
*Variables Associated with Postoperative Deep Vein Thrombosis**

Diagnosis/Variable	% Deep Venous Thrombosis	*P* Value
Benign	6	
Cancer	17.7	
Recurrent cancer	39	<.001
Past history of deep venous thrombosis	56	<.001†
Prior radiation therapy	36	<.001†
Nonwhite races	25	.03†
Ankle edema	40	.005†
Leg stasis changes	45	.002
Severe varicose veins	86	.001†
Radical vulvectomy	32	.001†
Pelvic exenteration	88	.001†
Duration of surgery (min)		
<120	5	
120–300	14	
>300	32	.001†
Estimated blood loss (mL)		
<200	17.7	
200–600	12	
>600	23.5	.01
Weight		.02
Age		<.001†

*Overall incidence of deep venous thrombosis in 411 gynecologic surgery patients was 17.5%.
†Factors significant in logistic regression model.
Reprinted with permission of The American College of Obstetricians and Gynecologists (Obstetrics and Gynecology, 1987, 69:146–150).

gery should allow the clinician to stratify patients into low-, moderate-, and high-risk groups and thereby apply appropriate prophylactic methods while at the same time not exposing a low-risk group of patients to the potential complications and expense of some prophylactic treatment regimens.

NATURAL HISTORY

Before venous thromboembolism prophylaxis is considered, an understanding of the natural history of postoperative deep venous thrombosis and pulmonary embolism is necessary because the time sequence and site of deep venous thrombosis is relevant to the most effective use of prophylactic methods. The advent of noninvasive methods to detect deep venous thrombosis, especially ^{125}I-fibrinogen counting, has allowed a clear understanding of the natural history of postoperative deep venous thrombosis. Reports of general surgery patients have shown that most deep venous thromboses arise in the calf veins.[14, 15] These thrombi might lyse spontaneously, remain in the calf, or propagate to the proximal deep venous system of the leg. It is these more proximal thrombi that are the major source of pulmonary emboli and cause long-term sequelae and morbidity of the post-thrombotic stasis syndrome.

The natural history of thromboembolic complications after gynecologic surgery has some similarities and some differences when compared with that of general surgery. Three-hundred eighty-two gynecologic surgery patients were studied in a prospective fashion using ^{125}I-fibrinogen counting throughout their postoperative hospitalization.[16] This group of patients had undergone major abdominal and pelvic surgery and included a high proportion of patients with gynecologic malignancies. Seventeen percent of patients developed postoperative venous thromboembolic complications; 85% of the thrombi were located in the veins of the calf, and most were of little clinical significance. Nearly one third of these calf thrombi lysed spontaneously, 4% propagated to the proximal leg veins, and 4% became symptomatic pulmonary emboli. The remaining 65% of thrombi in the calf did not propagate beyond the calf throughout postoperative surveillance, and long-term follow-up showed there were no clinically significant complications of these thrombi. These findings are similar to those reported from general surgery patients and further emphasize that calf

vein thrombosis, while a frequent event, is of minimal clinical significance. The 4% incidence of pulmonary emboli originating from calf veins is similar to reports by Doouss[17] and Moser and DeMoine[18] and conflict with the report of Kakkar and colleagues,[14] who found an incidence of 10% of pulmonary emboli associated with calf vein thrombosis.

The 4% of gynecologic patients who developed deep venous thrombosis proximal to the calf are a much more significant group of patients in that these thrombi may progress to potentially life-threatening pulmonary emboli. In my experience, these proximal thrombi often arose in conjunction with calf vein thrombosis, but in approximately half the patients no calf vein thrombosis was found. It is also important to emphasize that 40% of gynecology patients who developed symptomatic pulmonary emboli postoperatively had no evidence of deep venous thrombosis on noninvasive ^{125}I-fibrinogen counting. This finding suggests that thrombi and subsequent pulmonary emboli arising from pelvic veins are much more frequent in the gynecology patient than the general surgery patient. Unfortunately, a satisfactory test for the detection of pelvic vein thrombosis has not been established, although preliminary work with Indium-111–labeled platelets, which are incorporated into acutely forming thrombi and emboli, may be a reasonably noninvasive technique to image pelvic veins.[19, 20]

The time of occurrence of venous thromboembolic events is important to recognize so that effective prophylaxis may be applied during the interval the patient is at greatest risk to develop deep venous thrombosis or pulmonary emboli. Of all venous thromboembolic complications, 50% occur within the first 24 hours postoperatively and 75% are detected by the third postoperative day.[16] It seems then that the surgical procedure itself, including venous stasis in the legs after induction of general anesthesia as well as the release of tissue thromboplastins secondary to surgical trauma, leads to the immediate formation of occult postoperative thrombi. The early postoperative occurrence of most thromboembolic events therefore requires the application of prophylaxis in the operating room and throughout the perioperative period to achieve maximal reduction in thromboembolic complications. The later occurrence of thromboembolic complications, however, must not be forgotten because 15% of venous thromboembolic complications after gynecologic surgery were diagnosed after the seventh postoperative day.[16]

The patient who remains at risk for thromboembolic complications because of immobility, prolonged postoperative recovery, or possibly a hypercoagulable state secondary to advanced malignancy should continue to receive prophylaxis beyond the conventional perioperative recommendations.

DIAGNOSIS

The early recognition of deep venous thrombosis and pulmonary embolism and immediate treatment are critical to successful recovery from these serious postoperative complications. Most pulmonary emboli arise from the deep venous system of the leg, although after gynecologic surgery the pelvic veins are also a recognized source of fatal pulmonary emboli. The diagnosis of lower extremity deep venous thrombosis requires a high level of suspicion and the appropriate use of diagnostic tests. The signs and symptoms of deep venous thrombosis of the lower extremity include pain, edema, erythema, and a prominent vascular pattern of the superficial veins. These signs and symptoms are relatively nonspecific in that 50% to 80% of patients with these symptoms will not actually have deep venous thrombosis.[21] Conversely, approximately 80% of patients with symptomatic pulmonary emboli have no signs or symptoms of thrombosis in the lower extremities.[22] Because of the lack of specificity of these signs and symptoms, additional diagnostic tests should be performed to establish the diagnosis of deep venous thrombosis. The "gold standard" for diagnosis of deep venous thrombosis has been contrast medium–enhanced venography. Unfortunately, this study is modestly uncomfortable, requires the injection of a contrast medium that may cause allergic reaction or renal injury, and may result in phlebitis in approximately 5% of patients.[23] Newer diagnostic tests have been developed that are less invasive yet have a high accuracy rate in most patients. Impedance plethysmography is a noninvasive study that measures the change in electrical impedance of the lower extremity when venous blood flow and volume are altered by an occlusive cuff on the thigh. This study may be performed at the patient's bedside and be repeated as often as necessary without any risk to the patient. Correlation with venography in symptomatic patients approaches 95%.[24, 25] The test is very good for the identification of deep venous thrombi in the popliteal, femoral, and external iliac segments. It is less accurate (30%) in identifying calf vein

thrombosis and does not identify thrombi occurring in the internal iliac venous system. False-positive results are primarily due to extrinsic venous compression. In gynecology, this might include a large pelvic mass compressing the external iliac or common iliac vein.

Doppler ultrasonography has also been used for the noninvasive diagnosis of deep venous thrombosis, although its accuracy is slightly less than that of impedance plethysmography. The reason for this is primarily due to the variable interpretation of audible venous flow patterns, which is somewhat subjective.[26] B-mode duplex Doppler imaging has been found to be more effective in the diagnosis of symptomatic venous thrombosis, especially when it arises in the proximal lower extremity. With duplex Doppler imaging, the femoral vein can be visualized and clots may be seen directly.[27] Compression of the vein with the ultrasound probe tip allows for assessment of venous collapsibility; the presence of a thrombus diminishes vein wall collapsibility. Color flow studies have also been added to this imaging technique. Doppler imaging is less accurate when evaluating the calf venous system and the pelvic veins. Magnetic resonance imaging can also accurately identify thrombi in the deep venous system.[28] The primary drawback to magnetic resonance imaging is the time involved in examining the lower extremity and pelvis as well as the expense of this study. All of these diagnostic studies are accurate when performed by a skilled technologist and in most patients may replace the need for routine contrast medium–enhanced venography.

The diagnosis of pulmonary embolism also requires a high index of suspicion, because many of the signs and symptoms are associated with other, more common pulmonary complications after surgery. The classic findings of pleuritic chest pain, hemoptysis, shortness of breath, tachycardia, and tachypnea should alert the physician to the possibility of a pulmonary embolism. Many times, however, the signs are much more subtle and may only be suggested by a persistent tachycardia or a slight elevation in the respiratory rate. Patients suspected of pulmonary embolism should be evaluated initially by chest radiography, electrocardiography, and arterial blood gas analysis. Any evidence of abnormality should be further evaluated with a ventilation-perfusion lung scan in a search for evidence of decreased perfusion in areas of adequate ventilation. Unfortunately, a high percentage of lung scans may be interpreted as "indeterminant." In this setting, careful clinical evaluation and judgment are required to decide whether pulmonary arteriography should be obtained to document or exclude the presence of a pulmonary embolism.

TREATMENT

The treatment of postoperative deep venous thrombosis requires the immediate institution of anticoagulant therapy. Heparin should be initiated as a bolus of 5000 units intravenously, followed by a continuous intravenous infusion of 1000 units/h. Approximately 4 hours after initiation of heparin therapy, an activated partial thromboplastin time should be obtained to assess the adequacy of the anticoagulant effect. In general, prolongation of the activated partial thromboplastin time to one and one-half to two times the control level achieves appropriate anticoagulant therapy. The goals of anticoagulant therapy include the prevention of clot propagation or embolization and the prevention of rethrombosis in a high-risk patient; the risks are primarily bleeding complications.[29] Oral maintenance therapy using sodium warfarin (Coumadin) is advised for at least 3 months. Standard treatment regimens call for the use of intravenous heparin for 10 days, followed by continuation of warfarin for 3 months.[30] However, a randomized trial evaluated a 10-day regimen of heparin compared with a 5-day regimen of heparin and found the 5-day regimen to be equally effective in treating the acute thrombosis and preventing rethrombosis.[31] Therefore, it is recommended that intravenous heparin be maintained for 5 days and during that time oral warfarin therapy be initiated. The goals of warfarin therapy are to achieve an oral dose of medication that will prolong the prothrombin time to approximately one and one-half times control value. Initially, prothrombin time values should be obtained on a daily basis until a stable dose of warfarin is established. Thereafter, the prothrombin time is checked at intervals of every 1 to 2 weeks for the duration of 3 months' therapy. Anticoagulant therapy may be discontinued in 3 months if the cause of the deep venous thrombosis episode (such as an acute surgical event or trauma) has been eliminated.

The major hazard of anticoagulant therapy in the postoperative patient is an increased risk of bleeding complications. Therefore, it is important that the activated partial thromboplastin time, prothrombin time, platelet count, and hematocrit be followed carefully and that the anticoagulant does not drastically alter the patient to a hypocoagulable state. Heparin-induced thrombocytopenia is a rare complication and has been reported in association with the use of both low-dose prophylactic heparin and standard anticoagulant doses.[32] Therefore, periodic checks of platelet count while the patient is on heparin therapy are advised.

Thrombolytic therapy (with streptokinase or urokinase) has been advocated by some investigators for the treatment of acute deep venous thrombosis. However, the risk of bleeding complications in a surgical site contraindicates thrombolytic therapy in the postoperative patient.

The management of pulmonary embolism also requires immediate anticoagulant therapy, identical to that outlined for the treatment of deep venous thrombosis. Respiratory support including oxygen and bronchodilators and an intensive care setting may be necessary. Massive pulmonary emboli are usually quickly fatal, although on rare occasion pulmonary embolectomy has been successfully performed. The use of pulmonary artery catheterization with the administration of thrombolytic agents bears further evaluation and may be important in the patient with massive pulmonary embolism. In situations in which anticoagulant therapy is ineffective in the prevention of rethrombosis and repeated embolization from the lower extremities or pelvis, vena cava interruption may be necessary. This may be accomplished through the percutaneous placement of a vena cava umbrella or a filter or the use of a large clip to obstruct the vena cava above the level of the thrombosis. In most cases, however, anticoagulant therapy is sufficient to prevent repeat thrombosis and embolism and to allow the patient's own endogenous thrombolytic mechanisms to lyse the pulmonary embolus.

PREVENTION OF DEEP VENOUS THROMBOSIS

An awareness of the risk factors associated with venous thromboembolic complications as well as the natural history of these complications allows us to develop strategies for the prevention of thromboembolic complications. Over the past two decades a number of prophylactic techniques have been evaluated in randomized clinical trials. Many trials have shown a significant reduction in the incidence of postoperative deep venous thrombosis, and a few trials have shown a reduction in fatal pulmonary embolism. There are no studies in the gynecology patient population that have

TABLE 14–2
Prophylactic Techniques Appropriate for Patients Having Major Gynecologic Surgery

Risk Category	Prophylactic Techniques
Low	Graduated compression stockings
Moderate	Intermittent pneumatic compression (24 hours)
	Low-dose heparin (q12 h)
	Graduated compression stockings
High	Intermittent pneumatic compression (5 days)
	Low-dose heparin (q8 h)
Very high risk	Combination of methods (e.g., intermittent pneumatic compression and graduated compression stockings or intermittent pneumatic compression and low-dose heparin)
	Inferior vena cava interruption

demonstrated a reduction in fatal pulmonary emboli. Of the prophylactic techniques reported, each has its advantages and disadvantages (Table 14–2). The ideal prophylactic method would be effective, free of significant side effects to the patient, well accepted by the patient and nursing staff, applicable to most patient groups, available to inpatients and outpatients, and inexpensive.

Pharmacologic Methods

LOW-DOSE HEPARIN

Small doses of subcutaneously administered heparin for the prevention of deep venous thrombosis and pulmonary embolism is the most widely studied of all prophylactic methods. The most significant of these studies was a randomized trial of surgery patients that demonstrated a significant reduction in fatal postoperative pulmonary embolism.[33] Subsequently, more than 80 controlled trials in 16,000 patients have demonstrated that low-dose heparin given subcutaneously 2 hours preoperatively and every 8 to 12 hours postoperatively is effective in reducing the incidence of postoperative venous thrombi.[34, 35] Controlled trials performed in gynecologic surgery patients also show a benefit in reducing postoperative deep venous thrombosis, although results vary depending on the risk of the patient.[6, 7, 36, 37]

Benign Gynecologic Surgery

There are two controlled randomized trials in the English literature of low-dose heparin used predominantly in surgery for benign gynecologic conditions.[6, 7] Both studies used the same regimen of low-dose heparin administration: 5000 units subcutaneously 2 hours preoperatively and every 12 hours for 7 days postoperatively. ^{125}I-fibrinogen counting for the detection of thrombosis was used for final diagnosis. All patients were older than 40 years of age, and follow-up was discontinued at the time of discharge from the hospital.

The results of the trial by Taberner and associates of 97 patients showed a 23% incidence of deep venous thrombosis in the patients treated with low-dose heparin.[7] This difference was statistically significant ($P < .05$). Unfortunately, although this was a randomized trial, the control group contained a larger number of patients with malignancy. When the cancer patients were excluded from the trial analysis, there remained no significant value to the use of low-dose heparin in patients with benign conditions. Subsequently, Ballard and associates evaluated a group of 110 patients who also had a predominance of benign gynecologic diseases.[6] The nontreated control group had a 29% incidence of deep venous thrombosis compared with a 3.6% incidence in the group treated with low-dose heparin ($P < .001$). In this trial, none of the patients developed deep venous thrombosis proximal to the calf and none developed a pulmonary embolus.

Gynecologic Oncology

Despite the apparent benefit of low-dose heparin prophylaxis in general surgery and gynecologic surgery patients with benign disease, my colleagues and I have found that low-dose heparin given every 12 hours postoperatively to patients with gynecologic cancer is ineffective.[36] In a randomized controlled trial of 185 patients undergoing major abdominal and pelvic surgery for gynecologic malignancy, there was no difference in the incidence of thromboembolic complications between the control group (12.4%) and the group treated with low-dose heparin (14.8%). When analysis of thromboembolic complications was confined to the first 7 postoperative days (while the patient received prophylaxis), the incidence of deep venous thrombosis was 12.4% for the control group compared with 6.8% in the group treated with low-dose heparin. Although this suggests a trend to the benefit of low-dose heparin, this difference was not statistically significant ($P = .2$). Patients with malignancy or poor functional status due to age or extent of surgery may remain at risk longer and may require a longer duration of low-dose heparin prophylaxis to truly benefit from this regimen.

In a subsequent controlled trial, a more intense low-dose heparin regimen (5000 units subcutaneously every 8 hours postoperatively or in three doses preoperatively at 8-hour intervals and every 8 hours postoperatively) significantly reduced the incidence of deep venous thrombosis in gynecologic oncology patients.[37] The incidence of ^{125}I-fibrinogen scan–detected deep venous thrombosis was 18.4% for the control group, 8.7% for those receiving heparin as a single dose preoperatively, and 4.1% for those receiving at least three doses of heparin preoperatively. Although not statistically significant when compared with patients receiving the other heparin regimen, the group receiving three doses preoperatively appeared to have the best outcome.

Low-Dose Heparin Complications

Complications associated with bleeding induced by low-dose heparin must also be considered in evaluating the risks of this prophylactic regimen. In most series, excessive bleeding is reported in patients receiving low-dose heparin prophylaxis, although the absolute excess in bleeding is only about 2%.[10] In a study of 182 patients undergoing major surgery for gynecologic malignancy, clinical and laboratory complications associated with low-dose heparin were evaluated. That study found a trend toward increased intraoperative blood loss, transfusion requirements, and wound hematomas associated with the use of low-dose heparin.[38] More intense regimens of low-dose heparin in gynecologic surgery patients are associated with an increased need for postoperative blood transfusion.[39]

Low-dose heparin alters the activated partial thromboplastin time in 10% to 15% of patients given 5000 units of sodium heparin subcutaneously.[38, 40] In patients who had prolongation of the activated partial thromboplastin time greater than one and one-half times the control value, hemorrhagic complications were significantly increased.[38] Thrombocytopenia has also been associated with the use of low-dose heparin,[41] although it is much more frequently noted during the use of therapeutic anticoagulant doses of heparin.[22]

Of particular relevance to the gynecologic surgeon performing pelvic, para-aortic, and inguinal lymphadenectomy for treatment or staging of malignancy are reports of increased lymphocyst formation and increased lymph fluid drainage attributed to the use of low-dose heparin.[38, 39, 42, 43] Although our prospective randomized studies have not found an increased incidence of lymphocysts, the volume of suction drainage from the retroperitoneal surgical site was increased nearly twofold.[38, 39]

LOW-MOLECULAR-WEIGHT HEPARIN

Low-molecular-weight heparin is composed of fragments of unfractionated heparin that differ in molecular weight, production methodology, and biologic and chemical function. In general, these agents are different from standard heparin in that they have nearly 100% bioavailability, a longer biologic half-life, and less variable anticoagulant response. Clinical trials in Europe have evaluated a number of these substances. In general, low-molecular-weight heparin has a lower frequency of bleeding, is effective with once-a-day dosing, and is at least equally effective to standard heparin.[44] Two randomized trials in the English literature of low-molecular-weight heparin in gynecologic surgery patients have similar results to those found in general surgery patients.[45, 46] Because each of the low-molecular-weight heparins has a distinct pharmacologic profile, each should be evaluated for safety and efficacy in clinical trials.

At present, only one low-molecular-weight heparin is approved by the Food and Drug Administration for use in the United States.[47] Although there are some potential benefits of low-molecular-weight heparins, the excess cost probably does not warrant that low-molecular-weight heparin be used widely for prophylaxis.

Mechanical Methods of Prophylaxis

Stasis in the veins of the legs has been clearly demonstrated on the operating table and during the postoperative hospital recovery. Many authors believe that the combination of stasis occurring in the capacitance veins of the calf during surgery or pregnancy plus the hypercoagulable state induced by surgery, pregnancy, and cancer are the prime factors contributing to the development of acute deep venous thrombosis. Prospective studies of the natural history of postoperative venous thrombosis after gynecologic surgery show that the calf veins are the predominant site of thrombi and that most thrombi develop within 72 hours of surgery.[16] Even though reduction of venous stasis in the perioperative period by various methods has been less extensively investigated (when compared with pharmacologic methods), a growing body of literature supports the important role that these mechanical prophylactic methods may play in the prevention of postoperative deep venous thrombosis.

Although probably of only modest benefit, reduction of stasis by short preoperative hospital stays, early postoperative ambulation, and elevation of the foot of the bed should be encouraged in all patients. More active forms of mechanical prophylaxis that have been evaluated in the gynecologic surgery patient include graded compression stockings and intermittent pneumatic leg compression.

GRADED COMPRESSION STOCKINGS

In a survey of general surgeons in the United States, graded compression elastic stockings were second only to low-dose heparin as the prophylactic method of choice in high-risk and moderately high-risk surgical patients.[48] The simplicity of elastic stockings and the absence of significant side effects are probably the two most important reasons that they are part of the routine postoperative orders of many surgeons. To be effective, the stockings must be designed and used properly. Early studies of static uniform compression stockings demonstrated no benefit from this style of stocking.[49, 50] Further evaluation of venous flow dynamics found better venous emptying and increased venous flow from stockings that had a gradient of pressure higher at the ankle and diminishing at the thigh.[51, 52]

The effectiveness of graded compression stockings in moderate-risk general surgery patients is most clearly demonstrated in a meta-analysis that evaluated 11 randomized trials.[53] The authors found a 68% reduction in deep venous thrombosis in patients who wore graduated compression stockings ($P < .001$).

There is only one study of graded compression stockings in gynecologic surgery patients who were at relatively low risk to develop deep venous thrombosis.[54] Cancer patients, diabetics, and those who had a past history of deep venous thrombosis or pulmonary embolism were excluded from the study. When evaluated by ^{125}I-fibrinogen scanning, none of the 104 patients in the compression stocking group developed deep venous thrombosis, while 4 of 92 patients (4.3%) in the control group developed calf vein deep venous thrombosis ($P = .48$). Although compression stockings lowered the incidence of deep venous thrombosis, the authors questioned whether this prophylaxis

was cost effective in a low-risk group of patients.[54]

Ensuring a proper fit of the compression stockings is very important as to avoid a tourniquet effect at the knee or mid thigh by poorly fitted stockings. Variations in human anatomy do not allow perfect fit of all patients to stocking sizes manufactured. As an example of this problem, a retrospective study of 281 patients undergoing radical hysterectomy or total abdominal hysterectomy found a fourfold increase in the incidence of clinically significant postoperative deep venous thrombosis and pulmonary embolism in patients weighing more than 90 kg who wore thigh-length elastic stockings perioperatively. It was suggested that a tourniquet effect of these stockings may have led to increased stasis in this group of patients already at high risk owing to obesity, age, malignancy, and major surgery.[3]

Overall, graded compression stockings are effective in preventing deep venous thrombosis in moderate-risk patients, and given their lack of side effects and low cost, they are considered the most cost-effective prophylactic technique in moderate-risk patients.[53] Furthermore, graded compression stockings may also be worn after hospital discharge, providing continued prophylaxis.

INTERMITTENT PNEUMATIC COMPRESSION

The largest body of literature evaluating the benefit of the reduction of postoperative venous stasis deals with intermittent compression of the leg by pneumatically inflated sleeves placed around the calf, or entire leg, during the intraoperative and postoperative periods. These sleeves provide cyclic compression to the leg for about 10 seconds (approximately 45 mm Hg) every minute and result in a pulsatile return of venous blood as well as stimulate the endogenous fibrinolytic system.[55] Clagett and Reisch have performed a meta-analysis of the results of intermittent pneumatic compression trials through 1988 and found a significant reduction of postoperative deep venous thrombosis in moderate-risk patients who were treated with intermittent pneumatic compression.[35]

Various pneumatic compression devices and leg sleeve designs are available, but the current literature has not demonstrated superiority of one system over another. Although the sequential full-leg sleeves appear to improve hemodynamics and enhance fibrinolysis, a randomized comparison with a single-chamber calf compression sleeve and a sequential multichamber sleeve showed no clinical difference in the incidence of deep venous thrombosis.[56]

The duration of postoperative intermittent pneumatic compression has been different in various trials. Because the onset of most deep venous thromboses occurs intraoperatively and in the first 48 hours postoperatively, it would seem that this time interval should be a minimum length for intermittent pneumatic compression. Several investigators have found intermittent pneumatic compression to be effective when used only in the operating room or for the first 24 hours postoperatively.[57–59] Salzman and associates[58] reported that intraoperative intermittent pneumatic compression was as beneficial as that applied for longer periods of time in patients after urologic surgical procedures.[58] On the other hand, Turpie and coworkers found continuing benefit in the use of intermittent pneumatic compression for up to 14 days postoperatively.[60, 61]

Intermittent pneumatic compression has not been evaluated in a controlled trial of patients undergoing surgery for benign gynecologic disease. In patients with gynecologic malignancy, however, it has been found to reduce the incidence of postoperative venous thromboembolic complications by nearly threefold.[62] Calf compression was applied intraoperatively and for the first 5 postoperative days. The maximum benefit was realized during the 5 days of compression and diminished after intermittent pneumatic compression was discontinued. A subsequent trial evaluated whether intermittent pneumatic compression might achieve similar benefits when used only intraoperatively and for the first 24 hours postoperatively. However, there was no reduction of deep venous thrombosis when compared with the control group.[63] It appears that patients with gynecologic malignancies remain at risk because of stasis and hypercoagulable states for a longer period of time than the general surgical or urology patients; and if compression is to be effective, it must be used for at least 5 days postoperatively.

Intermittent pneumatic leg compression has no significant side effects or risks, although patient tolerance has been cited as a drawback to the use of this equipment. However, we have had only 7 patients of nearly 1000 treated with this modality request removal because of discomfort. The equipment is easily managed by the nursing staff; and although initial capital outlay for intermittent pneumatic compressors may seem large, Salzman and Davies calculated that the cost per patient of this prophylactic method is slightly less than that of low-dose heparin given for 7 days postoperatively.[64]

INFERIOR VENA CAVA INTERRUPTION

Interruption of the vena cava with a percutaneously inserted filter or a surgically placed clip will effectively prevent pulmonary embolism in situations where other prophylactic techniques are either contraindicated or are ineffective. The Greenfield filter, inserted percutaneously, is the most widely studied and has excellent results in high-risk groups such as cancer patients.[65] Heaps and Lagasse used a surgically placed inferior vena cava clip in very high-risk gynecologic oncology patients with no untoward complications and no deaths from pulmonary embolism.[66] The strategy of inferior vena cava interruption for venous embolism prophylaxis is infrequently necessary because the great majority of patients will achieve effective prophylaxis through standard techniques.

Comparison of Low-Dose Heparin and Intermittent Pneumatic Compression

Three studies have directly compared low-dose heparin and intermittent pneumatic compression in gynecologic surgery. Jobson and colleagues[67] reported intermittent pneumatic compression to be superior to low-dose heparin in a randomized trial of 330 patients undergoing major gynecologic surgical procedures. The clinical endpoint was the diagnosis of symptomatic pulmonary emboli. Of 164 patients in the low-dose heparin group, 7 developed postoperative pulmonary emboli, including two that were fatal. None of the 139 patients with intermittent pneumatic compression prophylaxis developed pulmonary emboli ($P = .006$). This large trial would have been more significant had a prospective method been used to screen all patients for postoperative deep venous thrombosis or pulmonary emboli. Without such prospective screening, one might argue that bias in the clinical detection of pulmonary emboli may have occurred.

In a smaller group of gynecologic surgery patients, Borow and Goldson found the incidence of ^{125}I-fibrinogen–detected thrombi to be lower in an intermittent pneumatic compression treatment group (9.1%) than in the untreated control group (16.6%).[68] However, there was no statistical difference in the incidence of deep venous thrombosis between the intermittent pneumatic compression– and low-dose heparin–treated groups.

My associates and I have reported a trial that compared low-dose heparin and intermittent pneumatic compression in a group of high-risk gynecologic oncology surgery patients.[39] Based on the results of prior trials,[37, 62] they used a low-dose heparin regimen of 5000 units every 8 hours for three doses preoperatively and for 7 days postoperatively. Intermittent pneumatic compression was started intraoperatively and continued for 5 days postoperatively. Surveillance for deep venous thrombosis was performed by the ^{125}I-fibrinogen scanning method. The incidence of deep venous thrombosis was not significantly different between the two groups. However, the postoperative transfusion requirements, the number of patients with prolonged partial thromboplastin times, and the retroperitoneal suction drainage volume were significantly increased in the low-dose heparin group. It was concluded that although both methods may be effective to prevent deep venous thrombosis in this high-risk patient group, intermittent pneumatic compression was superior because of its lack of significant side effects.

Combination Prophylaxis

Most prophylactic techniques achieve efficacy through addressing one arm of Virchow's triad: hypercoagulability, venous stasis, or endothelial injury. Combining prophylactic techniques, therefore, might result in even further reduction of thromboembolic complications. The results of trials of combined prophylaxis are reviewed by Wille-Jorgensen.[69] In general, combined techniques result in better prophylaxis, especially in high-risk patients. However, any advantage is gained at an increased cost. In a detailed analysis of cost-effectiveness, Oster and colleagues found that the combination of intermittent pneumatic compression and graduated compression stockings would be the most effective and least expensive of the combination therapies available.[70]

REFERENCES

1. Jeffcoate TNA, Tindall VR. Venous thrombosis and embolism in obstetrics and gynecology. Aust NZ J Obstet Gynaecol 1965;5:119–130.
2. Kimball AM, Hallum AV, Cates W. Deaths caused by pulmonary thromboembolism after legally induced abortion. Am J Obstet Gynecol 1978;132:169–174.
3. Clarke-Pearson DL, Jelovsek FR, Creasman WT. Thromboembolism complicating surgery for cervical and uterine malignancy: incidence, risk factors and prophylaxis. Obstet Gynecol 1983;61:87–94.
4. Creasman WT, Weed JC Jr. Radical hysterectomy. In: Schaefer G, Graber EA, eds. Complications in Obstetrics and Gynecologic Surgery. Hagerstown, MD, Harper & Row, 1981, pp 389–398.
5. Venesmaa P, Ylikorkala O. Morbidity and mortality associated with primary and repeat operations for ovarian cancer. Obstet Gynecol 1992; 79:168–172.
6. Ballard M, Bradley-Watson PJ, Johnstone ED, et al. Low doses of subcutaneous heparin in the prevention of deep venous thrombosis after gynecologic surgery. J Obstet Gynaecol Br Commonw 1973;80:469–472.
7. Taberner DA, Poller L, Burnstein RW, et al. Oral anticoagulants controlled by British comparative thromboplastin versus low dose heparin prophylaxis of deep venous thrombosis. Br Med J 1978;1:272–274.
8. Walsh JJ, Bonnar J, Wright FW. A study of pulmonary embolism and deep leg thrombosis after major gynecologic surgery using labeled fibrinogen phlebography and lung scanning. J Obstet Gynaecol Br Commonw 1974;81:311–315.
9. Crandon AJ, Koutts J. Incidence of post-operative deep vein thrombosis in gynecologic oncology. Aust NZ J Obstet Gynecol 1983;23:216–219.
10. Goldhaber SZ, Morpurgo M, for the WHO/ISFC Task Force on Pulmonary Embolism. Diagnosis, treatment, and prevention of pulmonary embolism. JAMA 1992;268:1727–1733.
11. Clarke-Pearson DL, DeLong ER, Synan IS, et al. Variables associated with postoperative deep venous thrombosis: a prospective study of 411 gynecology patients and creation of a prognostic model. Obstet Gynecol 1987;69:146–150.
12. Clayton JK, Anderson JA, McNicol GP. Preoperative prediction of postoperative deep venous thrombosis. Br Med J 1976;2:910–916.
13. Crandon AJ, Peel KR, Anderson JA, et al. Prophylaxis of postoperative deep venous thrombosis: selective use of low-dose heparin in high-risk patients. BMJ 1980;2:345–347.
14. Kakkar VV, Flanc C, Howe C, et al. Natural history of postoperative deep vein thrombosis. Lancet 1968; 2:230–233.
15. Nicolaides AN, O'Connell JD. Origin and distribution of thrombi in patients presenting with clinical venous thrombosis. In: Nicolaides AN, ed. Thromboembolism: Etiology, Advances in Prevention and Management. Baltimore: University Park Press, 1975, pp 167–180.
16. Clarke-Pearson DL, Synan IS, Coleman RE, et al. The natural history of postoperative venous thromboembolism in gynecologic oncology: a prospective study of 382 patients. Am J Obstet Gynecol 1984;148:1051–1054.
17. Doouss TW. The clinical significance of venous thrombosis of the calf. Br J Surg 1976;63:377–378.
18. Moser KM, DeMoine JR. Is embolic risk conditioned by location of deep venous thrombosis? Ann Intern Med 1981;94:439–444.
19. Clarke-Pearson DL, Coleman RE, Petry N, et al. Postoperative pelvic vein thrombosis and pulmonary embolism detected by indium-111–labeled platelet imaging: a case report. Am J Obstet Gynecol 1984; 149:796–798.
20. Clarke-Pearson DL, Coleman RE, Siegel R, et al. [111]Indium-labeled platelet imaging for the detection of deep venous thrombosis and pulmonary embolism in pa-

tients without symptoms after surgery. Surgery 1985;98:98–103.

21. Haegger K. Problems of acute deep vein thrombosis. Angiology 1968;20:219.

22. Palko PA, Namson EM, Fedonik SO. The early detection of deep venous thrombosis using ^{131}I-tagged fibrinogen. Can J Surg 1964;7:215.

23. Athanasoulis CA. Phlebography for the diagnosis of deep leg vein thrombosis, prophylactic therapy of deep venous thrombosis and pulmonary embolism. DHEW publication No. (NIH) 76-866, Washington, DC, US Government Printing Office, 1975.

24. Wheeler HB, O'Donnell JA, Anderson FA. Occlusive cuff impedance phlebography: a diagnostic procedure for venous thrombosis and pulmonary embolism. Prog Cardiovasc Dis 1974;17:199–204.

25. Clarke-Pearson DL, Creasman WT. Diagnosis of deep vein thrombosis in obstetrics and gynecology by impedance phlebography. Obstet Gynecol 1981;58:52.

26. Yao JST, Gourmos C, Hobbs JT. Detection of proximal vein thrombosis by Doppler ultrasound flow-detection method. Lancet 1972;1:1.

27. Anthonie WA, Lensing MD, Paolo P, et al. Detection of deep-vein thrombosis by real-time B-mode ultrasonography. N Engl J Med 1989;320:342.

28. Mintz MC, Levy DW, Axel L, et al. Puerperal ovarian vein thrombosis: MR diagnosis. AJR 1987;149:1273.

29. Clarke-Pearson DL, Synan IS, Creasman WT. Anticoagulation therapy for venous thromboembolism in patients with gynecologic malignancy. Am J Obstet Gynecol 147:369, 1983.

30. Moser KM, Fedullo PR. Venous thromboembolism: three simple decisions. Chest 1983;83:246.

31. Hull RD, Raskob GE, Rosenbloom D, et al. Heparin for 5 days as compared with 10 days in the initial treatment of proximal venous thrombosis. N Engl J Med 1990;322:1260.

32. Bell WR, Royal RM. Heparin induced thrombocytopenia: a comparison of three heparin regimens. N Engl J Med 1980;303:902.

33. Kakkar VV. Prevention of fatal postoperative pulmonary embolism by low-dose heparin: an international multicenter trial. Lancet 1975;2:45–51.

34. Collins R, Scrimgeour A, Yusuf S, et al. Reduction in fatal pulmonary embolism and venous thrombosis by perioperative administration of subcutaneous heparin. N Engl J Med 1988; 318:1162–1173.

35. Clagett GF, Reisch JS. Prevention of venous thromboembolism in general surgical patients: results of meta-analysis. Ann Surg 1988; 208:227–240.

36. Clarke-Pearson DL, Coleman RE, Synan IS, et al. Venous thromboembolism prophylaxis in gynecologic oncology: a prospective controlled trial of low-dose heparin. Am J Obstet Gynecol 1983;145:606–613.

37. Clarke-Pearson DL, DeLong ER, Synan IS, et al. A controlled trial of two low-dose heparin regimens for the prevention of deep vein thrombosis. Obstet Gynecol 1990;75:684–689.

38. Clarke-Pearson DL, DeLong ER, Synan IS, et al. Complications of low-dose heparin prophylaxis in gynecologic oncology surgery. Obstet Gynecol 1984;64:689–695.

39. Clarke-Pearson DL, Synan IS, Dodge R, et al. A randomized trial of low-dose heparin and intermittent pneumatic calf compression for the prevention of deep venous thrombosis following gynecologic oncology surgery. Am J Obstet Gynecol 1993;168:1146–1153.

40. Gurewich V, Numm T, Thazhathekudyil T, et al. Hemostatic effect of uniform, low-dose subcutaneous heparin in surgical patients. Arch Intern Med 1978; 138:41–46.

41. Galle PC, Muss HB, McGrath KM, et al. Thrombocytopenia in two patients treated with low-dose heparin. Obstet Gynecol 1978;52:95–99.

42. Catalona WJ, Kadmon D, Crane DB. Effect of minidose heparin on lymphocele formation following extraperitoneal pelvic lymphadenectomy. J Urol 1979;123:890–894.

43. Piver MS, Malfetano JH, Lele SB, et al. Prophylactic anticoagulation as a possible cause of inguinal lymphocyst after radical vulvectomy and inguinal lymphadenectomy. Obstet Gynecol 1983;62:17–21.

44. Jorgensen LN, Wille-Jorgensen P, Hauch O. Prophylaxis of postoperative thromboembolism with low molecular weight heparin. Br J Surg 1993;80:689–704.

45. Fricker J-P, Vergues Y, Schach R. Low-dose heparin versus low-molecular weight heparin (Kabi 2165, Fragmin) in the prophylaxis of thromboembolic complications of abdominal oncological surgery. Eur J Clin Invest 1988;18:561–567.

46. Borstad E, Urdal K, Handeland G, Abildgaard U. Comparison of low molecular weight heparin vs. unfractionated heparin in gynecological surgery. Acta Obstet Gynecol Scand 1988;67:99–103.

47. Carter CA, Skoutakis VA, Spiro TE, et al. Enoxaparin: the low-molecular-weight heparin for prevention of postoperative thromboembolic complications. Ann Pharmacol 1993;27:1223–1230.

48. Conti S, Daschback M. Venous thromboembolism prophylaxis: a survey of its use in the United States. Arch Surg 1982;117:1036–1040.

49. Browse NL, Jackson BT, Maye ME, et al. The value of mechanical methods of preventing postoperative calf vein thrombosis. Br J Surg 1974;60:319–323.

50. Rosengarten DS, Laird J, Jeyasingh K, et al. The failure of compression stocking (Turbigrip) to prevent deep venous thrombosis after operation. Br J Surg 1970; 57:296–299.

51. Sigel B, Edelstein AL, Savitch L, et al. Type of compression for reducing venous stasis. Arch Surg 1975; 110:171–175.

52. Lawrence D, Kakkar VV. Graduated, static, external compression of the lower limb: a physiological assessment. Br J Surg 1980;67:119–121.

53. Wells PS, Lensing AWA, Hirsh J. Graduated compression stockings in the prevention of postoperative venous thromboembolism: a meta-analysis. Arch Intern Med 1994;154:67–72.

54. Turner GM, Cole SE, Brooks JH. The efficacy of graduated compression stockings in the prevention of postoperative deep venous thrombosis after major gynecologic surgery. Br J Obstet Gynaecol 1984;91:588–591.

55. Guyton DP, Khayat A, Schreiber H. Pneumatic compression stockings and prostaglandin synthesis: a pathway of fibrinolysis. Crit Care Med 1985;13:266–269.

56. Saltzman EW, McNanama GP, Shapiro AH, et al. Effect of optimization of hemodynamics on fibrinolytic activity and antithrombotic efficacy of external pneumatic calf compression. Ann Surg 1987;206:636–641.

57. Roberts VC, Cotton LT. Prevention of postoperative deep venous thrombosis in patients with malignant disease. BMJ 1974;1:358–360.

58. Salzman EW, Ploet J, Bettlemann M, et al. Intraoperative external pneumatic calf compression to afford long-term prophylaxis against deep vein thrombosis in urological patients. Surgery 1980;87:239–242.

59. Nicholaides AN, Fernandes e Fernandes J, et al. Intermittent sequential pneumatic compression of the legs in the prevention of venous stasis and postoperative deep venous thrombosis. Surgery 1980;87:69–76.

60. Turpie AGG, Gallus AS, Beattie WS, et al. Prevention of venous thrombosis in patients with intracranial dis-

ease by intermittent pneumatic compression of the calf. Neurology 1977;27:435–438.

61. Turpie AGG, Delmore T, Hirsh J, et al. Prevention of venous thrombosis by intermittent sequential calf compression in patients with intracranial disease. Thromb Res 1979;15:611–615.

62. Clarke-Pearson DL, Synan IS, Hinshaw W, et al. Prevention of postoperative venous thromboembolism by external pneumatic calf compression in patients with gynecologic malignancy. Obstet Gynecol 1984;63:92–98.

63. Clarke-Pearson DL, Creasman WT, Coleman RE, et al. Perioperative external pneumatic calf compression as thromboembolism prophylaxis in gynecologic oncology: report of a randomized controlled trial. Gynecol Oncol 1984;18:226–230.

64. Salzman W, Davies GC. Prophylaxis of venous thromboembolism: analysis of cost effectiveness. Ann Surg 1980;191:207–218.

65. Cohen JR, Grella L, Citron M. Greenfield filter instead of heparin as primary treatment for deep venous thrombosis or pulmonary embolism in patients with cancer. Cancer 1994;70:1993–1996.

66. Heaps J, Lagasse LD. Use of the inferior vena cava clip in patients at high risk of pulmonary embolism. Gynecol Oncol 1990;39:227–231.

67. Jobson VW, Homesley HD, Welander CE. Comparison of heparin and intermittent calf compression for prevention of pulmonary embolism. Gynecol Oncol 1983;15:143–146.

68. Borow M, Goldson H. Postoperative venous thrombosis: evaluation of five methods of treatment. Am J Surg 1981;141:245–251.

69. Wille-Jorgensen P. Prophylaxis of postoperative thromboembolism with combined methods. Semin Thromb Hemost 1991;17:272–279.

70. Oster G, Tuden RL, Colditz GA. Prevention of venous thromboembolism after general surgery: cost-effectiveness analysis of alternative approaches to prophylaxis. Am J Med 1987;82:889–899.

15

Vicki V. Baker

CHAPTER

Management of Wound Complications

Even with detailed attention to perioperative care and optimization of the patient's medical condition, wound complications occasionally occur after gynecologic surgery. Wound complications are a significant cause of postoperative morbidity that contribute to prolongation of the hospitalization, the cost of patient care, and patient anxiety and distress.

Review of the recent literature reveals marked variation in the incidence of wound complications after gynecologic surgery. Confounding variables such as comorbid illness, obesity, complexity of the surgical case, duration of surgery, experience of the surgeon, and differences in patient populations are not consistently dealt with and undoubtedly contribute to this variation.

FACTORS THAT INFLUENCE WOUND HEALING

A number of factors have been identified that influence the likelihood of wound complications after surgery (Table 15–1). Systemic factors include obesity, small vessel disease, anemia, malnutrition, infection at a site remote from the surgical site, and cancer. Interestingly, treatment with combination chemotherapy has not been conclusively demonstrated to adversely affect wound healing.[1]

Nutritional deficiencies also influence wound healing. The adverse effects of protein–calorie malnutrition (marasmus) are readily apparent,

TABLE 15–1
Factors That Increase the Likelihood of Wound Complications After Surgery

Systemic Factors

Obesity
Small vessel disease (secondary to hypertension, aging, prior radiation therapy)
Anemia
Malnutrition
Infection
Cancer

Surgical Factors

Excessive use of cautery
Tissue trauma
Excessive suture tension

Postoperative Factors

Abdominal distention
Vomiting
Coughing
Straining
Seroma/hematoma
Wound infection

but the contribution of micronutrient deficiencies may be overlooked. Vitamin C plays a role in maintaining capillary wall integrity. Vitamin A counteracts the effects of corticosteroids on wound healing. The B complex of vitamins permits the effective cross-linking of collagen fibers required for the progressive increase in tensile strength of a healing incision. Iron supports oxygen transport and is a cofactor for collagen synthesis. Zinc, which can be quickly depleted by stress, small bowel fistula drainage, and weight loss, is a cofactor for collagen formation and protein synthesis. Tissue deficiencies of one or more micronutrients may predispose to postoperative wound complications, although clinical data are limited.

Factors related to surgery also influence the likelihood of postoperative wound complications. Operative procedures that require more than 2 hours to complete and the number of units of blood administered have been associated with an increased risk of wound complications. Although anecdotal experience may suggest otherwise, the *method* of wound closure per se is not a predictor of wound complications. Both internal retention and single-layer continuous en bloc closures appear comparable in terms of the likelihood of wound infection, immediate postoperative disruption, and herniation.[2, 3] In contradistinction, *surgical technique* is an important determinant of both immediate and delayed wound complications. Excessive use of the cautery, which results in thermal injury of normal tissue, should be avoided. Wounds should not be closed under excessive tension. Israelsson and Jonsson have shown that the best long-term wound healing results are achieved when the suture to incision length ratio is greater than 4.[4] This ratio reflects the size of the tissue bites, the distance between bites, and the tension of the closure. A ratio less than 4 is associated with a 2.5-fold higher incidence of hernia as compared with wounds closed with a suture to wound length ratio greater than 4.

Postoperative factors that influence the occurrence of wound complications include abdominal distention, vomiting, vigorous coughing, straining (prolonged Valsalva), wound seroma, hematoma, and infection of the incision.

NORMAL WOUND HEALING

Regardless of the severity of the injury or the anatomic location, wounds heal in only one of two ways: regeneration or connective tissue repair. The type of repair is influenced by the type of the tissue that has been injured and the ability of the injured tissue to regenerate. Wounds limited to the epithelium and dermal layers heal by regeneration. Wounds that extend through the dermis, such as gynecologic surgical incisions, heal by replacement.

Like any full-thickness wound, abdominal surgical incisions exhibit three distinct yet overlapping phases of healing. In wounds that are closed primarily, these phases are not necessarily obvious as discrete events on physical examination. The *inflammatory phase* involves hemostasis and inflammation. The overall result is control of bleeding and the establishment of a clean wound bed. In a clean wound, this phase lasts for 3 to 5 days.

The *proliferative* or *fibroblastic phase* occurs next and is characterized by filling in of the wound defect with new connective tissue and covering of the wound with epithelium. In wounds that have been closed primarily, minimal tissue synthesis is required. In wounds that heal by secondary intention, this phase is marked by the appearance of granulation tissue. Granulation tissue is composed primarily of capillaries, which explains its red color and propensity to bleed after minimal surface trauma.

After the appearance of granulation tissue, the wound begins to epithelialize. Epithelialization involves the proliferation and migration of epithelial cells from the skin edges to resurface the wound defect. A moist, warm, uninfected environment is necessary for epithelial cell migration. Conditions that promote drying of the wound retard healing.

The *maturation phase* of wound healing occurs after completion of connective tissue synthesis and epithelial cell migration. With normal wound healing, a ridge of induration surrounding the incision is normally palpated on the sixth through the tenth postoperative days. This reflects the accumulation of collagen. The absence of a palpable ridge of indurated tissue indicates an increased risk of superficial wound separation.

The maturation phase of wound healing continues for up to 1 year or even longer after injury. Collagen maturation and remodeling provide strength to the scar. The erythema of a recent scar fades with time because the capillaries that once supplied oxygen and nutrients to the healing wound are no longer needed.

POSTOPERATIVE WOUND CARE

After primary closure of the surgical incision, a dressing is applied. The purpose of this dressing is to absorb drainage, maintain a sterile environment, and serve as a barrier to trauma. A nonadherent, absorptive dressing should be used. Gauze is not a good dressing material because it becomes incorporated into the suture line as the exudate dries, and it may damage the epithelium when it is removed. Ideally, a sterile, dry bandage should remain in place for approximately 48 hours. This allows for uninterrupted epithelial cell migration, which in turn decreases the likelihood of bacterial contamination and infection.

Skin clips are removed when epithelial migration across the incision is complete. Premature removal can result in superficial wound separation and a wide scar. Delayed skin clip removal can result in a "railroad track" scar as a consequence of epithelial downgrowth into the skin clip puncture sites.

After removal of the skin clips, Steri-strips are placed on the incision. Pepicello and Yavorek have suggested that Steri-strips can be used in place of skin clips.[5] The wound infection rate was 1.4%, and the advantages of this method of skin reapproximation include the absence of foreign body granulomas and superficial cellulitis.

Normal wound healing is an orderly process that follows a typical time course. An increase in incisional pain, peri-incisional erythema, drainage, or an elevated temperature suggests the possibility of a wound complication. Recognition of an impending wound complication is important to obviate more serious complications that may, in turn, result in prolonged hospitalization, increased health care costs, and potential disability.

POSTOPERATIVE WOUND COMPLICATIONS

Postoperative wound complications may be categorized in a number of ways. Overlap is common, and one type of complication is often associated or predisposes to another. The three most common postoperative wound complications encountered by the gynecologist are superficial separation, dehiscence, and infection. Hernia formation and excessive scarring are delayed wound complications and are not discussed.

Superficial wound separation refers to separation of the skin and subcutaneous tissue to varying depths. By definition, the fascia is intact in a superficial wound separation. This complication may be a consequence of hematoma, seroma, premature removal of the skin clips, excessive distracting forces on the wound edges, and/or infection.

Soisson and associates have reported that use of subcutaneous sutures for wounds that are greater than 5 cm in depth will decrease the occurrence of superficial separation.[6] Approximation of Camper fascia in patients who have had a cesarean section has been associated with a statistically significant reduction in the occurrence of superficial wound separation.[7]

Wound dehiscence refers to separation of the fascia with variable separation of the superficial tissues. It is an uncommon complication with an overall incidence of less than 1% in large series.[8] Many factors have been identified that increase the likelihood of dehiscence (Table 15–2). These factors, alone or in combination, contribute to ischemia and necrosis of the fascia. Interestingly, the type of incision, type of closure, presence of diabetes, and anemia have not been uniformly identified as contributing risk factors.[9]

The sentinel warning sign of fascial dehiscence is serosanguineous drainage from the wound after the first postoperative day. Occasionally, the diagnosis is delayed until the skin clips are removed, at which time the skin separates. Omentum and occasionally small bowel are visible and may eviscerate above the level of the fascia. When the superficial tissues do not separate, the patient is left with a large ventral hernia.

When dehiscence is diagnosed, the wound should be immediately covered with sterile bandages and arrangements made to return the patient to the operating room as soon as possible. After suitable anesthesia, the wound

TABLE 15–2
Factors That Increase the Risk of Wound Dehiscence

Age greater than 65
Wound infection
Pulmonary disease
Hemodynamic instability
Ostomy in the incision
Hypoproteinemia
Systemic infection
Obesity
Uremia
Malnutrition
Cancer
Ascites
Corticosteroid use
Hypertension
Excessive tension on the suture line
Sutures placed within 0.5 cm of the cut fascial edge

should be carefully explored. Any devitalized tissue should be sharply debrided. The fascial margins are often ischemic or frankly necrotic and should be excised. Irrigation of the wound to remove bacteria and adherent, nonviable tissue should be performed.

Several techniques have been described for the reapproximation of a wound dehiscence. The muscle and fascia can be reapproximated with interrupted figure-of-eight sutures, although many surgeons prefer some type of retention closure. The internal retention Smead-Jones closure or through-and-through external retention closure using permanent, monofilament suture offers comparable short-term and long-term results.

Postoperative ileus and ascites may cause excessive abdominal distention that causes dehiscence of the incision. Direct reapproximation of the fascia in this situation may result in a significant increase in intra-abdominal pressure. Significant elevations of intra-abdominal pressure may cause respiratory compromise, decreased cardiac output, oliguria, decreased blood flow to the mesenteric and splanchnic beds, and decreased blood flow to the anterior abdominal wall. The association between elevated intra-abdominal pressure and these pathophysiologic effects is referred to the abdominal compartment syndrome.[10–12] When direct reapproximation of the fascia will result in excessive tension on the suture line or if the patient is at risk of developing the abdominal compartment syndrome, mesh closure should be considered. Mesh closures allow for the egress of peritoneal fluid and permits closure of the wound without undue tension on the suture line.

The use of both absorbable and nonabsorbable mesh has been described.[13–15] The mesh is sutured to the fascial edge using running or interrupted number 1 polypropylene suture. Potential problems with the use of permanent mesh material include enterocutaneous fistula formation and foreign body reaction. Absorbable mesh is less likely to cause these problems, but the incidence of late hernia formation is much greater.

An alternative to the mesh closure has been described by Saxe and associates.[16] These investigators used an abdominal wall pack technique for delayed wound closure for those circumstances in which massive distention precluded a more conventional closure. Sutures of number 2 nylon were placed through the abdominal wall at least 4 cm from the cut fascial edge and no more than 2 cm apart. An effort was made to place these sutures extraperitoneally. The exposed viscera were covered with rayon gauze, which was covered by fluff gauze. The retention sutures were tied with minimal tension. The wound packing was covered with burn gauze to absorb the serous drainage and was changed as needed to keep the dressing dry. In 3 to 4 days, the patient was returned to the operating room after the intestinal distention had resolved and wound closure could be accomplished without placing excessive tension on the retention sutures. If abdominal closure could not be achieved because of continued distention, the rayon gauze packing and retention sutures were replaced and attempted closure was considered in the subsequent 72 hours.

Infection is the most common reported wound complication and is often the cause of wound disruption and herniation. The diagnosis of a wound infection is obvious in the presence of erythema, purulent drainage, leukocytosis, and fever. However, the immunocompromised host may not exhibit these signs and prolonged wound healing may be the only indication of infection.

Bacteroides species are the most common anaerobes that infect necrotic wounds. In the absence of nonviable tissues, *Pseudomonas* and *Staphylococcus aureus* are the most common wound pathogens.

The likelihood of a clinical wound infection is influenced by the balance between colony count and local host resistance. In general, more than 10,000 organisms per gram of tissue are necessary for the clinical diagnosis of a wound infection. However, wound infection secondary to beta-hemolytic streptococci warrants specific mention. This organism is particularly virulent and causes wound infection at a much lower innoculum than other organisms such as *Staphylococcus*, *Bacteroides*, and *Pseudomonas*. Wound infection secondary to beta-hemolytic streptococci causes incisional pain that is out of proportion to the findings on physical examination. Bullae and superficial erythema of the surrounding skin are late findings and are invariably accompanied by signs of systemic sepsis. Prompt recognition and intravenous penicillin are crucial therapeutic interventions. Wound debridement to remove necrotic tissue and permit drainage of tissue edema fluid is an important adjunct.

Postoperative bacterial gangrene presents as a wound that is edematous, erythematous, and tender that progresses to central necrosis with a surrounding margin of erythematous tissue. The patient is febrile and appears toxic. The treatment includes broad-spectrum antibiotics

followed by excision of the necrotic tissue and debridement to healthy tissue. The wound is left open to establish a bed of healthy granulation tissue before grafting.

Necrotizing fasciitis may be clostridial or nonclostridial although the clinical presentations are similar. This condition is most commonly seen in the gynecology patient who is a diabetic and presents with a Bartholin gland abscess, although it has been reported after abdominal and perineal surgery.[17] The wound exhibits crepitus on palpation and edema that extends *beyond* the area of erythema (unlike postoperative bacterial gangrene). The fascia is gray and necrotic, but there is little purulent drainage or blood in the wound. Radiographs exhibit soft tissue gas, and clinical studies reveal markedly elevated creatine phosphokinase and lactate dehydrogenase values. Necrotizing fasciitis is a life-threatening condition that requires prompt recognition, vigorous hydration, broad-spectrum antibiotic coverage, and aggressive surgical resection of the involved tissues.

CLINICAL MANAGEMENT OF WOUND COMPLICATIONS

Regardless of the type of wound complication, the fundamental management strategy is to reduce or eliminate factors that delay healing (Table 15–3). Systemic factors must be addressed in parallel with local wound factors. The patient's cardiorespiratory function, nutritional status, and fluid status must be optimized. The local environment of the incision must be restored to normal so that it supports and facilitates the wound healing process. The

TABLE 15-3
Basic Strategies for the Management of Postoperative Wound Complications

Reduce or eliminate causative factors
    Correct anemia
    Eliminate excess moisture
Provide systemic support
    Nutritional supplementation if indicated
    Adequate hydration
    Optimize general medical condition
Provide topical therapy
    Debride necrotic and nonviable tissue
    Eliminate infection
    Obliterate dead space
    Remove exudate but maintain moist environment
    Maintain wound surface temperature

TABLE 15–4
Antiseptic Solutions That May Be Used for Topical Wound Care

Solution	Indications	Precautions
Dakin's solution (0.25%)	Dissolves necrotic tissue	Toxic to fibroblasts—cytotoxic
	Kills *Streptococcus* and *Staphylococcus*	May damage normal skin (irritating)
Betadine (1% povidone-iodine)		Toxic to fibroblasts—cytotoxic
		Questionable effectiveness in infected wounds
		Stains tissues
		May cause iodine toxicity if used over large surface
Acetic acid	Effective against *Pseudomonas*	Toxic to fibroblasts
Chlorhexidine	Good for yeast and mold	Cytotoxic and allergenic
Topical antibiotics	Antimicrobial	Allergenic
	Not cytotoxic	
Sulfadiazine	Broad-spectrum antimicrobial	Cytotoxic
Hydrogen peroxide	Provides some degree of mechanical debridement	Can ulcerate granulation tissue
		Toxic to fibroblasts
		Can mimic gas gangrene when forceful irrigation causes subcutaneous emphysema
		May cause allergies

optimal local wound environment is one that is clean, moist, and warm.

Debridement

Debridement of necrotic and nonviable tissue is the first step in eradicating infection from the wound. After aggressive but not indiscriminate debridement, the wound should then be irrigated with normal saline to further decrease the bacterial count. Irrigation using a 20-mL syringe and 16-gauge needle or a Water Pik provides sufficient hydrostatic pressure to dislodge adherent bacteria and residual necrotic tissue. Bulb syringe irrigation is of little efficacy as a means to debride a wound.

Wet to dry dressings are also used to assist initial wound debridement. These dressings should be changed three to four times every 24 hours. Each time the dry dressing is removed, the adherent fibrinous debris from the wound is also removed. However, the *prolonged* use of wet to dry dressings results in desiccation of the wound microenvironment and normal healing is delayed. For this reason, wet to dry dressings should be used only for a brief period of time followed by the application of wound dressings that optimize the local wound environment.

Control of Infection

Once the wound has been mechanically debrided and the gross infection removed, the selective use of surfactant cleansers or topical antiseptics may be indicated depending on the severity of the complication. The wound can be packed with gauze soaked in one of a number of solutions to minimize wound bacterial colonization (Table 15–4). Most of the agents, including povidone-iodine, chlorhexidene, acetic acid, hydrogen peroxide, and Dakin's solution, inhibit fibroblast proliferation and should only be used until infection is controlled and evidence of granulation tissue is apparent. At this point, saline-soaked wet-to-wet gauze packing of the wound works well. The prolonged use of these solutions should be avoided because there are data to suggest that they are toxic to fibroblasts.[18]

The role of topical antibiotics in eradicating wound infection has not been established. Antibiotics that do not interfere with wound healing include silvadene, polysporin, neosporin, benzoyl peroxide, and bacitracin. In animal models, silver sulfadiazine and mafenide acetate impede wound contraction.[19]

Support of the Local Wound Environment

The choice of wound dressing is equally important to the type of cleansing regimen. The incision dressing should maintain a moist and warm local wound environment. Excessively moist wounds do not heal normally. Wound exudates macerate surrounding healthy skin, dilute wound healing factors and nutrients that are present at the wound surface, and provide an excellent culture media for bacterial infection. Dead space in the wound exacerbates this problem by allowing the accumulation of exudate. At the other end of the spectrum, dry wounds do not heal normally. Desiccation of the wound surface and crust formation delay the appearance of granulation tissue and retard epithelial cell migration.

Thermal insulation of the wound is also important. Maintenance of a normal wound temperature improves blood flow and enhances epidermal migration.

Unfortunately, there is no single dressing material that is uniformly applicable. The surgeon must assess the need for debridement, the presence or absence of infection, the presence of dead space, and the amount of exudate. The dressing that best addresses all of these factors simultaneously is then chosen.

Perhaps the most familiar dressing used for an uncomplicated superficial wound separation is wet-to-dry gauze packing. With this dressing, gauze is moistened with normal saline, packed lightly into the incision to obliterate dead space, and removed and replaced after it dries. From the perspective of wound healing, a wet-to-dry dressing is one of the least desirable management strategies. Allowing the gauze to dry ensures that it will stick to the granulation tissue and subsequently disrupt it when the dressing is changed. In contra-

distinction, moist gauze packing that is removed and changed before it dries is of benefit by maintaining a moist, warm environment in a wound that is healing by secondary intention.

Occasionally, straight-forward interventions such as wet-to-wet gauze packing and tissue debridement are not effective and other products should be used. There are a number of commercial dressings available for the management of complicated wounds (Table 15–5).

Transparent adhesive dressings are semipermeable membranes that permit gaseous exchange between the wound bed and the atmosphere but prevent bacterial invasion because of the membrane pore size. Their transparency permits visual monitoring of wound healing without requiring removal of the dressing. However, these dressings are nonabsorptive, and a fluid environment over the wound is rapidly created and maintained in the presence of an exudate. A border of dry skin is necessary for a secure seal. The frequency of dressing changes is based on the accumulation of exudate or loss of the dressing seal.

Hydrocolloid water dressings contain hydroactive particles in a matrix that can be molded to fit the wound. These dressings maintain a moist wound environment and insulate the wound. The edges of the dressing are secured with tape. The dressing is changed every 3 to 5 days. A yellow, malodorous exudate is usually

TABLE 15–5
Wound Dressings That Are Commercially Available for Managing Complicated Wounds

Dressing Type	Examples	Indications	Contraindications
Transparent adhesive	OpSite, Tegaderm	Partial-thickness wounds, dry necrotic wounds that require debridement	Exudative wounds, wounds with sinus tracts, friable skin margins
Hydrocolloid wafer dressing	DuoDerm, Intrasite, Tegasorb	Partial-thickness wounds, venous ulcers, granulating wounds with moderate exudate at most	Heavy exudate, sinus tracts, infection
Absorption dressing	Sorbsan, DuoDerm paste, Debrisan	Moderate to heavy exudate, sinus tracts, necrosis	Minimal exudate present, dry eschar that must be debrided, partial thickness wounds
Synthetic barrier dressing	Hydron	Partial-thickness wound full-thickness wound with exudate	Wounds with dry eschar or sinus tracts
Gel dressing	Vigilon, Intrasite gel	Partial-thickness wound, full-thickness wound	None
Gauze		Exudates, dead space, sinus tracts, combination of exudate and necrotic tissue	Partial-thickness wound, dry wound with necrotic tissue

present when the dressing is removed. Most of these dressings are occlusive and do not permit oxygen diffusion to the wound surface. However, these dressings do prevent secondary infection and are associated with reduced infection rates when compared with conventional dressings. This type of dressing should not be used in the presence of infection.

Nonadhesive semipermeable polyurethane foam dressings are nonadherent wafers with hydrophobic surfaces that absorb exudate from the wound. They are useful in the management of full-thickness, deep wounds that have moderate amounts of exudate.

Absorption dressings are designed for wounds with large amounts of exudate. These dressings include copolymer starch dressings, Dextran bead dressings, and calcium alginate dressings. Because they are packed into the wound, they also eliminate dead space and are especially useful when sinus tracts are present. These dressings require a cover dressing to provide protection from external contamination and to provide insulation.

Gauze dressing creates a dry environment and is generally contraindicated for this reason. However, it is useful as an absorbant of exudate and as a way to fill sinus tracts. Mesh gauze rather than cotton-filled sponges should be placed against the wound surface. In addition, fine mesh is preferable to coarse mesh because there is less damage to the epithelium when the dressing is changed.

Gel barriers are used to maintain moist wound environments.

Synthetic barrier dressings are designed to absorb exudate and maintain a moist environment. When mixed, these dressings form a paste that conforms to the wound contour.

The care of normal skin surrounding an infected wound must also be considered. Stripping of the epithelial surface often occurs in patients who require prolonged wound care as tape dressings are frequently applied and removed. To minimize this problem, porous tape should be applied without tension. Alternatively, wound dressings can be secured with roll gauze, tubular stockinette, or Montgomery straps. Skin sealants or solid-wafer skin barriers can also be placed on the skin and tape placed on the barrier to secure the dressing.

When satisfactory healing has been restored, the wound can be secondarily closed.[20, 21] Wounds should not be secondarily closed until the bacterial count is reduced to less than 10,000 organisms per gram of tissue. Attempts to close wounds before a reduction in bacterial count are associated with failure in over 75% of cases. Conversely, wound closure is successful in over 90% of cases when the bacterial counts are reduced below the critical threshold of 10,000 organisms per gram of tissue.[22] An exception to this generalization is made for wound infections due to beta-hemolytic streptococci. Because this is such a virulent organism, wound closure should not be attempted until the wound is culture negative.

When delayed closure is not an option, continued attention to the local wound environment will permit healing by secondary intention. When this occurs, the wound undergoes contracture, pulling the surrounding skin toward the center of the defect. As wound contracture occurs, granulation tissue fills the defect. The speed with which wounds heal by secondary intention is influenced by many factors. The logarithm of wound area is an important determinant.[23] Other factors that influence wound healing time include wound depth, location, and skin temperature. The shape of the wound per se is not an important determinant of healing time. Other factors being comparable, healing time is influenced by the diameter of the largest circle that can be contained within the wound margins (Fig. 15–1).

Hyperbaric Oxygen Therapy

The amount of oxygen delivered to the tissues can be increased by increasing the amount of oxygen dissolved in the plasma when patients breathe 100% oxygen under conditions of in-

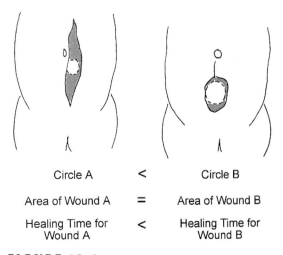

Circle A	<	Circle B
Area of Wound A	=	Area of Wound B
Healing Time for Wound A	<	Healing Time for Wound B

FIGURE 15–1
The speed of wound healing by secondary intention is influenced by the area of the defect rather than the length of the incision or the shape of the wound margins.

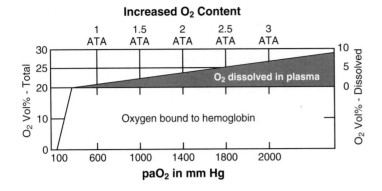

FIGURE 15-2
As the partial pressure of oxygen is increased, the amount of oxygen dissolved in the plasma increases.

creased atmospheric pressure (Fig. 15–2). Therapeutically, hyperbaric oxygen therapy increases tissue oxygenation in patients with small vessel disease, including those with diabetes, long-standing hypertension, and obliterative endarteritis after radiation therapy. Hyperbaric oxygen therapy can also increase tissue oxygenation in healthy patients, but there is little evidence that it is of any benefit in accelerating normal wound healing. However, hyperbaric oxygen therapy may be of benefit in the management of nonhealing wounds that do not improve after debridement, eradication of infection, and optimization of the local wound environment. The physiologic benefits of hyperbaric oxygen therapy with respect to wound healing include correction of tissue hypoxia, stimulation of fibroblast proliferation and angiogenesis, and enhanced leukocyte function.

SUMMARY

Complicated wounds that exhibit prolonged healing must be followed closely and the findings clearly documented. Clinical parameters that reflect wound healing are listed in Table 15–6. The keys to the management of complicated surgical wounds include early recognition, appropriate intervention, and optimization of the patient's medical condition.

REFERENCES

1. Kolb BA, Buller RE, Connor JP, et al. Effects of early postoperative chemotherapy on wound healing. Obstet Gynecol 1992;79:988–992.
2. Hoffman MS, et al. Mass closure of the abdominal wound with delayed absorbable suture in surgery for gynecologic cancer. J Reprod Med 1991;36:356.
3. Sutton G, Morgan S. Abdominal wound closure using a running, looped monofilament polybuster suture: comparison to Smead-Jones closure in historic controls. Obstet Gynecol 1992;80:650–654.
4. Israelsson LA, Jonsson T. Suture length to wound length ratio and healing of midline laparotomy incisions. Br J Surg 1993;80:1284–1286.
5. Pepicello J, Yavorek H. Five-year experience with tape closure of abdominal wounds. Surg Gynecol Obstet 1989;169:310–314.
6. Soisson AP, Olt G, Soper JT, et al. Prevention of superficial wound separation with subcutaneous retention sutures. Gynecol Oncol 1993;51:330–334.
7. Del Valle GO, et al. Does closure of Camper fascia reduce the incidence of post-cesarean superficial wound disruption? Obstet Gynecol 1992;80:1013.
8. Riou JP, Cohen JP, Johnson H Jr. Factors influencing wound dehiscence. Am J Surg 1992;163:324–330.
9. Savolainen H, et al. Early laparotomy wound dehiscence: a randomized comparison of three suture materials and two methods of fascial closure. Ann Chir Gynaecol 1988;77:111–113.
10. Schein M, Wittman PH, Aprahamian CC, Condon RE.

T A B L E   1 5 – 6
Wound Assessment Parameters That Should Be Recorded to Document the Progress of Wound Healing

Pain

None, mild, moderate, severe

Exudate

None, bloody, serosanguineous, serous, purulent

Amount of Exudate

Minimal, moderate, heavy

Odor

None, slight, moderate, strong

Necrotic Tissue

None, gray-white, yellow slough, black eschar

Wound Edges

Even with wound bed, well defined, rolled under, and thickened

Edema

None, nonpitting, pitting

Erythema

None, slight, moderate, marked

The abdominal compartment syndrome: the physiological and clinical consequence of elevated intra-abdominal pressure. J Am Coll Surg 1995;180:745–753.

11. Eddy VA, Key SP, Morris JA Jr. Abdominal compartment syndrome: etiology, detection and management. J Tenn Med Assoc 1994;87:55–57.

12. Morris JA Jr, Eddy VA, Blinman TA, et al. The staged celiotomy for trauma, issues in unpacking and reconstruction. Ann Surg 1993;217:576–586.

13. Jones JW, Jurkovich GJ. Polypropylene mesh closure of infected abdominal wounds. Am Surg 1989;55:73–76.

14. Fabian TC, Croce MA, Pritchard FE, et al. Planned ventral hernia: staged management for acute abdominal wall defects. Ann Surg 1994;219:643–653.

15. Greene MA, Mullins RJ, Malangoni MA, et al. Laparotomy wound closure with absorbable polyglycolic acid mesh. Surg Gynecol Obstet 1993;176:213–218.

16. Saxe JM, Ledgerwood AM, Lucas CE. Management of the difficult abdominal closure. Surg Clin North Am 1993;73:243–251.

17. Nolan TE, King LA, Smith RP, Gallup DC. Necrotizing surgical infection and necrotizing fasciitis in obstetrics and gynecologic patients. South Med J 1993;86:1363–1367.

18. Lineaweater W, McMorris S, Soucy D, et al. Cellular and bacterial toxicities of topical antimicrobials. Plast Reconstr Surg 1985;75:394–396.

19. Leitch IOW, Kucukcelebi A, Robson MC. Inhibition of wound contraction by topical antimicrobials. Aust NZ J Surg 1993;63:289–293.

20. Dodson MK, et al. A randomized comparison of secondary closure and secondary intention in patients with superficial wound dehiscence. Obstet Gynecol 1992;80:321.

21. Dodson MK, et al. Extrafascial wound dehiscence: deep en bloc closure versus superficial skin closure. Obstet Gynecol 1994;83:142.

22. Robson MC, Heggers JP. Delayed wound closure based on bacterial counts. J Surg Oncol 1970;2:379.

23. McGrath MH, Simon RH. Wound geometry and the kinetics of wound contraction. Plast Reconstr Surg 1983;72:66–72.

16

Patricia Braly

Abscess, Hematoma, and Lymphocyst

Postoperative complications usually have their origins in the preoperative or intraoperative time frame, and efforts to prevent these complications must therefore begin before and during the surgical procedure. Before the start of any surgical procedure it is imperative that the responsible surgeon review the pertinent aspects of the patient's past history, including the presence of significant systemic disease such as diabetes, past surgical history, and aspects of the planned surgical procedure that could potentially increase the risk of infection. Careful review of preoperative laboratory results should be performed to rule out the presence of urinary tract, genital tract, or distant infection, such as upper respiratory tract involvement. Few pelvic infections develop after gynecologic surgery if there has been no significant introduction of pathogens into the operative site from the lower genital tract or other colonized areas. Additionally, adherence to proper surgical technique, such as atraumatic handling of tissues, decreasing the size of pedicles to minimize the amount of necrotic debris, limiting the amount of foreign material such as suture materials and drains, achieving hemostasis, and eliminating dead space all contribute to minimizing the incidence of surgical site infection. Optimal wound healing and outcome may also be dependent on factors such as incision placement.

PROPHYLACTIC ANTIBIOTICS

The introduction of antibiotics into clinical practice has been associated with the effective treatment of infection and has also allowed the development of regimens to prevent surgical site infection. The definition of a prophylactic antibiotic regimen is the administration of antibiotics to a patient who is free of signs or symptoms of infection. When prophylactic antibiotic regimens were first introduced, typical treatment began when the patient entered the hospital and systemic administration of antibiotics was often continued throughout the hospitalization. Because of the observation that this prolonged antibiotic regimen could lead to superinfection with resistant organisms, it soon became evident that the continuous administration of antibiotics was not the optimal method of decreasing the risk of surgical site infection. Numerous clinical studies have documented that not all surgical procedures require antimicrobial prophylaxis, and, when indicated, the most effective regimens are limited to one or a few doses of antibiotic. After evaluating a large number of patients and various types of surgical procedures, surgical wounds have been classified as to infectious risk[1]:

Clean surgical procedures include those operative procedures in which there is no break in sterile technique, no evidence of inflammation, and no entry into the gastrointestinal or genitourinary tract. In these cases, the use of prophylactic antibiotics does not appear to be justified because the risk of postoperative surgical site infection in control patients is only 1% to 2%. Examples of this category include myomectomy and most adnexal surgery.

Clean-contaminated surgical procedures include those operative procedures in which there is no break in sterile technique and no evidence of inflammation, but either the gastrointestinal or genitourinary tract was entered. Postoperative infection in these patients ranges from 10% to 20% and is reduced to an average of 7% when prophylactic antibiotics are administered. Hysterectomy should be considered in this category.

Contaminated surgical procedures are those in which there is a break in sterile technique, in which there is gross spillage from the gastrointestinal tract, or in which surgery is performed in an inflamed site. The infection rate in these patients ranged from 20% to over 35% without prophylactic antibiotics and is reduced to 10% to 15% with the use of antibiotics.

Dirty procedures are those done in patients with a history of trauma, with a perforated viscus, or in the presence of purulent material. The infection rate in these patients ranges from 25% to 50% without antibiotics, and the use of perioperative antibiotics reduces this infection rate by approximately half.

Most gynecologic surgical procedures are elective and can be scheduled at a time when the patient is free from significant infection, including urinary tract, pelvic, or respiratory tract infection. The timing of prophylactic antibiotic administration is critical, with the most effective time being within the 2 hours immediately before the incision.[2] Infection rates were statistically significantly higher when prophylactic antibiotic regimens were administered more than 2 hours before the start of surgery.

Numerous studies, including retrospective studies, prospective placebo-controlled and blinded studies, and prospective comparative studies, have evaluated multiple prophylactic antibiotic regimens for patients undergoing hysterectomy. Many investigators have tried to identify consistent risk factors associated with the development of postoperative surgical site infection, including patient age, menopausal status, obesity, diabetes, anemia, lower socio-economic group, history of previous pelvic inflammatory disease, history of recent preceding surgery, surgeon experience, length of the surgical procedure, and excessive blood loss. Between studies, none of these factors has been consistently shown to increase the risk of postoperative surgical site infection, with the implication being that determination of the high-risk patient must be done on an individual basis. For patients undergoing vaginal hysterectomy, there are few negative studies that have not confirmed that the use of prophylactic antibiotics decreases the need for systemic antibiotic administration in the postoperative period for the treatment of surgical site infection. Because there is consensus regarding the use of prophylactic antibiotics in patients undergoing vaginal hysterectomy, the next question becomes which drug or drugs to use and how many doses to use. When compared with an antibiotic having a narrow antibacterial spectrum, an antibiotic with broad coverage should provide better prophylaxis, but no clinical trials have confirmed that theory. Similarly, there is no uniform evidence that multiple-dose regimens are more effective than the use of a single-dose antibiotic regimen. There is information to suggest that the preoperative local application of an antibiotic preparation, either as a vaginal suppository or spray, may be effective in preventing infection after hysterectomy.[3, 4] Conversely, preoperative vaginal preparation seems to have little effect on the numbers of endocervical bacteria, which are the most likely bacteria inoculated into the surgical site.

Two studies published in the mid 1970s indicated that suction drainage was an effective alternative to antibiotic administration in the prevention of postoperative infection.[5, 6] Other subsequent studies, however, failed to confirm the efficacy of drainage and even suggested the association of increased pelvic abscess formation with drain utilization.[7, 8] There appears to be little benefit to the use of routine suction drainage after vaginal hysterectomy. Instead, a common recommendation is to administer cefazolin (a first-generation cephalosporin) or cefoxitin (a second-generation cephalosporin) intravenously as a single 1-g dose 30 minutes before making the incision. Although some surgeons continue to give the antibiotics every 8 hours for up to 24 hours after surgery, there

is no proof that these additional doses are more effective.

In general, it is thought that women undergoing abdominal hysterectomy experience more postoperative morbidity than after vaginal hysterectomy, presumably because of the additional risk for abdominal incision infection and the increase in immobility after abdominal hysterectomy. Many studies have also been performed to evaluate the efficacy of prophylactic antibiotics in patients undergoing abdominal hysterectomy. At least two studies identified an increased risk of postoperative surgical site infection of up to 35% in patients who were diagnosed preoperatively with either bacterial or *Trichomonas* vaginitis.[9, 10] As with studies of vaginal hysterectomy antibiotic prophylaxis, when studies of abdominal hysterectomy patients are combined, a statistically significant decrease in postoperative surgical site infection is found in patients who have been given preoperative prophylactic antibiotics. This finding does not necessarily suggest that all patients undergoing abdominal hysterectomy should be given antibiotics, but it does suggest that high-risk patients should be identified who would benefit from prophylaxis. As was seen for patients undergoing vaginal hysterectomy, neither multiple-dose regimens nor the administration of an agent with an expanded spectrum of coverage has been shown to be more effective in patients undergoing abdominal hysterectomy compared with a single dose of a first- or second-generation cephalosporin. Also similar is the fact that there is no consensus regarding the efficacy of routine placement of suction drains in patients who have undergone abdominal hysterectomy. Some preliminary information suggests that the use of a povidone-iodine–soaked pack left in the vagina until its transection at hysterectomy decreases the postoperative infection rate to that seen with the use of prophylactic antibiotics.[11] Another small pilot study suggests that less bacterial contamination occurred when the vaginal vault was kept closed using an automatic stapling device compared with closure with the routine suture material.[12] In summary, the recommendation for patients undergoing abdominal hysterectomy is similar to that for those scheduled for vaginal hysterectomy (i.e., the administration of a single intravenous dose of 1 g of a first- or second-generation cephalosporin 30 minutes before the first incision).

The incidence of pelvic infection requiring systemic antibiotic therapy after radical hysterectomy varies from 1.5% to more than 20%, with a wound infection rate of 2.8% to 18.8%.[1]

When data are combined from many prospective studies, it appears that the overall incidence of major operative site infection is significantly reduced with the administration of prophylactic antibiotics, although this did not always translate to shortened hospitalization. In one study by van Lindert and coworkers, antibiotic concentrations were measured serially in fat, serum, and pelvic tissues; these authors found that effective concentrations continued for more than 3 hours of surgery.[13] Interestingly, these investigators noted that a blood loss of more than 1500 mL resulted in a significantly lower concentration when measured in the fat and serum 1 to 2 hours after antibiotic administration. Somewhat surprisingly, duration of surgery was not found to be a risk factor for postoperative surgical site infection. The recommendation for prophylactic antibiotics before radical pelvic surgery is similar to that for vaginal and abdominal hysterectomy (i.e., a single intravenous dose of a first- or second-generation cephalosporin), with a second dose being administered to patients sustaining a blood loss of more than 1500 mL.

USE AND ABUSE OF SURGICAL DRAINS

The use of surgical drains, which has been reported since the fifth century BC, presumably is based on the observations of clinical improvement after spontaneous wound or abscess drainage ("laudable pus"). Centuries later, it seemed prudent to prophylactically drain areas prone to infection. In the past few decades, however, changing surgical practices including the use of prophylactic antibiotics have raised questions regarding the optimal use of drains. Furthermore, new radiographic imaging and percutaneous drainage techniques have dramatically changed the way in which deep fluid collections are diagnosed and treated.[14, 15]

Despite their widespread use, many issues regarding surgical drains remain controversial, including when to use drains, which drains to use, techniques for the placement of the drain, how long to maintain drainage, and how much suction to use. Most of the clinical data that are available in this area consists of retrospective, uncontrolled studies that often do not describe types of drains used, the method of drain placement, and the duration of drainage. Because of this, the contemporary use of surgical drains is usually based on personal bias and tradition rather than pertinent data.

INTRA-ABDOMINAL INFECTION

Clinically apparent infection in the postoperative period is determined by numerous factors, including the numbers of microorganisms introduced and their intrinsic virulence, the microenvironment of the contaminated tissue, and the responsiveness of the host. The type of anatomic injury is also of paramount importance, whether it be the planned surgical incision or an inadvertent perforation of the gastrointestinal tract. Regardless of the source of pathogens introduced into the peritoneal cavity, a complex series of local and systemic host defense mechanisms are mobilized, all aiming at controlling the infection. The primary task of the local host defense mechanisms is the immediate removal of the microorganisms from the peritoneal cavity with concurrent control of the pathogens at the site of entry, thus preventing disseminated peritonitis and sepsis.

Intra-abdominal infection begins as the process of peritonitis, or inflammation of the mesenchymal cell lining of the peritoneal cavity. The process of peritonitis has been studied extensively and has been determined to consist of several distinct phases, including contamination, dissemination, inflammation, and resolution or loculation of the infection. When pathogens enter the peritoneal cavity, there is almost immediate clearance of these microorganisms by absorption through the diaphragmatic stomata to the lacunae and then through the thoracic duct to the systemic circulation, where they are then attacked by phagocytic cells. The dissemination of contaminants within the peritoneal cavity and their eventual absorption by the diaphragmatic lymphatics is largely accomplished by the natural forces of peritoneal fluid movement. Peritoneal fluid accumulates secondary to normal hydrostatic tissue forces with increased clearance of the fluid in patients who are largely recumbent. In this position, there is a natural movement of the peritoneal fluid toward the diaphragm, facilitated by a pressure gradient with each expiration that draws fluid toward the diaphragm. Bacteria appear in the thoracic duct within 6 minutes and in the general circulation 12 minutes after they gain access to the peritoneal cavity.[15] Factors that have been shown to have a negative impact on the clearance capacity of the diaphragm include increased intrathoracic pressure, such as with mechanical ventilation or positive end-respiratory pressure (PEEP)[15]; depression of spontaneous respiration as is seen with the use of narcotics[16]; a decrease in the normal circulation of peritoneal fluid, as with ileus or the reverse Trendelenburg position; and blockage of the diaphragmatic stomata, as can be seen with platelet-fibrin-microbial organism complexes.[17] Similarly, hyperventilation that often occurs with sepsis and peritoneal inflammation facilitates the absorptive capacity of the diaphragm. Even though this mechanism of diaphragmatic clearance appears to be the first line of defense against the development of peritonitis, it is doubtful that this is beneficial to the patient unless the peritoneal inoculum is minimal.[18]

The second major mechanism used to clear bacterial contamination from the peritoneal cavity is through the activation of macrophages and neutrophils. The phagocytic function of the macrophages is immediately triggered by the presence of the microorganisms and facilitated by complement activation from antigen–antibody complexes, bacterial products, or endotoxins.[19] Under the influence of the lipopolysaccharide components of the gram-negative bacterial cell wall, the macrophages are activated to secrete large amounts of cytokines such as tumor necrosis factor-α, interleukins (IL-1 and IL-6), and prostaglandin E_2.[20, 21] The release of these cytokines along with platelet-activating factor and metabolites of arachidonic acid initiates a series of events that aid local entrapment of bacteria within fibrin deposits,[22, 23] facilitate neutrophil chemoattraction directly[24] or indirectly[25] by complement complexes, facilitate the ingestion of opsonized bacteria,[25] and increase capillary permeability and enhance the production of acute phase proteins from hepatocytes.[20, 26] The triggered neutrophils respond in an all-or-none manner and are found within the peritoneal cavity within 2 hours of the injury, reaching a peak within 6 to 8 hours, and continue the influx for the next 2 to 3 days. They attack the opsonized microorganisms and destroy them by releasing their proteolytic enzymes, oxygen free radicals, and peroxide. The presence of foreign material such as drains, barium, and talc, or other substances such as blood, bile, gastric mucus, necrotic tissue, and fibrin, impairs the function of the neutrophils. These substances cause the neutrophils to release proteolytic enzymes early in an attempt to neutralize the foreign material and, as a result, the ability of the neutrophils to control and eradicate the intraperitoneal microorganisms is impeded.[19]

The third mechanism by which the peritoneal cavity attempts to control infection is through the localization of the infectious organisms by fibrin formation. This complex phenomenon requires the participation of several types of peritoneal cells. Under normal conditions, the mesothelial cells that compose the peritoneum and have the same common origin as endothelial cells, secrete tissue plasminogen activator, a substance that converts plasminogen to plasmin, thus inducing fibrin lysis.[25, 27] With any trauma such as ischemia or infection, the mesothelial cells are exfoliated, thus decreasing the fibrinolytic activity of the mesothelium drastically. The uncovered submesothelial cells release thromboplastin, thus further promoting clot formation by the intrinsic pathway.[23] At the same time, the permeability of the subperitoneal vessels increases and more fibrinogen-rich exudate is released into the peritoneal cavity. The net effect of these events is fibrin formation, with resulting encasement of peritoneal bacteria and adhesion formation with eventual progression to abscess formation in some cases. Because neutrophils and other phagocytes cannot penetrate the fibrin, the entrapped bacteria multiply and, in many instances, contribute to abscess formation.[25]

Infection within the peritoneal cavity is usually polymicrobial with a synergistic relationship between aerobic and anaerobic organisms. Growth of the aerobic organisms is associated with oxygen consumption in the microenvironment, therefore producing an anaerobic condition that facilitates the growth of the anaerobic bacteria. Some bacteria including *Escherichia coli* are facultative and can proliferate with or without oxygen.

DIAGNOSIS OF ABDOMINAL AND PELVIC ABSCESS

An abscess is a well-defined collection of pus that is walled off from the rest of the peritoneal cavity and represents the success of the peritoneal defense mechanism. For an abscess to be formed, both aerobic and encapsulated anaerobic microorganisms must be present.[19] The abscess usually forms in dependent locations in the peritoneal cavity, within an abdominal viscus, or retroperitoneally. The diagnosis and management of intra-abdominal abscess requires that the surgeon have a certain understanding of the epidemiology and clinical presentation of this problem. Surgical patients have many causes for postoperative fever and infectious morbidity, with abdominal abscess formation being just one of the causes. It is imperative for the surgeon to have an appropriate index of suspicion based on the clinical probability that a given patient has an intra-abdominal abscess. In clinical practice, the development of peritonitis is the most common and important risk factor responsible for subsequent abscess formation. Every clinician must consider the patient with postoperative peritonitis to be at risk for abscess formation, and each of these patients with clinical evidence of persistent infection after the initial treatment must be evaluated systematically for the presence of a postoperative abscess. All patients who have had multiple abdominal procedures during one hospitalization are at increased risk for abscess formation. The patient who requires a second emergent surgery for bleeding complications will have the risks of contamination from the second surgery as well as the negative effects of hematoma formation.[28]

For several reasons, the diagnosis of postoperative abscess within the abdominal cavity can be one of the most difficult of any in medicine. First, the signs and symptoms of postoperative infection are not specific for the site of origin of the infection, with fever and leukocytosis being common to infections of the urinary tract, lungs, surgical site, or abscess. Second, the presence of an incision makes abdominal examination by palpation or even by ultrasound more difficult and less revealing. Third, patients with fever and leukocytosis are often promptly placed on empiric antibiotic therapy, thus obscuring early signs and symptoms of abscess formation.[28]

In patients who develop a pelvic abscess after hysterectomy, it is usually localized to the retroperitoneal space above the vaginal apex.[29] In the postoperative period, it is common for up to 200 mL of blood and lymphatic fluid to collect in this area and, because of its proximity to the vaginal apex, this is an ideal site for infection to develop. Two studies from one group[5, 6] suggest that draining this space with suction drains prevented infection as effectively as prophylactic antibiotics, but other studies[8, 29] have concluded that drainage alone is ineffective in preventing postoperative infection and abscess formation.

Two distinct clinical presentations are possible for patients with pelvic abscess after hysterectomy.[29] In one case, the patient develops recurrent temperature elevations along with central pelvic pain on or after the second or third postoperative day. Examination often reveals a tender mass above the vaginal apex. Opening of the cuff allows drainage of the abscess, often associated with rapid defervescence of the fever. In the other situation, a patient is noted to have a falling hematocrit and hemoglobin after hysterectomy. These women are typically asymptomatic with a normal examination except for persistent temperature elevations related to an infected pelvic hematoma. Even though the hematoma may not be palpable, either because of location or consistency, ultrasonography is helpful for delineation of the hematoma. Even though the majority of pelvic abscesses after hysterectomy are diagnosed before discharge of the patient, on occasion the patient has a normal early postoperative recovery but then presents 10 to 14 days after surgery with sudden onset of severe abdominal and pelvic pain. It is uncommon for a postoperative abscess to present more than 3 weeks after discharge from the hospital.

Conventional radiographic studies are often employed for patients in whom there is a clinical suspicion of postoperative abscess. The three-view abdominal study (flat, upright, and lateral views) is commonly performed but may be of limited value because diffuse intestinal distention as is seen with ileus may obscure the classic findings of displacement of the gastric bubble, retroperitoneal gas collections, and extraluminal air–fluid interface. Even though, as noted earlier, the routine use of abdominal drains in the postoperative patient has questionable value, the drainage of purulent material or bowel contents from the tract can be an early sign of abscess or fistula formation. The tract can also be useful to administer water-soluble contrast material to document the extent of an abscess cavity or to document the fistula site.

Several studies have concluded that ultrasound examination of the abdomen is as accurate as other imaging studies such as computed tomography (CT scanning). Ultrasonography does have several clear advantages, including being relatively inexpensive and portable to the bedside so that patients in the intensive care unit can be examined. Disadvantages of this technique include difficulty examining patients with open wound or stomas because of the requirement for direct contact of the transducer on the skin. In addition, the resolution of ultrasound is suboptimal in obese patients and those with marked intestinal gaseous distention.

Another technique that has been extensively studied for the imaging of intra-abdominal abscess is radioisotope scanning. Although theoretically both gallium citrate– and indium-111–labeled leukocytes can be used to diagnose and delineate abscess formation, neither method is effective in the immediate postoperative period because the peritoneal inflammation resulting from surgical dissection will also attract the isotope. In general, these techniques become more specific in patients more than 2 weeks after any surgical procedure.

Because of its improved ability to determine anatomic relationships in the abdominal cavity, the diagnostic procedure of choice for patients in whom postoperative abscess is suspected is the CT scan. Especially with the use of oral and intravenous contrast media, CT scans have the capacity to identify abscess formation within the parenchyma of the liver and other visceral structures, in the retroperitoneal areas, and in dependent areas of the peritoneal cavity, such as the pelvis, the pericolic gutters, and the subdiaphragmatic spaces. On occasion, it is difficult to differentiate between abscess formation and other noninfectious fluid collections such as hematomas. Air bubbles can be found in 30% to 50% of abscesses and are helpful for identifying these structures. The precision of CT scans is such that percutaneous abscess drainage under CT scan guidance has become a common intervention that can often save the patient a more invasive surgical procedure for drainage.

Magnetic resonance imaging has been proposed by some investigators as a further refinement in technique for the diagnosis of intra-abdominal abscess but so far real improvement in sensitivity and specificity has been demonstrated.

MANAGEMENT OF ABDOMINAL OR PELVIC ABSCESS

If the patient is not on antibiotics at the time of diagnosis of an abscess, the decision between a single-agent versus combination therapy must be made. Unfortunately, little definitive data are available to guide this decision. Because abscesses are typically polymicrobial, the use of an antibiotic regimen requires activity against a variety of organisms, including streptococci, enterococci, members of the Enterobacteriaceae, and obligate anaerobes including *Bacteroides.* Among single-agent antibiotic regimens, the three most commonly used agents that provide adequate coverage include ticarcillin/clavulanic acid, ampicillin/sulbactam, and imipenem/cilastatin.[30] If the patient fails to respond to this therapy, the options include discontinuation of this agent and institution of combination therapy or, more logically, to

expand the spectrum of activity by adding specific Enterobacteriaceae and other facultative gram-negative anaerobic coverage (such as aminoglycosides and second- and third-generation cephalosporins). If initial therapy consists of combination antibiotic therapy, or the patient does not respond within 72 hours, the abscess will require surgical intervention, such as drainage.

Once the diagnosis of intra-abdominal or pelvic abscess has been established and it has not rapidly responded to antibiotics, the treatment of choice is drainage of the abscess contents without leakage into the adjacent uncontaminated peritoneal cavity. In the past, this drainage was typically accomplished by reoperation but gradually percutaneous abscess drainage under radiographic guidance has replaced surgery in many circumstances. When first described, initial criteria for percutaneous abscess drainage specified that the collection be unilocular, easily accessible without passing through vital structures, and not associated with bowel anastomosis, fistulas, or complicating factors such as an immunosuppressed patient. Immediate surgical backup was also considered to be mandatory. In the past 10 years, however, the criteria for percutaneous abscess drainage have gradually been expanded to include multiple or multilocular abscesses, abscesses located deep to vital structures, abscesses associated with gastrointestinal fistula or anastomotic leak, and in critically ill patients.[31] A standby surgical backup is necessary only in exceptional cases.

Percutaneous abscess drainage initially was performed as a two-step procedure by first localizing the abscess with either ultrasonography or CT scan after which the patient was transferred to a fluoroscopy suite for catheter placement. The current recommendation is to perform the percutaneous abscess drainage as a one-stage procedure, thereby eliminating both the need to move the patient during the procedure and the possibility of needle or guide wire dislodgment while the patient is moved. Imaging provides an indication as to whether multiple catheters are required with scanning immediately after drainage of the abscess, giving immediate feedback on the adequacy of evacuation. The use of multiple catheters should be considered appropriate and essential for the successful management of extensive or complex abscesses.

Diagnostic aspiration and Gram stain of a specimen from a presumed abscess cavity is critical for future treatment planning. Fluid from an abscess cavity usually reveals both bacteria and leukocytes, although specimens from a patient on antibiotics often have only white blood cells (the "sterile abscess"). On the other hand, a Gram stain that demonstrates bacteria without white blood cells suggests either bowel contents or a severely immunocompromised patient who cannot mount an appropriate response.

Once the abscess has been localized and confirmed by diagnostic aspiration and Gram stain of the fluid, a catheter is placed, usually through a trocar or by the Seldinger technique. Most abscess cavities can be adequately drained with a 12F to 14F catheter but, on occasion, a larger catheter may be necessary to drain an infected hematoma or an abscess with necrotic tissue. Smaller 7F to 9F catheters may be adequate to drain simple cysts, seromas, and lymphocysts. Although suturing can be used to secure the catheter to the skin, most contemporary systems include adhesive and locking devices to minimize the risk of dislodgment. Postplacement catheter care is usually the responsibility of the physician placing the catheter and often includes regular irrigation with a small volume of saline and low suction. Criteria for removal of the catheter include clinical parameters including improvement in fever and white blood cell count, minimal or no drainage from the catheter, resistance to injection of even small amounts of saline, and radiographic evidence of abscess cavity or fistula closure.

In situations in which percutaneous drainage is either not advisable or not readily available, a surgical approach may be necessary. When the abscess is documented to be centrally located within the abdomen or pelvis or when it is likely to be the result of a failed bowel anastomosis, reexploration through the original incision is preferable. If the abscess is documented to be laterally located in the pericolic gutter or high in the lateral pelvis, a flank or limited lateral abdominal incision may allow for a retroperitoneal approach for drainage. As discussed previously, the use of drains in the setting of reoperation for postoperative abscess has little scientific basis. In general, however, closed suction drains are preferable to sump or passive drains and should be used to drain confined spaces as opposed to open intraperitoneal space.[28]

As soon as the diagnosis of intra-abdominal or pelvic abscess is established and concurrently with the planning for drainage, attention should be turned toward evaluation of the nutritional status, electrolyte and acid–base balance, and antimicrobial coverage. Because of the associated catabolic effect of sepsis and likelihood of persistent ileus, enteral nutrition should be strongly considered whenever technically feasible. Nutritional support should include the following substrates: carbohydrates up to 5 g/kg/d; 45% branched-chain amino acids enriched with high-leucine solutions up to 2 g/kg/d; and medium-chain triglycerides up to 1 g/kg/d. The total calorie supply should not exceed 40 kcal/kg/d.[19] Antimicrobial therapy reduces the bacterial concentrations in the blood and tissues and reduces the frequency of complications related to drainage of the abscess. The selection of the appropriate drug or drug combination is usually empiric because this therapy most often must be started before culture results are available. Because of the polymicrobial nature of intra-abdominal infections, the use of combination or triple antibiotic regimens to cover both aerobic and anaerobic organisms has been the standard for the past 20 years. More recently, in an attempt to reduce toxicity and lower costs, the trend has been to replace combination antimicrobial therapy with equally effective single-agent regimens. It is important that the antibiotic selected for treatment of intra-abdominal infection should be administered intravenously before, during, and after the drainage procedure for 5 to 7 days. Depending on clinical response, the empiric antibiotic therapy may be changed based on the results of culture and sensitivity results from the abscess specimens.[19]

POSTOPERATIVE HEMATOMA AND LYMPHOCYST

Postoperative hematomas are a consequence of intermittent or slow, continuous venous bleeding in the operative site. Because the pressure of the expanding hematoma eventually exceeds the venous pressure, it tends to be self-limiting, with the eventual formation of a stable clot. The size of the hematoma is at least partly determined by the capacity of the compartment into which the bleeding occurs, with retroperitoneal and broad ligament hematomas containing up to several units of blood.

The diagnosis of postoperative hematoma is typically made after the finding of a lower than expected hematocrit when checked on the third or fourth postoperative day. Patients may complain of pain or tenderness to palpation in the area surrounding the hematoma. Depending on the location and discreteness of the hematoma, most can be palpated with careful abdominal and rectovaginal examination. When a hematoma is suspected but cannot be documented by physical examination, radiologic imaging studies including ultrasonography and CT scanning are helpful to confirm the diagnosis. It is often difficult or even impossible without sampling the fluid to determine if a hematoma is secondarily infected, because even a sterile hematoma is often associated with tenderness and fever. In the absence of these symptoms, hematomas that are less than 5 cm in diameter may be treated conservatively. In most instances, hematomas that are larger than 5 cm should be evacuated once liquefaction has occurred (approximately the fifth postoperative day). When large hematomas are not evacuated, most eventually become secondarily infected, even when the patient is being treated with antibiotics. Whenever a hematoma is confirmed by needle aspiration, definitive incision and drainage or percutaneous drainage with large-bore catheter placement should be performed soon afterward because the introduction of the needle into the hematoma often results in the inoculation of pathogens.

A lymphocyst is a local collection of lymphatic fluid that collects postoperatively as a result of retrograde drainage of lymph and is a rare complication unless a lymph node dissection has been performed. The incidence of pelvic lymphocysts detected clinically is typically 3% to 5% but varies widely in the literature from 1% to greater than 50%,[32] with a significant decrease in lymphocyst documentation over the past few decades. This decreased incidence is often attributed to improved surgical techniques, the use of prophylactic antibiotics, and the decreased frequency of performing lymphadenectomy after pelvic irradiation. Risk factors most commonly attributed to postoperative lymphocyst formation include extent of operative lymphadenectomy, prior radiation therapy, use of minidose heparin, diuretic usage, pregnancy, and lymph node metastases. The symptoms of the lymphocyst are related to its size and location, with most lymphocysts being quite small and asymptomatic. When symptoms of a pelvic lymphocyst are present, they usually become apparent several weeks after the surgical procedure and include pelvic fullness, urinary frequency, and constipation. Depending on the size and location, a pelvic lymphocyst may be palpable on pelvic or abdominal examination as either a vague fullness or a discrete, nontender mass, often noted cephalad to the inguinal ligament. Most lymphocysts resolve spontaneously over several weeks to several

months through the process of resorption of the lymphatic fluid and sealing off of the afferent lymphatic channels. As this resolution proceeds and the lymphocyst becomes smaller, a smaller mass of firmer consistency is often noted that may be difficult to differentiate from recurrent carcinoma.[32]

The diagnostic workup and differential diagnosis of a pelvic lymphocyst must be made in the appropriate clinical context and is usually suggested by the finding of a unilocular or multilocular cystic pelvic mass on ultrasonography or CT scan. This finding is not specific for a lymphocyst, however, and other disorders such as hematoma, pelvic abscess, thrombophlebitis, urinoma, seroma, adnexal mass, and carcinoma must be excluded. A definitive diagnosis generally requires needle aspiration with chemical and cytologic examination of the aspirated fluid to exclude infection, urinoma, and tumor. Once the diagnosis of postoperative lymphocyst has been made, the treatment of choice is usually expectant management because the majority of these are asymptomatic and will resolve spontaneously over a few weeks. An exception to this recommendation includes the situation of ureteral obstruction and progressive hydronephrosis or pyelonephritis. In this situation, needle aspiration and drainage of as much fluid as possible usually relieves the ureteral obstruction but often the lymphocyst will refill rapidly (within 24 to 72 hours). Repeated aspirations may be associated with secondary infection and abscess formation, so, in this situation, percutaneous placement of a 7F to 14F pigtail catheter under radiographic guidance allows for prolonged drainage. This technique of catheter placement is the most definitive but may require long-term catheter drainage, averaging 14 to 18 days.[33] Lymphocysts larger than 10 cm tend to require even longer drainage times. An alternative to long-term percutaneous catheter drainage exists that includes introduction of a sclerosing agent such as tetracycline. This procedure requires prior documentation of no direct vascular communication with the cavity by instilling a radiographic dye to confirm that there is no spillage from the cavity. Once this has been confirmed, a solution of tetracycline consisting of 1 g mixed into 500 mL of sterile saline is slowly injected into the lymphocyst cavity until resistance is met, the catheter is clamped for 1 hour, and then the fluid is drained.[34] Occasionally, repeated instillations of the sclerosing agent are needed to obliterate the lymphocyst cavity. If these conservative methods fail, surgical exploration with marsupialization of the lymphocyst cavity may be required so that lymphocyst fluid can drain internally into the peritoneal cavity.

In theory, any technique such as lymphatic vessel ligation that decreases lymphatic fluid leakage should be associated with a reduction in the incidence of lymphocyst formation. Despite the fact that retroperitoneal suction drains were first advocated to decrease the frequency of postoperative lymphocyst formation in 1961 by Symmonds and Pratt,[35] there is little agreement as to whether routine placement of retroperitoneal drains is helpful. Some authors suggest that placement of retroperitoneal drain actually stimulates lymphatic drainage.[36] If drains are used, they are typically removed 3 to 6 days postoperatively, depending on the amount of drainage. Another technique that has been advocated to decrease lymphocyst formation in the postoperative period is the practice of not closing the retroperitoneal space at the end of the procedure, thus allowing for drainage of the lymphatic fluid into the peritoneal space. Some authors suggest that discontinuation of minidose heparin and diuretics will also be associated with a decreased incidence of lymphocyst formation.[37] There are no data to address the question of the role of prophylactic antibiotics in lymphocyst formation.

REFERENCES

1. Hemsell DA. Infection. In: Orr JW, Shingleton HM, eds. Complications in Gynecologic Surgery: Prevention, Recognition and Management. Philadelphia, JB Lippincott, 1994.
2. Classen DC, Evens RS, Pestotnik SL, et al. The timing of prophylactic administration of antibiotics and the risk of surgical-wound infection. N Engl J Med 1992; 326:281.
3. Turner SJ. The effect of penicillin vaginal suppositories on morbidity in vaginal hysterectomy and on the vaginal flora. Am J Obstet Gynecol 1950;60:806.
4. Wright VC, Lanning NM, Natale R. Use of a topical antibiotic spray in vaginal surgery. Can Med Assoc J 1978;118:1395.
5. Swartz WH, Tanaree P. Suction drainage as an alternative to prophylactic antibiotics for hysterectomy. Obstet Gynecol 1975;45:305.
6. Swartz WH, Tanaree P. T-tube suction drainage and/or prophylactic antibiotics: a randomized study of 451 hysterectomies. Obstet Gynecol 1976;47:655.
7. Galle PC, Urban RB, Homesley HD, et al. Single-dose carbenicillin versus T-tube drainage in patients undergoing vaginal hysterectomy. Surg Gynecol Obstet 1981;153:351.
8. Wijma J, Kauer FM, van Saene HKF, et al. Antibiotics and suction drainage as prophylaxis in vaginal and abdominal hysterectomy. Obstet Gynecol 1987;70:384.
9. Soper DE, Bump RC, Hurt WG. Bacterial vaginosis and trichomoniasis vaginitis risk factors for cuff cellulitis after abdominal hysterectomy. Am J Obstet Gynecol 1990;163:1016.
10. Larsson P-G, Platz-Christensen J-J, Forsum U, et al. Clue cells in predicting infections after abdominal hysterectomy. Obstet Gynecol 1991;77:450.
11. Zakat H, Lotan M, Bracha Y: Vaginal preparation with povidone-iodine before abdominal hysterectomy. Clin Exp Obstet Gynecol 1987;14:1.
12. Beresford JM, MacKenzie AMR. Bacterial contamination at abdominal hysterectomy: a comparison of staple closure with regular suture closure of the vaginal vault. J Gynecol Surg 1991;7:233.
13. van Lindert ACM, Giltaij AR, Derksen MD, et al. Single-dose prophylaxis with broad-spectrum penicillins (piperacillin and mezlocillin) in gynecologic oncology surgery with observations on serum and tissue concentrations. Eur J Obstet Gynecol Reprod Biol 1990;36:137.
14. Dougherty SH, Simmons RL. The biology and practice of surgical drains: I. Curr Probl Surg 1992;29:560.
15. Skau T, Nystrom PO, Ohnam L. Bacterial clearance and granulocyte response in experimental peritonitis. J Surg Res 1986;40:13.
16. Mengle HA. Effect of anesthetics on lymphatic absorption from the peritoneal cavity in peritonitis: an experimental study. Arch Surg 1937;34:839.
17. Dumont AE, Robbins E, Martelli A, et al. Platelet blockade of particle absorption from the peritoneal surface of the diaphragm. Proc Soc Exp Biol Med 1981;167:137.
18. Dumont AE, Maas WK, Ileoca H, et al. Increased survival from peritonitis after blockade of transdiaphragmatic absorption of bacteria. Surg Gynecol Obstet 1986;162:248.
19. Pissiotis CA, Klimopoulos S. Recent advances in the management of intra-abdominal infections. Surg Ann 1993;25:59.
20. Dunn DL, Barke RA, Knight NB, et al. Role of resident macrophages, peritoneal neutrophils, and translymphatic absorption in bacterial clearance from the peritoneal cavity. Infect Immunol 1985;49:257.
21. Ertel W, Morrison MH, Wang P, et al. The complex pattern of cytokines in sepsis: association between prostaglandins, cachectin, and interleukins. Ann Surg 1991;214:141.
22. Ahrenholz DH, Simmons RL. Fibrin in peritonitis: I. Beneficial and adverse effects of fibrin in experimental *E. coli* peritonitis. Surgery 1980;88:41.
23. Hau T, Payne WD, Simmons RL. Fibrinolytic activity of the peritoneum. Surg Gynecol Obstet 1979;148:415.
24. Movat H, Cybulsky MI. Neutrophil emigration and microvascular injury: role of chemotoxins, endotoxin, interleukin-1, and tumor necrosis factor alpha. Inflammation 1987;6:153.
25. Hau T, Haaga JR, Aeder MI. Pathophysiology, diagnosis and treatment of intra-abdominal abscess. Curr Probl Surg 1984;21:24.
26. Fong Y, Moldawer LL, Shires GT, et al. The biological characteristics of cytokines and their implication in surgical injury. Surg Gynecol Obstet 1990;170:363.
27. Raftery AT. Effect of peritoneal trauma on peritoneal fibrinolytic activity and intraperitoneal adhesion formation. Eur Surg Res 1981;13:397.
28. Fry DE, Clevenger FW. Reoperation for intra-abdominal abscess. Surg Clin North Am 1991;71:159.
29. Hemsell DL. Gynecologic postoperative infections. In: Pastorek JG, ed. Obstetric and Gynecologic Infectious Disease. New York, Raven Press, 1994.
30. Faro S. Pelvic abscess. In: Mead PB, Hager WD, eds. Infection Protocols for Obstetrics and Gynecology. Montvale, NJ, Medical Economics Publishing, 1992.

31. VanSonnenberg E, D'Agostino HB, Casola G, et al. Percutaneous abscess drainage: current concepts. Radiology 1991;181:617.

32. Shingleton HM, Siller BS. The lymphatic system. In: Orr JW, Shingleton HM, eds. Complications in Gynecologic Surgery: Prevention, Recognition, and Management. Philadelphia, JB Lippincott, 1994.

33. VanSonnenberg E, Wittich GR, Casola G, et al. Lymphoceles: imaging characteristics and percutaneous management. Radiology 1986;161:593.

34. Mann WJ, Vogel F, Patsner B, et al. Management of lymphocysts after radical gynecologic surgery. Gynecol Oncol 1989;33:248.

35. Symmonds RE, Pratt JH. Prevention of fistulas and lymphocysts in radical hysterectomy. Obstet Gynecol 1961;17:57.

36. Ilancheran A, Monaghan JM. Pelvic lymphocyst: a ten-year experience. Gynecol Oncol 1988;29:333.

37. Catalona WJ, Kadmon D, Crawe DB. Effect of mini-dose heparin on lymphocele formation following extraperitoneal pelvic lymphadenectomy. J Urol 1980; 123:890.

Allan J. Jacobs

Bleeding and Anemia in the Surgical Patient

Next to abdominopelvic pain, blood loss is the most common symptom of gynecologic conditions that are treated operatively. In 1981, menorrhagia was the major complaint in 30% of women with leiomyomas[1] and was often accompanied by anemia. With more conservative contemporary indications for surgery, the proportion of women with leiomyomas whose surgery is performed because of bleeding undoubtedly is even higher. Endometrial hyperplasia, various gynecologic carcinomas, and dysfunctional uterine bleeding all may require operation. Hemorrhage is the pathophysiologic mechanism common to the majority of gynecologic emergencies requiring surgery. Spontaneous abortions and ruptured ectopic pregnancy both present as hemorrhage, which may result in anemia or hypovolemia. Excessive blood loss is the second most common complication of gynecologic surgery, next to infection. It is the most common life-threatening complication in a woman undergoing a pelvic procedure. Clearly, coagulation, hemorrhage, anemia, and hypovolemia are phenomena important to every gynecologic surgeon.

Hematologic problems are best diagnosed and managed preoperatively. The patient's description of her presenting illness, as well as the review of systems, will document whether gross bleeding is present. Family history of coagulopathy may be useful. The patient's history should document known coagulopathies and whether there is a tendency for the patient to experience purpura, gingival bleeding, and epistaxis spontaneously or with gentle trauma. A history of tolerating prior operation or trauma without bleeding complications reassures the gynecologic surgeon that the patient does not have a clinically important inherited coagulopathy. The history should also document the presence of any hepatic or renal disease and recent medication history, especially whether there was recent use of aspirin, nonsteroidal anti-inflammatory drugs, or alcohol. In the patient with chronic anemia, the physician must establish the etiology, and determine whether and how to correct the anemia preoperatively. Conjunctival pallor suggests that anemia is present. Severe anemia may result in cardiovascular changes of increased cardiac output and high output failure. These manifest as increased pulse pressure, tachycardia, and a third heart sound. Physical examination may reveal vaginal or rectal bleeding. If this bleeding arises from the vulva, vagina, exocervix, anus, or distal 8 cm of the rectum, physical examination should localize the lesion.

Routine laboratory studies should include complete blood cell count in all patients, and serum urea nitrogen, creatinine, and hepatic enzyme studies in women older than 40 and those with chronic illness. If bleeding is documented by history or on physical examination, or there is any reason to suspect coagulopathy, then prothrombin time (PT), partial thromboplastin time (PTT), and quantitative platelet count are obtained. Bleeding time is obtained in patients with suspected coagulopathy with normal platelets, PT, and PTT, to document disorders of platelet function such as von Willebrand's disease. If the hemoglobin concentration is less than 10 g/dL, serum iron, iron-binding capacity, and ferritin values are evaluated, as well as a reticulocyte count. Reference values are contained in Table 17–1. The cause of any active bleeding from the urinary, genital, gastrointestinal, and respiratory tracts should be documented using the appropriate noninvasive and invasive studies before a major operation. This involves cervical cytology, endometrial biopsy, and endocervical curettage for supracervical bleeding. Rectal bleeding warrants colonoscopy or barium enema. Hematuria is evaluated with urine culture (to exclude hemorrhagic bacterial cystitis), cystoscopy, and either intravenous urography or renal ultrasound study.

COAGULATION

Coagulopathies may cause hemorrhage and often result from excessive hemorrhage as well. The physiology and pathophysiology of the clotting mechanism is integral to a discussion of surgically important hemorrhage. Discussion of surgically significant hemorrhage may begin with the mechanisms that control coagulation. Intact capillaries normally inhibit coagulation by production of prostacyclin (to inhibit platelet clumping), by inactivating adenosine diphosphate (a promoter of platelet aggregation), and by allowing adherence to the endothelium of a heparin–antithrombin III complex that inhibits activation of the coagulation cascade. Disruption of capillary endothelium releases tissue thromboplastins, which activate the clotting mechanism. Subepithelial collagen, exposed after disruption of the capillary endothelium, initiates platelet aggregation when high blood flow is present.[2] Activation of surface platelet receptors causes morphologic changes in the platelets and initiates the synthesis of thromboxane A_2.[3] These changes lead to platelet aggregation and formation of a platelet plug. Meanwhile, collagen and tissue thromboplastins initiate sequential changes in

TABLE 17–1
*Reference Ranges for Tests Useful in Evaluation of Anemia and Coagulopathies**

Laboratory Study	Normal Range	Limit for Elective Operation
Hemoglobin	12.0–16.0 g/dL	>8†–10‡ g/dL (see text)
Hematocrit	36%–48%	>24†%–30‡% (see text)
Mean corpuscular hemoglobin	27–31	N/A§
Mean corpuscular hemoglobin concentration	33%–37%	N/A§
Mean corpuscular volume	76–100	N/A§
Platelets	150,000–450,000/mm³	>100,000/mm³
Prothrombin time	10.5–13 s	<14 s
Partial thromboplastin time	28–38 s	>40 s
Bleeding time	2.5–7.5 min	>10 min
Fibrinogen (plasma)	250–400 mg/dL	>100 mg/dL
Fibrin degradation products (plasma)	<10 μg/mL	N/A§
Iron (serum)	50–170 μg/dL	N/A§
Iron-binding capacity (serum)	250–450 μg/dL	N/A§
Ferritin (serum)	12–150 ng/mL	N/A§
Transferrin (serum)	200–400 mg/dL	N/A§
Reticulocytes	0.5%–1.5% × (Hct/45%)	N/A§
Folate		
Serum	2–15 ng/mL	N/A§
Erythrocytes	160–700 ng/mL	N/A§
Vitamin B₁₂ (serum)	200–900 pg/mL	N/A§

*All values refer to whole blood except as specified.
†Patients with normal cardiac, pulmonary, and vascular function.
‡Patients with limited cardiac, pulmonary, and vascular function.
§Abnormality of this measurement does not preclude surgery.

a number of plasma proteins (the "clotting cascade"), the end result of which is the conversion of fibrinogen into a fibrin clot at the site of vascular injury (Fig. 17–1). The so-called intrinsic system begins with factor XII, which is activated by contact with damaged epithelium. The extrinsic system involves the activation of factor VII by tissue thromboplastin, which is released by injured cells outside the capillaries. The intrinsic and extrinsic systems converge as factors VII, VIII, and IX and activate factor X. Eventually, prothrombin is converted to thrombin, which catalyzes the conversion of fibrinogen to fibrin. The latter forms a clot at the site of injury. This process is enhanced when blood is stagnant.[2] Thrombin also stimulates the production of thromboxane A_2 by platelets.

Fibrinolysis begins when the clot is first formed, as plasminogen is bound to fibrin and incorporated into the clot. Endothelial cells release tissue plasminogen activator, which itself is activated by thrombin. Tissue plasminogen activator catalyzes the conversion of plasminogen to plasmin. Plasmin is also activated by streptokinase and urokinase. Fibrin in the clot and factors V and VII are degraded by plasmin.

Disorders of Coagulation Antecedent to Operation

A defect in coagulation may produce anemia secondary to severe menorrhagia. Coagulopa-

thies may also lead to excessive bleeding at the time of operation. A number of conditions may be associated with clinically significant coagulopathy (Table 17–2); some of the more important syndromes are discussed below.

Blood vessel disorders are an unusual cause of bleeding. Infectious purpura, Cushing's syndrome, and vitamin C deficiency are the most common causes.

The most frequently encountered disorder of platelet aggregation results from use of aspirin or of other nonsteroidal anti-inflammatory drugs. These substances cause irreversible inhibition of platelet cyclooxygenase activity,[4] which blocks the platelet from synthesizing thromboxane A_2 for the duration of its 7- to 10-day life span. Bleeding time is prolonged for several days after a single dose of one of these drugs.[5] Dextran, some antibiotics, and tricyclic antidepressants can also cause disorders of platelet aggregation. Hepatic and renal failure also produce platelet dysfunction. Alcohol abuse is associated with both thrombocytopenia and qualitative platelet dysfunction.

The most common inherited coagulopathy is von Willebrand's disease. This autosomal dominant condition results from loss of, or mutational defect in, a plasma protein known as the von Willebrand factor. This factor serves at least two significant functions in normal coagulation: (1) it is necessary for platelet adhesion, and (2) it binds to factor VIII to protect it from

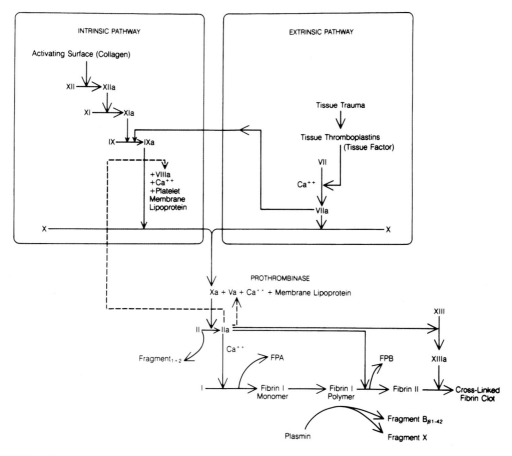

FIGURE 17–1
In the traditional view of coagulation, the intrinsic and extrinsic coagulation pathways converge at the step where factor X is activated. Activated factors are indicated by the letter "a." Dotted lines indicate that thrombin (factor IIa) enhances the activity of other factors. (Blaisdell WF From "Trauma Resuscitation" in *Scientific American Surgery,* edited by D. Wilmore, L. Cheung, A. Harken, J. Holcroft and J. Meakins. I Emergency Care, 7 Bleeding. Scientific American, Inc., New York, 1996. All rights reserved.)

degradation. Loss of function of this protein results in bleeding of variable severity from the epithelia of the nose, gums, and uterus. Some affected individuals have gastrointestinal hemorrhage as well. Bleeding time is usually prolonged, and is invariably prolonged after aspirin administration. This also aggravates the bleeding. Factor VIII antigen levels in plasma are usually reduced. Platelet count is normal. The coagulation defect of von Willebrand's disease can be corrected temporarily with cryoprecipitate. Ten to 15 units commonly are used, and therapeutic efficacy can be confirmed by observing partial correction of the bleeding time. Treatment is given at least every 12 hours, and more frequently if necessary to control clinically significant bleeding.

Thrombocytopenia has many causes (Table 17–3) and may require evaluation by a hematologist.

Any clotting factor may be deficient as a result of a genetic defect. The most common such defect is hemophilia A, or factor VIII deficiency, which is transmitted as an X-linked recessive disorder. Among acquired causes, liver disease and anticoagulant administration are most common. Intestinal malabsorption, or prolonged use of antibiotics with destruction of the normal colonic bacteria, may produce the same clinical picture. Warfarin is an inhibitor of vitamin K. It causes decreased synthesis of vitamin K–dependent clotting factors (factors VII, IX, X, and prothrombin), resulting in prolonged PT with little or no prolongation of the PTT. Heparin, on the other hand, binds to antithrombin to activate lysis of thrombin, factor IXa, and factor Xa.[6] If a patient on heparin requires a procedure that may produce bleeding, it is sufficient to discontinue the heparin, which is degraded in a few hours. On the other hand, warfarin is present for several days, so that mere discontinuation is insufficient to re-

TABLE 17-2
Some Conditions Responsible for Disorders of Coagulation

	Acquired	Inherited
Platelet Dysfunction	Aspirin	Wiskott-Aldrich syndrome
	Nonsteroidal anti-inflammatory drugs	Hereditary thrombocytopenia
	Alcohol abuse	Thrombesthenia
	Uremia	von Willebrand's disease
	Liver disease	
	Deficiency	
	Excessive bleeding with consumption and dilution	
	Splenomegaly—any cause	
	Idiopathic thrombocytopenic purpura	
	Drug reaction	
	Heparin	
	Neoplasms	
	Aplastic anemia	
	Disseminated intravascular coagulation	
Plasma Clotting Factors	Liver disease	Hemophilia B (factor IX)
	Heparin	Other clotting factor deficiencies
	Warfarin	
	Vitamin K deficiency	
Vascular	Vitamin C deficiency	Cushing's syndrome

store normal coagulation in a timely manner. Rather, sufficient fresh frozen plasma (FFP) is administered to lower the PT to less than 14 seconds, after which surgery may be safely performed. After the procedure, warfarin is restarted and heparin is used for anticoagulation until therapeutic PT levels are achieved.

Correction of Coagulopathies Using Blood Products

Platelet concentrate is derived from freshly donated whole blood. Each unit raises the platelet count by approximately 10,000/mm.[3, 7] Platelet transfusions are given to surgical patients with microvascular bleeding *and* a platelet count

TABLE 17-3
Some Causes of Thrombocytopenia

Thrombotic thrombocytopenia purpura
Sepsis
Viral infection
Human immunodeficiency virus infection
Heparin and other drugs (especially quinidine, antibiotics)
Aplastic anemia
Megaloblastic anemia (e.g., vitamin B_{12} deficiency)
Leukemia
Bone marrow metastases
Idiopathic thrombocytopenic purpura
Hypersplenism

Italics indicate those conditions that a gynecologist is most likely to encounter.

less than 50,000/mm.[3, 8] They may be indicated with counts 100,000/mm[3] in the face of uncontrollable small vessel hemorrhage.[9] They may be given with a count of less than 30,000/mm[3] in a patient likely to bleed (e.g., someone who is to undergo a minor procedure) or less than 5,000/mm[3] in someone whose situation does not otherwise predispose to bleeding.[8] The life span of platelets is less than 10 days, so that thrombocytopenia due to an episode of platelet depletion spontaneously corrects in a few days. Administration of allogeneic platelets frequently leads to sensitization to them. Consequently, platelets should not be administered unless absolutely necessary.

FFP is separated from whole blood and stored at $-18°C$ within 8 hours after collection. It contains all plasma clotting factors as well as naturally occurring inhibitors. The usual indications for the administration of FFP include deficiency of coagulation factors (inherited or acquired) with active bleeding, or before an invasive procedure[10]; coagulopathy secondary to massive blood transfusion[11]; and reversal of warfarin for an invasive procedure.[8] It may also be indicated in antithrombin III deficiency, in thrombotic thrombocytopenic purpura, and in the hemolytic-uremic syndrome. The usual starting dose is 2 units, with enough given to obtain the appropriate therapeutic and laboratory effect. Hazards are the same as those of erythrocyte transfusions.

Cryoprecipitate is derived from fresh plasma thawed below 6°C. It contains factor VIII, factor

XIII, von Willebrand factor, and fibrinogen.[8] Cryoprecipitate from numerous donors is pooled, and viruses are inactivated by heat. It is indicated in von Willebrand's disease and in hemophilia A. Hypofibrinogenemia is rarely found as an isolated entity and is usually best treated with FFP.

Disorders of Coagulation Associated With Surgery

Generalized bleeding during surgery is often due to depletion of platelets and protein coagulation factors as a result of extensive pathologic clotting. There are three causes for such depletion. The most common of these is dilutional coagulopathy. This occurs through a "washout" phenomenon—spontaneous or operative losses of whole blood are replaced by red cell concentrates and crystalloids, which dilute platelets and protein clotting factors. This, in turn, may lead to a coagulopathy.[12, 13] Clotting factors may be consumed by intracorporeal coagulation due to local causes, such as abruptio placenta; this is called consumption coagulopathy. A coagulopathy may, alternatively, have a systemic etiology, so that there is deposition of fibrin in small arteries throughout the body, together with pathologic bleeding. This is known as disseminated intravascular coagulation (DIC). The distinction among these syndromes is fuzzy, and all are frequently, and loosely called DIC. Table 17–4 lists some of the etiologic conditions that are seen in gynecologic practice.[14–17] The process of DIC can be initiated by a pathologic effect on a number of processes involved in normal hemostasis (Fig. 17–2). For example, abruptio placenta releases tissue thromboplastins, which activate factor VII, whereas endotoxins activate the intrinsic clotting system. Monocytes release substances[18] that promote coagulation[19, 20] and may trigger

TABLE 17–4
Causes of Disseminated Intravascular Coagulation Seen in Gynecologic Practice

Prolonged intrauterine fetal demise
Amniotic fluid embolism
Trophoblastic embolism
Septic abortion
Induced abortion by intra-amniotic saline infusion[14]
Postpartum hemolytic-uremic syndrome[15]
Septicemia
Ovarian carcinoma[16]
Extensive operation[17]

DIC in patients with sepsis, disseminated neoplasm, anaphylaxis, and major transfusion reactions.[21] Whatever the initiating mechanism, the end result is the elaboration of abnormal quantities of thrombin, with conversion of fibrinogen to fibrin throughout the circulation. Fibrinolysis is activated simultaneously, with the elaboration and presence in the circulation of fibrin degradation products. The deposition of fibrin in the microcirculation may lead to occlusion of small vessels by clot, which, in turn, can produce failure of oxygen-sensitive organs such as the kidney. The systemic coagulation reduces the circulating platelet and protein coagulation factors to a level that is insufficient to achieve normal hemostasis in response to microvascular injury. This, in turn, leads to massive hemorrhage and shock. Severe bacterial infection can also induce a generalized coagulopathy. Bacterial lipopolysaccharides can initiate the coagulation cascade by activating factor XII[22] and other procoagulants.[23]

Perioperatively, the coagulopathy can be recognized clinically by the presence of inappropriate small vessel bleeding. Patients on the ward will have purpura and bleeding from venipuncture and intravenous catheter sites. Patients on the operating table have diffuse oozing in the operative field. Postoperative patients may have intraperitoneal or retroperitoneal bleeding, which presents as hypovolemia. Epistaxis, hematemesis, and gingival bleeding may also occur. Compromise of renal and peripheral blood flow may lead to acute renal failure and peripheral thrombotic complications. Focal cutaneous infarction may be seen.

Laboratory studies are diagnostic. Findings include thrombocytopenia, hypofibrinogenemia, elevated fibrin degradation products, and prolonged PT and PTT. Thrombocytopenia is a consistent observation, and fibrinogen levels are almost always decreased. Other tests of the clotting cascade may not be depressed early in the course of DIC. In addition to DIC, other causes of perioperative coagulopathy include parenchymal liver disease and isolated fibrinolysis; in both of these conditions, the platelet count is normal.

The treatment of DIC is based on two principles: (1) elimination of etiologic factors and (2) restoration of deficient components of the clotting mechanism. Fibrinogen is replaced using cryoprecipitate or FFP. Platelet transfusions are given as needed to treat thrombocytopenia. In the context of acute hemorrhage, replacement of deficient clotting factors (as FFP or cryoprecipitate) or of platelets is indicated[12] if

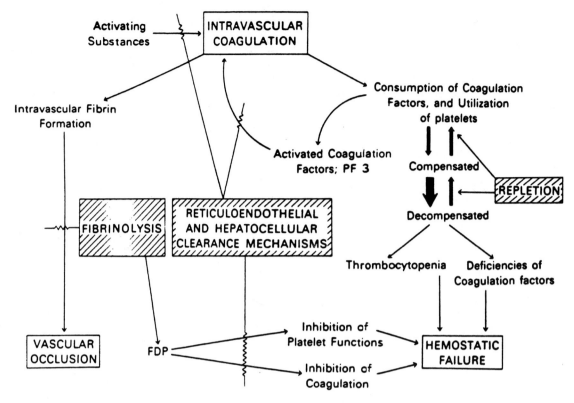

FIGURE 17–2
Factors that initiate disseminated intravascular coagulation. Known and possible factors are in boxes; elements of the normal coagulation mechanism are unboxed. (From Bithell TC. Acquired coagulation disorders. In: Lee GR, Bithell TC, Foerster J, et al, eds. Wintrobe's Clinical Hematology, 9th ed. Philadelphia, Lea & Febiger, 1993.)

and only if clinical coagulopathy is observed. The often-cited recommendation that 2 units of FFP be given for every 6 units of transfused erythrocytes is not valid, although many patients who lose this amount of blood will develop hypofibrinogenemia and will require FFP. Theoretically, heparin is beneficial in the treatment of DIC because it interrupts the pathologic coagulation. This theoretically prevents further adverse effects of generalized clotting and also allows restoration of normal levels of procoagulants. However, it is usually not given in the perioperative situation because it may promote bleeding. The use of protein C replacement is under investigation.[24]

ANEMIA

Acute blood loss is defined for purposes of this chapter as hemorrhage sufficient to produce hypovolemic changes. As hemorrhage progresses, signs of tissue hypo-oxygenation ensue. *Chronic blood loss* is defined as blood loss of a degree sufficient to produce anemia but not acute cardiovascular instability. Chronic blood loss may be physiologic, from menstrua-

tion, or may be the result of a pathologic process. If the rate of blood loss is less than the capacity of the marrow to replace erythrocytes but involves more than 1 mg of iron daily, the marrow iron stores will first be depleted, followed by development of anemia. Consequently, most chronic anemia is associated with iron deficiency. Blood loss occasionally may be greater than the ability of the marrow to synthesize erythrocytes (50 to 100 mL of blood daily), resulting in isovolemic anemia without iron deficiency. Exercise intolerance, malaise, and dyspnea are seen in otherwise healthy patients as blood hemoglobin falls below 7 g/dL; high output heart failure eventually ensues as the hemoglobin value falls. Patients with severe chronic anemia develop a bounding pulse and increased pulse pressure. Chronic anemia may unmask symptoms of latent disease such as coronary insufficiency or peripheral vascular insufficiency.

Medical Causes of Anemia

Many women undergoing a gynecologic operation have chronic metrorrhagia as their presenting complaint. The cause of anemia in this circumstance is usually either the blood loss per se or a combination of blood loss and iron deficiency. Nevertheless, the clinician must entertain the possibility that other factors may contribute to the pathophysiology of anemia, especially coagulopathy.

Anemia may be categorized according to whether the pathophysiology involves destruction or loss of erythrocytes or whether there is decreased production of erythrocytes (Table 17–5). In the former circumstance, a compensatory reticulocytosis is present, while decreased production of erythrocytes is associated with a low to normal reticulocyte count. Another way to classify anemia is according to erythrocyte size—as macrocytic, microcytic, or normocytic.

The major cause of anemia in women is blood loss with iron deficiency. One milliliter of erythrocytes contains approximately 1 mg of iron. The red cell volume of a woman is about 27 mL/kg. A 70-kg woman, therefore, has about 1.9 grams of iron in erythrocytes. Iron stores comprise up to 2.0 g. Dietary absorption of iron is quite inefficient, so that only 10% of the 10 to 15 mg in the average American diet is absorbed. Iron is normally lost through exfoliation of cells (up to 1 mg daily) and

through menstruation. Mean menstrual blood loss in normal women is 30 to 40 mL, with less than 60 mL lost per cycle in 95% of normal menstruating women.[25-27] It can readily be seen that the iron balance is tenuous in women of reproductive age. Iron deficiency leads to a microcytic, hypochromic anemia. Diagnosis is made by documenting serum iron less than 30 mg/dL. Total serum iron binding capacity rises, so that the transferrin saturation is less than 15%. The status of iron stores can be assessed by serum ferritin assay; values less than 30 μg/dL indicate abnormally low stores. Treatment consists of oral ferrous sulfate or ferrous gluconate, 325 mg two or three times daily. This dose elevates the blood hemoglobin level by about 1 g/dL each week in an iron-deficient patient, in the absence of ongoing loss of erythrocytes. Parenteral iron should be used only if a patient is unable to take oral iron, because it may produce severe hypersensitivity reactions. Iron dextran contains 50 mg/mL elemental iron. Up to 2 mL may be given daily by intramuscular or slow intravenous injection after an intramuscular test dose of 0.5 mL given as a precaution against anaphylaxis. Intramuscular injection must be given in the buttocks using a Z-track technique to prevent tat-

TABLE 17–5
Classification of Anemia

Erythrocyte Size	Decreased RBC Production	Increased RBC Production

Microcytic	Iron deficiency
	Chronic disease
	Thalassemias
		Blood loss
		  Gastrointestinal, genitourinary bleeding
		  Genital tract bleeding
		Coagulopathy associated with bleeding

Macrocytic	Megaloblastic
	  Folate deficiency
	  Vitamin B_{12} deficiency
	Nonmegaloblastic
	  Chemotherapy
	  Myxedema	

Normocytic	Chronic disease
	Red cell aplasia
	Myelodysplasia
		Blood loss (without iron deficiency)
		Hypersplenism
		  Hemolysis
		    Hemoglobinopathies (e.g., sickle cell disease)
		    Enzyme defects (e.g., deficiency in glucose-6-phosphate
		      dehydrogenase pyruvate kinase)
		    Methemoglobinemia
		    Structural (e.g., hereditary spherocytosis)
		    Hypersplenism
		    Tumor
		    Hemolytic-uremic syndrome
		    Disseminated intravascular coagulation
		    Infections (e.g., clostridial malaria)
		    Autoimmune disease
		    Vasculitis
		    Thrombotic thrombocytopenia purpura
		    Prosthetic valve

tooing of the local skin. Folic acid, 1 mg daily, may be given together with the iron. The cause of the bleeding should be eliminated. Discussion of operative therapy for specific gynecologic causes is beyond the scope of this chapter. To allow for a safer operation in women with benign chronic disorders and to avoid transfusion, it is common to administer a gonadotropin releasing hormone (GnRH) agonist such as depot leuprolide acetate (3.75 mg intramuscularly each month) for up to 3 months so that anemia can be corrected medically before operation. Combination oral contraceptives or progestins can be used to control dysfunctional uterine bleeding to avoid operation. If these are ineffective, GnRH agonists can be used for 3 months to allow medical correction of anemia before operation. GnRH agonists produce symptoms of climacteric, which are distressing to most patients. Also, they should not be used for longer than 6 months so as to avoid development of osteoporosis. Chronic bleeding sufficient to cause anemia without hypovolemia may also occur from the urinary or gastrointestinal tracts. Upper gastrointestinal bleeding is characterized by a history of melena, while colonic, rectal, or anal bleeding is accompanied by hematochezia. The site and etiology of the hemorrhage are determined through endoscopy with biopsy. Urinary tract bleeding sufficient to cause anemia is generally noticed by the patient as hematuria. Erythrocytes will be observed on urinalysis. The workup consists of urine cytology and culture. If infection is not present, or in case of persistent bleeding, cystoscopy and intravenous urography are performed. If these studies are negative, renal ultrasonography may show a renal tumor that does not distort the calices.

In the absence of a chronic disease state, the main differential diagnosis of microcytic anemia with low reticulocyte count is one of the thalassemias. These are hereditary conditions characterized by diminished synthesis of hemoglobin α chains (α-thalassemia) or β chains (β-thalassemia). α-Thalassemia is seen most commonly in persons of Chinese and southeast Asian origin but also occurs in those of African origin. Hemoglobin ordinarily has four copies of the α-globin chain. Individuals with three copies are asymptomatic. Those with two copies have thalassemia minor, a mild asymptomatic anemia. Those with only one copy have hemoglobin H disease, a chronic hemolytic anemia. Absence of α-globin chains is incompatible with life. Diagnosis is by exclusion in patients with mild anemia, severe microcytosis, and no hemoglobin A_2 or F, because

all of their hemoglobin is the normal adult hemoglobin A with 2 α-chains and 2 β-chains. β-Thalassemia is usually seen in persons of Mediterranean descent, but it may occur in those of Asian or African origin. Heterozygotes exhibit the thalassemia minor syndrome. They are distinguishable from individuals with α-thalassemia in that their hemoglobin distribution includes up to 8% hemoglobin A2 (2 α and 2 δ chains) and up to 5% hemoglobin F (2 α and 2 γ chains). This is established by hemoglobin electrophoresis. Homozygotes for β-thalassemia have thalassemia major, which results in early death. There is no treatment for thalassemia minor.

Many chronic diseases may also cause microcytic anemia. Affected individuals typically have low serum iron *and* total iron binding capacity. Ferritin and bone marrow iron stores may be normal or increased; if these stores are low, concomitant iron deficiency should be suspected. Treatment is by observation, transfusion, or erythropoietin. Recombinant erythropoietin (epoetin alfa) is used to stimulate erythrocyte production in patients with anemia due to chronic disease.[28] Iron, folate, and vitamin B_{12} deficiency should be corrected before starting this extremely expensive drug, and supplemental ferrous sulfate, 325 mg, two to three times daily, should be given simultaneously. The starting dose of epoetin alfa is 50 units/kg three times weekly for individuals with renal failure,[28] 100 units/kg three times a week in human immunodeficiency virus–infected patients on zidovudine, and 150 units/kg three times a week in those whose anemia is due to cancer chemotherapy. Doses are escalated if there is no reticulocyte response or if serum hemoglobin does not rise after 8 weeks of therapy. Epoetin alfa dose is adjusted in responding patients to maintain the serum hemoglobin between 10 and 12 g/dL. Anemia due to any other chronic disease may respond to epoetin.

Folic acid deficiency is caused by inadequate diet or small intestinal malabsorption. There is increased requirement for dietary folate in pregnancy and in chronic hemolytic anemia. Folate deficiency results in macrocytic, megaloblastic anemia. Hypersegmented neutrophils are seen on the peripheral smear. Diagnosis of folate deficiency is by demonstration of depressed erythrocyte folate levels; serum folate levels are acutely sensitive to recent diet. The deficiency is corrected by daily oral administration of 1 mg of folic acid. Normal serum vitamin B_{12} levels should be confirmed before beginning folate therapy, because folic acid therapy may correct the hematologic changes of vitamin B_{12} deficiency while allowing irreversible neurologic damage to progress. These changes usually begin with peripheral neuropathy and progress to imbalance and dementia. Vitamin B_{12} is absorbed in the terminal ileum. Its deficiency results from decreased production of intrinsic factor (its binding protein) by gastric parietal cells, due to a hereditary condition (pernicious anemia) or gastrectomy. Pernicious anemia occurs chiefly in individuals of northern European ancestry and becomes manifest after age 35. Vitamin B_{12} is absorbed in the terminal ileum, so that conditions interfering with its absorption there (e.g., surgical resection, regional enteritis, or blind loop syndrome) may also result in deficiency. Treatment is with parenteral vitamin B_{12}, because deficient patients cannot absorb the vitamin. For the first week, 200 μg is given daily intramuscularly, and then the same amount is given weekly until the anemia is corrected. The cause of the malabsorption is irreversible so that monthly injections must be continued indefinitely.

Treatment of iron, folate, and vitamin B_{12} deficiency should induce a reticulocytosis within a week.

Gynecologists may encounter anemia with decreased red cell production as a result of bone marrow ablation by extensive irradiation or of bone marrow infiltration by cancer. The diagnosis in each of these cases is readily suggested by the history and physical findings and can be confirmed by bone marrow biopsy if necessary. Additional causes for anemia with low reticulocyte count are found in Table 17–5.

Anemia with increased production of erythrocytes occurs as a result of either bleeding or hemolysis. The characteristic finding is an increased reticulocyte count, measuring more than 1.5% times the hematocrit divided by 45. This finding may not be present, however, if there is a secondary etiologic factor for the anemia (e.g., chronic disease or iron deficiency), which prevents a reticulocyte response. Anemia due to chronic hemorrhage has been discussed previously. The differential diagnosis of hemolysis is provided in Table 17–5; discussion of hemolysis is beyond the scope of this chapter.

The minimum blood hemoglobin concentration with which a patient should undergo operation depends in part on the nature of the operation, the anticipated blood loss, and the urgency of the procedure. Before a major elective procedure it is best to correct the anemia medically by administering the appropriate hematinics. For patients with anemia secondary to menorrhagia, hormonal suppression of bleeding is also helpful.

If possible, the hemoglobin concentration should be greater than 10.0 g/dL at the time of operation, but this no longer is considered an absolute requirement for elective surgery.[29] There is no general consensus for the guidelines for correction of hemoglobin before surgery in the stable patient, but it is clear that individualization is required. The two germane questions regarding use of blood products in the stable patient with chronic anemia are (1) whose anemia should be corrected by transfusion and (2) for whom should blood be crossmatched before operation? The answers to these questions depend on the oxygen-carrying capacity necessary to nourish vital structures. Transfusion for indications other than enhancement of tissue oxygenation is not indicated; it has been estimated that 20% to 70% of erythrocyte transfusions are unnecessary.[30] In most cases, this entails prevention of myocardial disease, although some patients may incur cerebral injury as a result of intraoperative hypoxia. Stehling and Simon[29] and Robertie and Gravlee[31] suggest guidelines for preoperative transfusion that are given in Table 17–6. Insofar as they apply to preoperative transfusions,

TABLE 17–6

Indications for Perioperative Transfusion in Gynecologic Patients

Hemoglobin <10 g/dL:
1. Conditions compromising ability to increase cardiac output sufficiently to offset the decrease in oxygen-carrying capacity resulting from intraoperative hemodilution (e.g., ischemic or valvular cardiac disease, cerebrovascular disease, chronic obstructive lung disease)
2. Age > 65 years
3. Anticipated mechanical ventilation longer than 48 hours
4. Postoperative conditions that increase oxygen demand (e.g., infection with fever; bronchospasm)
5. Postoperative conditions that decrease cardiac reserve (e.g., ischemia, arrhythmia)

Hemoglobin < 8 g/dL:
All above situations *and*
1. Anticipated blood loss >500 mL
2. ASA II or III status

Hemoglobin <6 g/dL:
All above situations *and*
1. Well-compensated patients with chronic anemia with hemoglobin <8 g/dL
2. Intraoperative hemodilution
3. Postoperative patients with symptomatic anemia (e.g., fatigue, dizziness, dyspnea)

Modified from Robertie PG, Gravlee GP. Safe limits of isovolemic hemodilution and recommendations for erythrocyte transfusion. Int Anesth Clin 1990;28:197–204.

these guidelines presuppose that the urgency of the clinical situation precludes medical correction of the anemia, or that such correction is impossible. I believe that women facing an operation likely to result in massive blood loss (as for cytoreduction of ovarian carcinoma, or for abdominal pregnancy) usually should have a hemoglobin value of 10g/dL before operation. Anemia should be corrected medically if possible. If medical correction is impossible due to ongoing bleeding, or if the urgency of the operation justifies the risks of transfusion, then transfusion of erythrocytes may be given to raise the blood hemoglobin to the threshold levels stated earlier. In the anemic patient, or in a patient likely to lose intraoperatively at least 500 mL of blood, it is best to crossmatch 2 units of blood. If massive blood loss is anticipated, it is wise to reserve additional units of blood.

ACUTE BLOOD LOSS

Intravascular water comprises 4% to 5% of total body weight of a nonobese woman. Cellular components and solutes present in blood add to its weight, so that blood comprises approximately 7% of the weight of a typical woman. The total weight of a 70-kg woman's blood then is approximately 4900 g. The density of blood is close to that of water, so that a woman of this weight has about 5 L of blood. Manifestations and management of acute blood loss is frequently expressed in terms of the percentage of blood volume lost. In clinical practice, it is difficult to estimate blood loss, however. The surgeon should manage acute hemorrhage on the basis of direct measurement of physiologic parameters; visual estimates of blood loss are too inaccurate to guide management.

The abrupt loss of large amounts of blood obviously will not result in immediate change in the hematocrit or blood hemoglobin concentration. Rather, the hematocrit declines over 4 to 6 hours by a percentage somewhat less than the percentage of blood that is lost. Full equilibration may not be complete for a few days after the episode of hemorrhage. This equilibration is accomplished by mobilization of extracellular fluid into the circulation as well as by fluid administration.

The three major problems caused by acute blood loss are hypovolemia, loss of oxygen-carrying capacity, and coagulation defect caused by washout of clotting factors and their dilution by infused fluids. These coagulation defects are discussed later in this chapter; other consequences of hemorrhage are discussed here.

Symptoms and signs of hypovolemia depend on the extent of blood loss (Table 17–7). Many normal blood donors experience a brief reflex syncope after the loss of 500 mL of blood, but true cardiovascular effects require loss of 20% to 30% of blood volume. Signs include postural hypotension followed by tachycardia, oliguria, and hypotension.[32] The extremities are cool because of generalized vasoconstriction. Late signs indicative of hypovolemic shock include pallor and agitation.

Severe blood loss results in tissue hypoxia as well as hypovolemia. The body's oxygen extraction ratio is normally 25%,[33] but it varies considerably among tissues. The extraction ratio of the heart is about 55%.[34] Thus, rapid loss of more than 50% of a healthy patient's blood produces anoxic cardiac changes. Persons with

TABLE 17–7
Effects of Acute Blood Loss in the Normal Individual

Volume Lost (mL)	Percent Total Blood Volume	Clinical Signs
500	10	Occasional vasovagal syncope
1000	20	Slight postural hypotension; increased tachycardia with exercise; no symptoms in resting individual
1500	30	Resting pulse may be normal or elevated; resting blood pressure may be normal or low; postural hypotension present; neck veins flat when supine
2000	40	Hypotensive, with rapid, thready pulse; air hunger; cold, clammy skin; decreased central venous pressure and cardiac output
2500	50	Lactic acidosis; severe shock

cardiovascular or pulmonary disease are especially susceptible to a sudden decrease in the oxygen-carrying capacity of blood. On the other hand, gradual blood loss is accompanied by compensatory changes. Thus, it is not possible to associate shock due to blood loss with a specific hemoglobin level. A young, healthy patient with chronic anemia can tolerate a hemoglobin of 3 to 4 g/dL, while an elderly patient with atherosclerosis or severe pulmonary disease may suffer ischemic changes with a hemoglobin of 10 g/dL. Such hypoxia rapidly damages various organ systems, compounding the pathologic state. The patient in shock demonstrates metabolic acidosis with an anion gap, due to lactic acidosis. Intestinal ischemia may result in endotoxemia from the gut flora, which causes vasodilatation and intravascular coagulation characteristic of septic shock. Gastric ischemia may lead to hemorrhage. The kidney may develop acute tubular necrosis. The lungs are susceptible to adult respiratory distress syndrome, which exacerbates the hypoxia (see Fig. 17–3). The terminal results of hypovolemia and shock are cerebral damage and death. The clinical manifestations

of shock and the hemoglobin value at which they occur reflect underlying cardiopulmonary reserve.

Treatment of hemorrhagic shock is directed toward two goals: (1) correction of the hemorrhagic process and (2) correction of hypoxia. Blood administration is important in restoring tissue oxygenation by increasing the oxygen-carrying capacity of the blood. Administration of oxygen is mandatory—by face mask if effective, but by endotracheal tube with mechanical ventilation if necessary. The effectiveness of treatment must be monitored by hourly measurement of vital signs, urine output, and pulmonary capillary wedge pressure. Coagulation studies, blood hemoglobin, electrolytes, cardiac output, and peripheral resistance must be measured frequently. Dopamine may be useful as an inotropic agent and for its positive effect on renal blood flow. Bicarbonate should be given only if the pH is less than 7.20. A full discussion of the treatment of shock is found elsewhere in this volume.

Development of dilutional coagulopathy usually requires loss of more than 50% of blood volume.

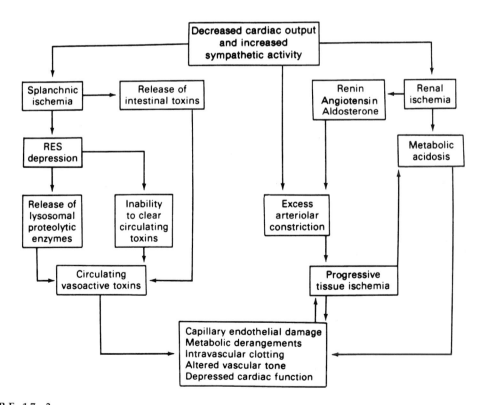

FIGURE 17–3
Pathophysiologic changes in shock. (From Thompson JT, Rock JA, and Wiskind A. Control of pelvic hemorrhage: blood component therapy and hemorrhagic shock. In: Thompson JT, Rock JA, eds. Te Linde's Operative Gynecology, 7th ed. Philadelphia, JB Lippincott, 1992.)

Management

Preoperative preparation of the patient with acute bleeding consists of replacement of blood and stabilization of the cardiovascular system. It is assumed for purposes of this discussion that the cause of the acute blood loss is known or being investigated and that the patient will need to undergo an emergency procedure. An indwelling bladder catheter is inserted to measure urine output. Vascular access is established, preferably with two intravenous 16-gauge catheters. One of these is used for administration of crystalloids and drugs and the other for blood products. A blood sample is sent to the laboratory for complete blood cell count, platelet count, electrolytes, serum creatinine and blood urea nitrogen, PT, PTT, plasma fibrinogen levels, and crossmatch. It is possible to derive the oxygen extraction ratio clinically with the use of invasive cardiopulmonary monitoring,[35] but this is not the usual practice. Rather, usual clinical parameters, including pulse, urine output, arterial pressure, visual estimation of blood loss, hemoglobin, and, when indicated, venous or pulmonary capillary pressure are monitored. Decisions on fluid and blood administration are made on the basis of these factors.

Hypovolemia is treated using volume expanders, decreased oxygen availability using erythrocyte transfusion, and coagulopathy using replacement of deficient platelets and/or coagulation factors. Isotonic electrolyte (crystalloid) solutions are inexpensive and relatively safe. Sufficient fluid is given to maintain the systolic blood pressure greater than 90 mm Hg and the diastolic pressure greater than 60 mm Hg. The most common preparations used for this purpose are 0.9% sodium chloride (normal saline) and Ringer's lactate solution (an aqueous solution in which each liter contains 130 mEq of sodium, 4 mEq of potassium, 3 mEq of calcium, 109 mEq of chloride, and 28 mEq of lactate). Human albumin solution has been used in the treatment of hypovolemia. Albumin has the theoretic advantage that its large molecular weight should tend to keep it within the vascular tree. Most authors believe that albumin appears to have no empiric advantage over crystalloid solutions.[36–38] Its high expense should preclude its use in the absence of a clear advantage. High-molecular-weight dextran has also been used in this clinical context. Its anticoagulant properties[39] militate against its use in hemorrhage. Its use is also associated with hypersensitivity reactions.[40]

With sufficient loss of blood oxygen-carrying capacity, volume replacement alone is inadequate. In this case, erythrocytes must be infused. Whole blood, containing about 35% erythrocytes by volume, is rarely used now, because the plasma, leukocytes, and platelets do not aid in oxygen transport and may result in problems. Furthermore, the most efficient use of donor blood is achieved by removing the nonerythrocyte components for use when specifically indicated.

More frequently, packed red blood cells are used. This preparation has a hematocrit twice that of whole blood and occupies half its volume. Like whole blood, it has a shelf life of about a month. This preparation contains large quantities of leukocytes and platelets. In patients with a history of febrile transfusion reactions or other problems related to leukocyte, platelet, or plasma sensitivity, leukocyte-poor packed red cells may be used. This is more expensive than ordinary packed erythrocytes and must be used within 24 hours of preparation. Persons with unusual blood types or multiple antibodies may benefit from reservation of frozen erythrocytes. These must be used within 24 hours of thawing.

Blood may be obtained from several sources (Table 17–8). Blood from volunteers is less likely to harbor infectious agents than blood from commercial donors. Directed donations from a patient's family and friends are no safer than those obtained from volunteer donors.[41] Indeed, blood from anonymous donors may be safer than that from known donors, because the latter may be under social pressure not to reveal known infectious diseases. Autologous blood is the safest source for transfusion, because a patient should not undergo an allergic reaction or acquire new infectious disease from administration of her own blood donated before operation. It is, however, possible for a patient to become septic from a contaminated unit of autologous blood, or to receive the wrong blood due to a systems error. Autologous blood, like allogeneic blood, must either be collected within 28 days of operation or else

TABLE 17–8
Sources of Blood for Transfusion From Allogeneic Donors

Commercial donation
Volunteer donation
Directed donation
Autologous donation
Donation before operation
Autotransfusion

frozen. A patient may donate at least one unit (500 mL) weekly but should take oral ferrous sulfate, 325 mg three times daily to replenish her erythrocyte volume. It is also possible during an operation to collect the patient's own erythrocytes and reinfuse them.[42] This may be done in clean cases but not in clean contaminated or contaminated procedures, because the blood then is no longer sterile. Thus, this technique is not applicable in operations in which the vagina, bladder, appendix, or intestine may have been entered. Autotransfusion has been used in clean abdominal cases.[43, 44]

In the face of vigorous bleeding in an emergency, it may be necessary to administer whole blood or packed erythrocytes without crossmatch. Simultaneous administration of erythrocytes and volume expanders is generally satisfactory, but whole blood may be given to patients with ongoing hemorrhage whose total loss exceeds 25% of blood volume.[45] In a situation of such urgency that there is insufficient time to prepare a crossmatch, type-specific whole blood or erythrocytes may be given. If the patient's blood type is unknown, she should receive type O-negative blood. This is as safe as type-specific non-crossmatched blood for emergency resuscitation.[46] The use of four or more units of O-negative blood may result in a hemolytic reaction, however, and may complicate later crossmatch. When time permits, or for elective operation, packed erythrocytes should be transfused, rather than whole blood, and complete crossmatch on these erythrocytes should be performed.

Attempts to enhance the oxygen-carrying capacity of blood by infusion of soluble oxygen-binding chemicals have not been successful. Perfluorocarbons have thus far proven to be ineffective[47] and toxic.[48, 49] The efficacy of stroma-free hemoglobin solutions has also been disappointing.[50]

Because of distribution of crystalloids through both the intravascular and extravascular compartments of the extracellular space, actively bleeding patients are given 1500 mL crystalloid with each 250-mL unit of packed erythrocytes to maintain the hemoglobin around 10 g/dL. (Although otherwise normal women will tolerate a lower hemoglobin, this level provides a reserve in case hemorrhage continues.) Solutions of crystalloids such as Ringer's lactate or 0.9% sodium chloride are used for fluid resuscitation. In a patient with acute blood loss who is not actively bleeding (e.g., at the conclusion of an operation), 1 to 2 L of crystalloid may be given rapidly; if the patient stabilizes, administration of erythrocytes is unnecessary.

In the presence of continuous bleeding, or of continued signs of hypovolemia after a crystalloid fluid challenge, crystalloids and blood are rapidly administered in the ratio of 1.5 L of solution to 1 unit of packed erythrocytes. Alternatively, whole blood may be given. The goal of fluid administration in a patient with heavy bleeding is to maintain normal vital signs without orthostatic changes, hourly urine output of at least 0.5 mL/kg and hemoglobin concentration greater than 10 g/dL. It must be stressed that under circumstances of acute blood loss such as major gynecologic hemorrhage or operative bleeding, measurement of hematocrit is inaccurate; several hours are required for the hematocrit to equilibrate after acute blood loss. At any instant of time the hemoglobin of a perioperative patient may reflect appropriate replacement of fluids, overreplacement, or underreplacement. Blood pressure, pulse, and urinary output are better indicators of need for resuscitation than are hematocrit or hemoglobin concentration. In the actively bleeding patient, measurement of central venous pressure or pulmonary capillary wedge pressure may be advisable.

The pneumatic antishock garment has been advocated for use in hypovolemic patients with abdominal hemorrhage to enhance cardiac function by increasing central circulation. It appears to be ineffective in this regard and probably should not be used.[51]

The timing of operation in a patient with acute hemorrhage may be difficult, because it may be beneficial to defer such an operation a few hours to allow correction of hypovolemia, decreased oxygen-carrying capacity, and coagulopathy. The benefits of such delay must be weighed against the risk of further deterioration due to the bleeding.

POSTOPERATIVE HEMORRHAGE

The diagnosis of postoperative hemorrhage, and the decision to reexplore or to intervene in another manner, are among the most difficult challenges facing the gynecologic surgeon. The ability to make a rational decision can be impaired by the surgeon's emotions, which easily lead to denial of the need to intervene. Pride and confidence in his or her own ability, fear of the consequences for the patient and of legal consequences, and possibly fatigue, all can cloud a surgeon's judgment. Paradoxically, the more difficult the procedure, the more difficult it is to conclude that a patient has hemorrhage that merits intervention. If a woman is hypotensive and oliguric several hours after a tubal ligation, she most likely has intra-abdominal hemorrhage. If the patient has undergone a complicated procedure, such as resection of ovarian carcinoma or severe endometriosis, in which she has lost several liters of blood through a large abdominal incision over several hours, and has received many liters of crystalloid and blood as replacement, it may be difficult to distinguish ongoing hemorrhage from other causes of hypovolemia, such as corrected intra-abdominal hemorrhage, fluid sequestration ("third spacing"), or evaporative intraoperative fluid loss.

Successful management of postoperative hemorrhage begins with its diagnosis as promptly as possible. Such diagnosis begins with appropriate monitoring. Patients who have undergone laparotomy or whose estimated blood loss from a vaginal procedure exceeds 500 mL should be kept as inpatients with measurement of vital signs and urine output (with the aid of an indwelling catheter) at least every 4 hours. Patients who have lost over 1000 mL of blood, who are older, or who have major underlying illness should be observed in a special care unit and have vital signs and urine output measured hourly, possibly with continuous pulse oximetry. Those who have been unstable, or who have had an especially extensive procedure, should have central venous or pulmonary capillary pressure monitoring as well. If at least 500 mL of blood have been lost, the hematocrit and hemoglobin concentration should routinely be measured 4 hours after the end of the operation. Other patients should have hematocrit and hemoglobin determined the morning after surgery. In a stable patient, 0.45% sodium chloride with 20 mEq/L of potassium chloride is used for fluid replacement. After a straightforward operation with no more than 1000 mL of blood loss, and good hemostasis at the conclusion of the procedure, an infusion of 100 to 125 mL/h should maintain an hourly urine output of more than 0.5 mL/kg.

Hypovolemia is the first consequence of blood loss. Postoperative hypovolemia may be due to persistent hemorrhage, to inadequate fluid replacement during surgery, or to fluid sequestration in the intestinal wall and lumen (third spacing). After a straightforward operation with minimal blood loss hypovolemia is likely to signify unrecognized bleeding. This may arise from intraperitoneal hemorrhage, retroperitoneal hematoma, or vaginal cuff bleeding. The latter can easily be determined by observing the passage of large amounts of blood per vagina. In the absence of this finding, blood is sent for hemoglobin and hematocrit. If the patient is oliguric, the bladder catheter is checked for patency. While this is pending, a fluid bolus of 500 to 1000 mL over 1 hour is given. If the hematocrit has fallen significantly from preoperative levels, or if the fluid bolus fails to restore urine output and vital signs to normal, reexploration should be considered. If the fluid bolus restores isovolemia, the patient may be observed carefully, with hourly vital signs and hematocrit determinations every 2 to 4 hours. Further deterioration suggests a need for reexploration.

The diagnosis of postoperative hemorrhage is more difficult after a major procedure with extensive loss of blood, handling of internal viscera, and insensible losses. In some cases, the operation might have left extensive denuded areas and hemostasis may have been incomplete. Fall of hematocrit after such an operation may alternatively represent equilibration following unrecognized blood loss, or hypovolemia may represent third spacing. Fluid sequestration after extensive cytoreduction of ovarian carcinoma may require replacement of crystalloid at a rate as high as 300 mL/h. Be that as it may, persistent hypovolemia, with falling hematocrit requiring transfusion of multiple units of blood suggests intra-abdominal hemorrhage. Increasing abdominal distention or passage of blood through the incision strongly suggests this diagnosis.

If the diagnosis of postoperative hemorrhage is suspected, hematocrit should be determined every 1 to 2 hours. Sufficient transfusion of packed erythrocytes should be administered to maintain the hemoglobin concentration at 10 g/dL. Because of the possibility of dilutional or consumptive coagulopathy, the platelet count, PT, and PTT should be determined. Platelet transfusions and infusions of FFP are given as appropriate, to attempt to correct any coagulopathy. Good peripheral venous access should be secured with large-gauge catheters and a central venous line or Swan-Ganz catheter should be inserted for monitoring.

When a patient with postoperative hemorrhage has attained maximum possible stability, laparotomy is performed. Possible maneuvers helpful in controlling intra-abdominal bleeding include identification and ligation of bleeding vessels and coagulation of oozing surfaces with electrocautery or an argon beam coagulator. Microvascular bleeding can often be controlled by applying a hemostatic substance such as microfibrillar collagen (Avitene) and applying a tight pack over the Avitene and the bleeding site for 10 minutes. I have found a slurry of Avitene and topical thrombin useful in this regard. If microvascular bleeding is widespread and otherwise uncontrollable, a tight pelvic pack of several Kerlix gauze tapes securely tied together may be inserted and either brought out of the abdomen or else brought out of the vagina as an "umbrella" pack. Such bleeding is usually associated with a coagulopathy. If hemostasis is obtained with such a pelvic pack, the pack is removed under anesthesia 24 hours later, provided the coagulopathy has been corrected.

Internal iliac artery ligation seldom corrects intra-abdominal hemorrhage. It is sometimes useful, because the resulting diminution in pressure may facilitate control of hemorrhage by direct ligation of bleeding vessels. The internal iliac artery should be ligated, when possible, below the level of the bifurcation of the anterior and posterior divisions. The posterior division nourishes skeletal structures rather than the pelvic viscera and need not be interrupted. Gluteal necrosis is a rare complication of ligation of the posterior division. Before ligation, the vessel is isolated by gentle blunt dissection with a right-angled clamp proceeding from lateral to medial to avoid injury to the internal iliac vein. A secure 1–0 permanent or absorbable suture is passed around the vessel and tied.

If an ovarian vessel is bleeding, the lateral retroperitoneal incision can be extended anteriorly along the paracolic gutter and the ovarian vascular bundle isolated and relegated above the pelvic brim. The ureter runs parallel to the ovarian vessels and 1 to 2 cm dorsal to it; ureteral identification should precede ovarian vessel ligation.

Temporary aortic occlusion using a vascular clamp or pressure with a stick sponge is another maneuver that reduces blood flow to the pelvis and facilitates identification of bleeding vessels, while diminishing the blood loss during the time required to correct the bleeding.

One other method for control of postoperative bleeding deserves mention. Hemorrhage from a single artery can be controlled using transcatheter embolization of that artery.[52–54] This technique can be used for spontaneous vaginal bleeding from cancer, as well as for postoperative patients. It ordinarily is performed by a specialist in invasive radiology. Percutaneous femoral artery catheterization under local anesthesia allows angiographic identification of the bleeding vessel, provided blood flow is at least 0.5 mL/min. Small pieces of an absorbable hemostatic material such as

gelatin sponge (Gelfoam) are passed through the catheter under angiographic control to occlude the vessel. Even if control of hemorrhage is unsuccessful, localization of the bleeding vessel may facilitate subsequent operative repair. The main complication of transcatheter embolization is pelvic infection.

Anemia is frequently noted in postoperative patients in the absence of active bleeding. In such cases, transfusion is given only for symptoms of hypovolemia or of hypo-oxygenation. Transfusion should not be given to promote wound healing, because it does not do so unless the blood hemoglobin value is less than 5 g/dL.[55] Rather, postoperative anemia arising from operative blood loss that is stable and does not pose an acute threat to the patient should be treated with oral administration of iron or (if the woman is asymptomatic and will have no further menstruation) be allowed to correct itself over time through ingestion of dietary iron.

SPECIAL CASES OF HEMORRHAGE

A patient may present with heavy vaginal bleeding from cervical, vaginal, or endometrial carcinoma. Such bleeding may often be controlled by packing the vagina for 24 hours. If the bleeding is visible from a cervical or vaginal lesion, Monsel's solution may be applied to the pack. If this does not control the hemorrhage, emergency radiation is indicated in the previously unirradiated patient. External radiation is given in 4.0-Gy fractions for 3 days; this dose, which is reckoned as part of the total external radiation dose, generally suffices to control the hemorrhage.[56] If this is ineffective, transcatheter embolization is the treatment of choice, followed by emergency resection of tumor. Such emergency operation, if done in a situation suboptimal from an oncologic standpoint, may jeopardize the patient's chance for a cure.

Heavy vaginal bleeding after vaginal surgery may be seen within 24 hours of a vaginal hysterectomy or within 10 days of conization. This can be controlled by suturing the bleeding vessel, which can generally be identified easily. It is unwise to try to control significant hemorrhage by simply packing the vagina, because this rarely works.

COMPLICATIONS OF TRANSFUSION

Transfusion of whole blood, of cellular elements of blood, or of fresh plasma has the

TABLE 17-9
Approximate Risk of Adverse Effects of Blood Transfusion

Effect	Risk per Unit $\times 10^{-1}$
Alloimmunization to leukocytes/ platelets	10
Alloimmunization to erythrocytes	100
Febrile	100–200
Allergic	100–300
Hepatitis C	2,000
Hemolytic (delayed)	5,000
Hemolytic (immediate)	25,000
Human T-lymphotropic virus type I	70,000
Anaphylactic reaction	100,000
Hepatitis B	100,000
Human immunodeficiency virus	100,000
Death	100,000

potential for numerous complications; there are excellent reviews of this topic.[57, 58] These complications may be very grave; there is one transfusion-related death per 100,000 recipients.[59] Most of these are caused by the transfused cells themselves. Others result from contamination with infectious agents or from elements in plasma. For the clinician, these complications may usefully be categorized as acute, subacute, and delayed. The incidence of various transfusion complications is summarized in Table 17–9.

Acute Transfusion Reactions

Transfusion with incompatible erythrocytes[60, 61] most commonly results in acute hemolysis. Eighty to 90% of these reactions are associated with ABO incompatibility.[59, 62] The pathophysiology involves complement-mediated lysis of the donor erythrocytes associated with IgM anti-A or anti-B immunoglobulins. The clinical context involves mismatching, clerical error, or atypical antibodies missed in the crossmatch process.[63] The incidence of hemolytic transfusions varies considerably and probably depends on the skill with which transfusion procedures are conducted, the index of suspicion during mild reactions, and the heterogeneity of the population of donors and recipients. In some centers this rate may be as high as 1 in 1000 transfusions. About half of all transfusion-associated fatalities involves an acute hemolytic reaction.[59] Thirteen percent of mismatched transfusions result from serologic mistake, 14% have no error associated, and the remaining 73% are associated with clerical errors or systems flaws.[59] Symptoms include sudden onset of fever, flushing, anxiety, and tachycardia. Dyspnea, chest pain, and hypotension may be present. Hemoglobinuria is soon observed. Serious sequelae may include DIC, acute renal tubular necrosis, and shock. Mortality from hemolytic reactions is as high as 1 in 10,000 transfusions.[63, 64]

Management begins with prevention, because most serious reactions are due to preventable errors. During a transfusion, nurses should observe the patient frequently. The transfusion should be stopped if any of the symptoms detailed in the previous paragraph should occur, because the severity of the reaction is related to the volume of infused blood. The remaining blood and an aliquot of the patient's own blood should be sent to the blood bank for investigation. PT, PTT, complete blood cell count with platelet count, serum urea nitrogen and creatinine, plasma fibrinogen, and plasma fibrin degradation product levels should be drawn and should be repeated as clinically indicated. Samples of the patient's blood and urine may be centrifuged; a reddish brown supernatant provides presumptive evidence of hemoglobinemia and hemoglobinuria, respectively. Blood culture should be considered to rule out an infection associated with hemolysis, such as *Clostridia perfringens*. Hydration with crystalloids should be vigorous. Enough fluid should be given (with furosemide if necessary) to maintain urine output at 100 mL/h. Further transfusion with other units of blood may be given if there is a strong clinical indication such as ongoing acute blood loss. If renal failure is present, fluid should be restricted. Any hypotension or coagulopathy should be managed appropriately. Exchange transfusion has been recommended for severe reactions,[65] but it would seem to be indicated only in extreme circumstances.

Nonhemolytic febrile reactions occur in up to 3% of transfusions.[66, 67] They usually arise as a result of prior sensitization to human leukocyte antigen or platelet-specific antibodies.[68, 69] The reaction occurs with infusion of blood that contains platelets or leukocytes against which the patient has antibodies. Sensitization usually occurs after prior transfusion but can occur from a fetal-maternal hemorrhage. Reactions are characterized by rigors and fever, often with malaise. Other symptoms of hemolytic reactions are absent, and the reaction is usually transient. Nevertheless, the transfusion should be discontinued and the blood returned to the blood bank with a sample of the patient's own blood, because immediate distinction between febrile and hemolytic reactions is not possible. Other elements of the workup for possible hemolytic reactions should be effected. It is common to try to prevent these reactions by premedicating patients with aspirin, 650 mg, orally and diphenhydramine (Benadryl), 50 mg orally or intravenously, before any transfusion, especially if a patient had a previous febrile reaction. The use of corticosteroids or of leukocyte-poor erythrocytes may be necessary in sensitized patients.

Volume overload may occur as a result of transfusion.[70] Acute pulmonary edema after transfusion accounts for about 10% of transfusion-related deaths.[59] The most common clinical scenario is transfusion for anemia of a patient with impaired cardiac reserve. If subtle signs of heart failure such as neck vein distention or a third heart sound are present, it may be prudent to administer a diuretic such as furosemide with the transfusion. The rate of red cell infusion in stable isovolemic women should be no more than 1 unit every 2 hours and should be closely supervised in elderly patients or in those with cardiac disease.

Allergic reactions, due in most instances to plasma components of the blood infusion, occur in up to 3% of transfusions.[67] Urticaria is the most common such reaction and does not necessitate discontinuation of the transfusion. Angioedema, bronchospasm, and anaphylaxis may also occur. In many instances, allergic reactions are associated with antibodies against IgA from the donor plasma.[71] Such antibodies occur in 2% of normal and in up to 21% of transfused individuals.[66, 72]

All problems described earlier may be associated with single transfusions. Some acute effects of transfusion occur only with massive transfusion. The most common of these is dilution of platelets and clotting factors.[73] Hypothermia is frequently seen in patients who undergo prolonged procedures through a large open incision. Infusion of large volumes of blood at room temperature may contribute to this. Therefore, blood warmers should be used for transfusions during surgery. Massive transfusion can also produce metabolic effects.[74] The high levels of potassium present in stored red blood cells and in their supernatant may produce clinical hyperkalemia if these cells hemolyze or in a patient with acidosis. Banked blood contains citrate as a preservative. This normally is rapidly metabolized by the liver. Patients with hepatic or renal failure, or of shock, may experience a coagulopathy from this citrate. They, or patients who receive massive transfusions through a central venous catheter, may undergo hypocalcemia with arrhythmias, because citrate binds ionic calcium.

Subacute Transfusion Reactions

Delayed hemolytic reactions, usually due to Rh and Jk incompatibility,[59] may occur 2 to 10 days after transfusion.[75] These are generally mild. They are usually due to anamnestic responses in individuals previously sensitized but occasionally may result from primary exposure to the incompatible blood.[76] Signs include fever and anemia; icterus and hemoglobinuria may be present. When such a reaction is suspected, an aliquot of the patient's blood should be sent to the blood bank for identification of the blood compatibility. If this is not present, more common causes of post-transfusion (and postoperative) hemolysis should be suspected. These include lysis and resorption of intraperitoneal blood, drug hemolytic reactions, severe infection, and nonimmune lysis of old donor blood. Severe delayed immune hemolytic reactions are rare and should be treated in the same manner as acute hemolytic reactions.

Noncardiogenic pulmonary edema associated with transfusion[67, 77] presents suddenly and is accompanied by fever, hypotension, and chest pain. It may occur within several hours of transfusion and resolves within 2 days. Pathogenesis may involve agglutination of transfused granulocytes in pulmonary capillaries, with complement-mediated endothelial damage[78] or an alloantibody reaction.[77] Diagnostic and evaluative measures are the same as for all cases of suspected pulmonary edema; pulmonary capillary wedge pressure will not be elevated. Supportive measures are similar to those used for other causes of pulmonary edema. In addition, high doses of corticosteroids have been advocated.[78] Over 80% of patients undergo rapid, complete recovery.[77]

Thrombocytopenia, which may be life threatening, may result from development of platelet-specific antibodies in response to the challenge of a transfusion containing allogeneic platelets.[79, 80] This rare condition is known as post-transfusion purpura. It may occur after a transfusion of whole blood or of packed erythrocytes, because both of these preparations invariably contain platelets. It may also occur after transfusion of platelet concentrate. The primary sensitization to platelets usually occurs during pregnancy, and thrombocytopenia occurs with an anamnestic response 2 to 10 days after transfusion. Treatment is with intravenous IgG,[81] plasma exchange,[82] and cortico-steroids.[83]

Delayed Transfusion Reactions

Infections are among the most common serious complications seen and are the most feared by the lay public. Table 17–10 provides a list of the infectious agents most likely to be found in blood in the United States and the life span of those agents in banked blood.

Infection with the human immunodeficiency virus by transfusion accounts for a small proportion (about 2%) of cases of the acquired immunodeficiency syndrome.[84] Conversely, the chances of infection from a unit of erythrocytes or whole blood is no more than 1 in 100,000 and may be less than 1 in 300,000.[58] During the 1980s, the most common cause of bloodborne human immunodeficiency virus infection was infusion of cryoprecipitate and other coagulation factor concentrates prepared from pooled plasma, especially to hemophiliacs, who often received many such infusions.[85] This no longer is a source of infection, because the virus in these preparations is now heat-inactivated before use.[86] This virus can still be transmitted with low frequency through transfusion of single units of cellular blood components and of FFP. Screening for the virus in blood is performed using an assay for anti–human immunodeficiency virus antibody. There is a latent period of 3 weeks to 6 months (usually less than 3 months) during which infected individuals remain antibody negative.[87, 88] If an infected person donates blood during this latent interval, he or she can transmit the virus. Furthermore, some infected individuals will not develop antibodies,[89] and false-negative test results may occur.

Human T-lymphotropic virus type I, which causes adult T-cell lymphoma, may also be transmitted by transfusion as determined by seroconversion.[90] Donated blood is routinely screened for this virus.

Viral hepatitis is, historically, the infection most associated with serious transfusion sequelae, but routine serologic testing of blood has markedly reduced the risk in recent years. Routine testing of donated blood has virtually eliminated transmission of hepatitis A by transfusion. Hepatitis B is more lethal than hepatitis A. Before 1985, it was responsible for at least 10% of all reported transfusion-related mortality,[59] although the long interval from transfusion to development of hepatitis may have led to major underreporting. This complication has largely been eliminated through routine testing of blood for the HbS antigen. About 80% of patients with non-A, non-B hepatitis harbor antibodies to hepatitis C proteins.[91, 92] Two thirds of these patients develop chronic liver disease. First-generation testing has reduced the risk of transmission of hepatitis C from 4% to 0.03% per unit[93, 94]; second-generation testing probably will reduce the risk further. There are at least three other forms of viral hepatitis that may be transmitted by blood exchange. The epidemiology and natural history of these illnesses are poorly understood.

Other serious infections may be present in transfused blood products. Syphilis may be transmitted by way of transfusion. This is unusual, however, because most blood banks perform serologic tests for syphilis on donated blood and because spirochetes rarely survive longer than 4 days in banked blood.[95] Malaria may also be transmitted through transfusion; all pathogenic *Plasmodium* species survive at least a week in banked blood.[96] Because there is no test for the presence of the parasite, the only means of prevention is by exclusion of donors who have recently traveled to epidemic areas. Bacterial sepsis can occur on rare occasions from blood contaminated with bacterial pathogens at the time of donation. Such sepsis accounts for almost 10% of transfusion-associated mortality.[59] Trypanosomiasis may be transmitted by transfusion but is not important in the United States. Epstein-Barr virus, cytomegalovirus, and parvovirus may be acquired

---

TABLE 17–10
Infectious Agents That May Be Transmitted by Transfusion*

Viruses

Human immunodeficiency virus (indefinite)
Viral hepatitis (hepatitis C > hepatitis B > hepatitis A) (indefinite)
Epstein-Barr virus (indefinite)
Cytomegalovirus (indefinite)
Parvovirus (indefinite)

Bacteria

Treponema pallidum (4 days)
Cutaneous bacteria (e.g., *Staphylococcus epidermidis*) (remain infectious; contamination generally apparent within 2 weeks)

Parasites

Plasmodium species (>7 days)
Toxoplasma gondii

---

*The approximate life span in banked blood of each agent is given in parentheses.

through transfusion, but infection in adults is usually mild. Other infections occasionally transmitted by blood transfusion include HTLV II infection, babesiosis, Chagas' disease, Colorado tick fever, Jakob-Creutzfeld disease, and various tropical virus infections.

Graft-versus-host disease is a rare complication of transfusions, especially of platelet and leukocyte concentrates, in immunosuppressed patients and is almost always fatal.[97] All blood products containing cellular elements should be irradiated before administration to patients at risk.[98]

REFERENCES

1. Buttram VC Jr, Reiter RC. Uterine leiomyomata: etiology, symptomatology, and management. Fertil Steril 1981;36:433–445.
2. Baumgartner HR. The role of blood flow in platelet adhesion, fibrin deposition, and formation of mural thrombi. Microvasc Res 1973;5:167–179.
3. Best LC, Holland TK, Jones PB, et al. The interrelationship between thromboxane biosynthesis, aggregation and 5-hydroxytryptamine secretion in human platelets in vitro. Thromb Haemost 1980;43:38–44.
4. Roth GJ, Majerus PW. The mechanism of the effect of aspirin on human platelets: I. Acetylation of a particulate fraction protein. J Clin Invest 1975;56:624–632.
5. Catalano PM, Smith JB, Murphy S. Platelet recovery from aspirin inhibition in vivo: differing patterns under various assay conditions. Blood 1981;57:99–105.
6. Jordan RE, Oosta GM, Gardner WT, et al. The kinetics of hemostatic enzyme–antithrombin interactions in the presence of low molecular weight heparin. J Biol Chem 1980;255:10081–10090.
7. Harrigan C, Lucas CE, Ledgerwood AM, et al. Primary hemostasis after massive transfusion for injury. Am Surg 1982;48:393–396.
8. Fresh-Frozen Plasma, Cryoprecipitate, and Platelets Administration Practice Guidelines Development Task Force of the College of American Pathologists. Practice parameters for the use of fresh frozen plasma, cryoprecipitate, and platelets. JAMA 1994;271:777–781.
9. Reed R, Ciavarella D, Heimback D, et al. Prophylactic platelet administration during massive transfusion. Ann Surg 1986;203:40–46.
10. Shanberg JN, Quattrochiocchi-Longe T. Analysis of fresh-frozen plasma administration with suggestions for ways to reduce usage. Transfus Med 1992;2:189–194.
11. Leslie SD, Toy PTCY. Laboratory hemostatic abnormalities in massively transfused patients given red blood cells and crystalloid. Am J Clin Pathol 1991;96:770–773.
12. Mannucci PM, Federici AB, Sirchia G. Hemostasis testing during massive blood replacement: a study of 172 cases. Vox Sang 1982;12:113–123.
13. Noe DA, Graham SM, Luff R, et al. Platelet counts during rapid massive transfusion. Transfusion 1982;22:392–395.
14. Sedaghat A, Ayromlooi J. Disseminated intravascular coagulation resulting in severe hemorrhage, following the intraamniotic injection of hypertonic saline to induce abortion. Am J Obstet Gynecol 1972;114:841–843.
15. Calvert GD. Postpartum haemolytic uraemic syndrome: case report and review. J Obstet Gynecol Brit Commonw 1972;79:244–249.
16. Mosesson MW, Coleman RW, Sherry S. Chronic intravascular coagulation syndrome. N Engl J Med 1968;278:815–821.
17. Cafferata HT, Aggeler PM, Robinson JA, et al. Intravascular coagulation in surgical patients: its significance and diagnosis. Am J Surg 1969;118:281–291.
18. Edgington TR. Recognition coupled responses of the monocyte: activation of coagulation pathways. Nouv Rev Fr Hematol 1983;25:1–6.
19. Geczy CL, Hopper KE. A mechanism of migration inhibition of delayed hypersensitivity reactions: II. Lymphokines promote coagulant activity in vitro. J Immunol 1981;126:1059–1065.
20. Muhlfelder TW, Niemitz J, Kreutzer D, et al. C5 chemotactic fragment induces leukocyte production of tissue factor activity: a link between complement and coagulation. J Clin Invest 1979;63:147–150.
21. Bithell TC. Acquired coagulation disorders. In Lee GR, Bithell TC, Foerster J, et al, eds. Wintrobe's Clinical Hematology, 9th ed. Philadelphia, Lea & Febiger, 1993, pp 1473–1514.
22. Morrison DC, Cochrane CG. Direct evidence for Hageman factor (factor XII) activation by bacterial lipopolysaccharides (endotoxins). J Exp Med 1974;140:797–811.
23. Thiagarajan P, Niemetz J. Procoagulant tissue activity of circulating peripheral blood leukocytes. Thromb Res 1980;17:891–896.
24. Okajima K, Imamura H, Kaga S, et al. Treatment of patients with disseminated intravascular coagulation by protein C. Am J Hematol 1990;33:277–278.
25. Cole SK, Billwicz WZ, Thomson AM. Sources of variation in menstrual blood loss. J Obstet Gynaecol Brit Commonw 1971;78:933–939.
26. Hallberg L, Hogdahl A-M, Nilsson L, Rybo G. Menstrual blood loss—a population study: variation at different ages and attempts to define normality. Acta Obstet Gynecol Scand 1966;45:320–351.
27. Hallberg L, Nilsson L. Constancy of individual menstrual blood loss. Acta Obstet Gynecol Scand 1964;43:352–359.
28. Eschbach JW, Kelly MR, Haley NR, et al. Treatment of the anemia of progressive renal failure with recombinant human erythropoietin. N Engl J Med 1989;321:158–163.
29. Stehling L, Simon TS. The red blood cell transfusion trigger: physiology and clinical studies. Arch Path Lab Med 1994;118:429–434.
30. Stehling LC, Esposito B. Appropriate intraoperative blood utilization (abstract). Transfusion 1987;27:545.
31. Robertie PG, Gravlee GP. Safe limits of isovolemic hemodilution and recommendations for erythrocyte transfusion. Int Anesth Clin 1990;28:197–204.
32. Addonizio VP, Stahl RF. Bleeding. In: Wilmore DW, Brennan MF, Harken AH, eds. American College of Surgeons Care of the Surgical Patient. New York, Scientific American, 1989.
33. Nunn JF, Freeman J. Problems of oxygenation and oxygen transport during haemorrhage. Anaesthesia 1964;19:206–216.
34. Chapler CK, Cain SM. The physiologic reserve in oxygen carrying capacity: studies in experimental hemodilution. Can J Physiol Pharmacol 1986;64:7–12.
35. Babineau TJ, Dzik WH, Borlase BC, et al. Reevaluation of current transfusion practices in patients in surgical intensive care units. Am J Surg 1992;164:22–25.
36. Lucas CE, Weaver D, Higgins RF, et al. Effects of albumin vs non-albumin resuscitation on plasma volume and renal excretory function. J Trauma 1978;18:564–568.

37. Moss GS, Lowe RJ, Jilek J, et al. Fluid therapy in shock. Prog Clin Biol Sci 1982;108:51–63.
38. Zadrobilek E, Hackl W, Sporn P, et al. Effect of large volume replacement with balanced electrolyte solutions on extravascular lung water in surgical patients with sepsis. Intens Care Med 1989;15:505–510.
39. Langdell RD, Adelson E, Furth FW, et al. Dextran and prolonged bleeding time: results of a sixty-gram one-liter infusion given to 163 normal human subjects. JAMA 1958;166:346–350.
40. Ring J, Mossmer K. Incidence and severity of anaphylactoid reactions to colloid volume substitutes. Lancet 1977;1:466–469.
41. AuBuchon JP. Autologous transfusions and directed donations: current controversies and future directions. Transfus Med Rev 1989;3:290–306.
42. Glover JL, Broadie TA. Intraoperative autotransfusion. Surg Annu 1984;16:39–56.
43. Dzik WH, Jenkins R. Use of intraoperative blood salvage during orthotopic liver transplantation. Arch Surg 1985;120:946–948.
44. Reul GJ, Solis RT, Greenberg SD, et al. Experience with autotransfusion in the surgical management of trauma. Surgery 1974;76:546–555.
45. American College of Obstetrics and Gynecology. Blood Component Therapy. Technical Bulletin #199. Washington, DC, November 1994.
46. Greenburg AG. Indications for transfusion. In: Wilmore DW, Brennan MF, Harken AH, eds. American College of Surgeons Care of the Surgical Patient. New York, Scientific American, 1989.
47. Gould SA, Rosen AL, Sehgal LR, et al. Fluosol-DA as a red-cell substitute in acute anemia. N Engl J Med 1986;314:1653–1656.
48. Waxman K, Tremper KK, Cullen BF, et al. Perfluorocarbon infusion in bleeding patients refusing blood transfusions. Arch Surg 1984;119:721–724.
49. Hoyt DB, Greenburg AG, Forbes S, et al. Rescuscitation with Fluosol-DA 20%—tolerance to sepsis. J Trauma 1986;26:713–716.
50. Rabiner SF, Helbert JR, Lopas H, et al. Evaluation of a stroma-free hemoglobin solution for use as a plasma expander. J Exp Med 1967;126:1127–1142.
51. Bickell WH, Pepe PE, Bailey ML, et al. Randomized trial of pneumatic antishock garments in the prehospital management of penetrating abdominal injuries. Ann Emerg Med 1987;16:653–658.
52. Nelson BE, Schwartz PE. Hemorrhage and shock. In: Nichols DH, ed. Gynecologic and Obstetric Surgery. St. Louis, CV Mosby, 1994, pp 208–221.
53. O'Hanlon KA, Trambert J, Rodriguez-Rodriguez L, et al. Arterial embolization in the management of abdominal and retroperitoneal hemorrhage. Gynecol Oncol 1989;34:131–135.
54. Schwartz PR, Goldstein HM, Wallace S, et al. Control of arterial hemorrhage using percutaneous arterial catheter techniques in patients with gynecologic malignancies. Gynecol Oncol 1975;3:276–288.
55. Jonsson K, Jenses JA, Goodson WH, et al. Tissue oxygenation, anemia, and perfusion in relation to wound healing in surgical patients. Ann Surg 1991;214:605–613.
56. Markoe AM. Radiation oncologic emergencies. In Perez CA, Brady LW, eds. Principles and Practice of Radiation Oncology. Philadelphia, JB Lippincott, 1987, pp 1267–1270.
57. Dodd RY. The risk of transfusion-transmitted infection. N Engl J Med 1992;327:419–421.
58. Dodd RY. Adverse consequences of blood transfusion: quantitative risk estimates. In Nance ST, ed. Blood Supply: Risks, Perceptions and Prospects for the Future. Bethesda, MD, American Association of Blood Banks, 1994.
59. Sazama K. Reports of 355 transfusion-associated deaths: 1976 through 1985. Transfusion 1990;30:583–590.
60. Greenwalt TJ. Pathogenesis and management of hemolytic transfusion reactions. Semin Hematol 1981;18:84–94.
61. Pineda AA, Brzica SM Jr, Taswell HF. Hemolytic transfusion reaction: recent experience in a large blood bank. Mayo Clin Proc 1978;53:378–390.
62. Honig CL, Bove JR. Transfusion-associated fatalities: review of Bureau of Biologics reports. Transfusion 1980;20:653–661.
63. Baker RJ, Moinichen SL, Nyhus LM. Transfusion reaction: a reappraisal of surgical incidence and significance. Ann Surg 1969;169:684–693.
64. Binder LS, Ginsberg V, Harmel LH. A six year study of incompatible blood transfusions. Surg Gynecol Obstet 1959;108:19–34.
65. Seager OA, Nesmith MA, Begelman KA, et al. Massive acute hemodilution for incompatible blood reaction. JAMA 1974;229:790–792.
66. Barton JC. Nonhemolytic, noninfectious transfusion reactions. Semin Hematol 1981;18:95–121.
67. Brubaker DB. Immunologically mediated immediate adverse effects of blood transfusions (allergic, febrile nonhemolytic, and noncardiogenic pulmonary edema). Plasma Ther 1985;45:6–19.
68. Decary F, Ferner P, Giaredoni L, et al. An investigation of non-hemolytic transfusion reactions. Vox Sang 1984;46:277–285.
69. De Rie MA, van der Plas-van Dalen CM, Engelfreit CP, et al. The serology of febrile transfusion reactions. Vox Sang 1985;49:126–134.
70. Duke M, Herbert VD, Abelman WH. Hemodynamic effects of blood transfusion in chronic anemia. N Engl J Med 1964;271:975–980.
71. Burks AW, Sampson HA, Buckley RH. Anaphylactic reactions after gamma globulin administration in patients with hypogammaglobulinemia: detection of IgE antibodies to IgA. N Engl J Med 1986;314:560–564.
72. Vyas GN, Perkins HA. Anti-IgA in blood donors. Transfusion 1976;16:289–290.
73. Collins JA. Problems associated with the massive transfusion of stored blood. Surgery 1974;75:274–295.
74. Collins JA. Massive transfusion in surgery and trauma. Prog Clin Biol Res 1982;108:5–16.
75. Moore SB. Delayed hemolytic transfusion reactions. Am J Clin Pathol 1980;74:94–97.
76. Patten E, Redd CR, Riglin H, et al. Delayed hemolytic transfusion reaction caused by a primary immune response. Transfusion 1982;22:248–250.
77. Popovsky MA, Moore SB. Diagnostic and pathogenetic considerations in transfusion-related acute lung injury. Transfusion 1985;25:573–577.
78. Jacob HS. Complement-mediated leucoembolization: a mechanism of tissue damage during extracorporeal perfusions, myocardial infarction, and in shock—a review. Q J Med 1983;52:289–296.
79. Abramson N, Eisenberg PD, Aster RH. Post-transfusion purpura: immunologic aspects and therapy. N Engl J Med 1974;291:1163–1166.
80. Pegels JG, Bruynes ECE, Engelfreit CP, et al. Posttransfusion purpura: a serological and immunological study. Br J Haematol 1981;49:521–530.
81. Hamblin TJ, Naoroso Abidi SM, Ness PA, et al. Successful treatment of post-transfusion purpura with high dose immunoglobulins after lack of response to plasma exchange. Vox Sang 1985;49:164–167.
82. Cimo PL, Aster RH. Post-transfusion purpura: success-

ful treatment by exchange transfusion. N Engl J Med 1972;287:290–292.

83. Slichter SJ. Post-transfusion purpura: response to steroids and association with red blood cell and lymphocytotoxic antibodies. Br J Haematol 1982;50:599–605.

84. Perkins HA. Transfusion-associated AIDS. Am J Hematol 1985;19:307–313.

85. AIDS-Hemophilia French Study Group. Immunologic and virologic status of multitransfused patients: role of type and origin of blood products. Blood 1985;66:896–901.

86. Schimpf K, Brackmann HH, Kreuz W, et al. Absence of anti-human immunodeficiency virus types 1 and 2 seroconversion after the treatment of hemophilia A or von Willebrand's disease with pasteurized factor VIII concentrate. N Engl J Med 1989;321:1148–1152.

87. Cooper DA, Maclean P, Finlayson R, et al. Acute AIDS retrovirus infection: definition of an acute illness associated with seroconversion. Lancet 1985;1:537–540.

88. Groopman JE, Hartzband PI, Shulman L, et al. Antibody seronegative human T-lymphotropic virus type III (HTLV-III) infected patients with acquired immunodeficiency syndrome or related disorders. Blood 1985;66:742–744.

89. Salahuddin, Markham PD, Redfield RR, et al. HTLV-III in symptom-free seronegative persons. Lancet 1984;2:1418–1420.

90. Okochi K, Sato H, Hinuma Y. A retrospective study on transmission of adult T cell leukemia virus by blood transfusion: seroconversion in recipients. Vox Sang 1984;46:245–253.

91. Esteban JI, Gonzalez A, Hernandez JM, et al. Evaluation of antibodies to hepatitis C virus in a study of transfusion-associated hepatitis. N Engl J Med 1990;323:1107–1112.

92. Alter MJ, Margolis HS, Krawczynski K, et al. The natural history of community-acquired hepatitis C in the United States. N Engl J Med 1992;327:1899–1905.

93. Alter MJ. Review of serologic testing for hepatitis C virus infection and risk of posttransfusion hepatitis C. Arch Pathol Lab Med 1994;118:342–345.

94. Donahue JG, Munoz A, Ness PM, et al. The declining risk of post-transfusion hepatitis C virus infection. N Engl J Med 1992;327:369–373.

95. Bove JR. Does it make sense for blood transfusion services to continue the time-honored syphilis screening with cardiolipin antigen? Vox Sang 1981;41:183.

96. Guerrero IC, Weniger BC, Schultz MG. Transfusion malaria in the United States, 1972–1981. Ann Intern Med 1983;99:221–226.

97. Brubaker DB. Human transfusion graft-versus-host disease. Vox Sang 1983;45:401–420.

98. Leitman SF, Holland PV. Irradiation of blood products: indications and guidelines. Transfusion 1985;25:293–300.

18

George J. Olt

Postoperative Bowel Complications

All gynecologists are faced with patients who develop postoperative bowel complications. Fortunately, most of these complications, such as postoperative ileus, are self limiting. Others, however, can be life threatening. Therefore, it is important to recognize and manage these problems rapidly and accurately to limit morbidity and mortality.

GASTROINTESTINAL BLEEDING

Gastrointestinal bleeding is an infrequent postoperative complication. However, when bleeding occurs it carries significant risk of morbidity and mortality and therefore must be rapidly and carefully evaluated and treated. Postoperative patients are susceptible to bleeding from any site within the gastrointestinal tract and are at increased risk of stress-related mucosal damage, particularly if they are debilitated or have undergone extensive surgical procedures. Symptoms, diagnosis, and treatment are dependent on the bleeding location. By convention, bleeding sites are divided into upper gastrointestinal, which occurs proximal to the ligament of Treitz, and lower gastrointestinal from distal sites. Acute upper gastrointestinal bleeding occurs more frequently than lower gastrointestinal bleeding, although precise relative incidences are unknown.

Upper Gastrointestinal Bleeding

Peptic ulcers (gastric and duodenal) are the most frequent sites of upper gastrointestinal bleeding, representing approximately 50% of all nonvariceal bleeding.[1] Other common causes that may be exacerbated by surgery are Mallory-Weiss tears and gastric erosions. The incidence of esophageal varices, which are related to alcohol intake, is much higher in inner-city hospitals than in community hospitals.

History and physical examination may be helpful in making a provisional diagnosis. For example, bleeding after retching may be caused by a Mallory-Weiss tear. Postoperative patients with shock or sepsis may have gastric mucosal erosions. Aspirin or nonsteroidal anti-inflammatory drug usage is associated with a 15% rate of gastric ulcers and increases the relative risk for upper gastrointestinal bleeding.[2, 3] The character of bleeding can be helpful to predict rebleeding.[4] Patients with coffee-grounds emesis are less likely to rebleed than those who vomit bright red blood. Repeated episodes of melena are predictive of continued bleeding. Vomiting of blood coupled with hematochezia indicates large amounts of bleeding from a probable arterial source. History and physical examination are not specific enough to make a reliable diagnosis, and therefore other diagnostic techniques must be performed.

Initial treatment of gastrointestinal bleeding must focus on stabilization of the patient. At least two sites of venous access with large-bore catheters should be obtained; and if the patient is hypovolemic, vigorous crystalloid fluid resuscitation should be initiated. Coagulation studies, hematocrit, and type and crossmatch of 4 units of packed red blood cells should be obtained. Placement of a large-bore nasogastric tube followed by irrigation with room temperature saline allows assessment of the rate of bleeding, prevention of aspiration, and removal of blood clots in preparation for endoscopy.

Flexible endoscopy should be performed as rapidly as feasible. The overall accuracy of endoscopy for detecting the site of bleeding is approximately 90% but decreases with time after bleeding.[5] Surgery remains the mainstay of treatment of upper gastrointestinal bleeding, although endoscopic therapy such as laser or electrocoagulation may be useful in selected patients with mild bleeding.

Lower Gastrointestinal Bleeding

Most lower gastrointestinal bleeding originates in the colon, but it may also arise from the small bowel or from an upper gastrointestinal source. In patients with lower gastrointestinal bleeding, the bleeding will stop spontaneously in 80%. However, 25% of these patients have recurrence of bleeding and 50% of these patients will bleed again.[6] The most common causes of lower gastrointestinal bleeding are diverticulosis and angiodysplasia, which are responsible for roughly 79% of cases.[7] Other causes of lower gastrointestinal bleeding include neoplasms, inflammatory bowel disease, radiation colitis, and hemorrhoids.

The appearance of the patient's stool may provide insight into the source of bleeding. Melanotic stools, which are black, sticky, and foul smelling are caused by bacterial degradation of hemoglobin and suggest an upper gastrointestinal source. The source may be in the small bowel or proximal colon if the bleeding is not brisk. Clotted blood may be confused with melena but will turn toilet water red. Gross blood is most frequently from lower gastrointestinal bleeding but may also occur with rapid upper gastrointestinal bleeding.

It is often difficult to diagnose and localize bleeding from the small bowel, but, fortunately, it occurs rarely and is frequently self limited. Often, bleeding is mild and intermittent. Upper and lower endoscopy cannot directly visualize the distal small bowel but should be performed to rule out sources of bleeding proximal to the ligament of Treitz and distal to the ileocecal valve.

Radionuclide scanning may be helpful in patients in whom a bleeding site cannot be identified by endoscopy. The most common method uses technetium-99m–labeled red blood cells injected intravenously, followed by abdominal nuclear scintigraphy. The advantages of this technique are its sensitivity and the ability to rescan patients for 24 hours after injection, which presents the opportunity to detect intermittent bleeding. The major disadvantage is the inability of precise localization of the bleeding site.

Angiography is also a valuable tool for evaluating lower gastrointestinal bleeding. Although angiography requires active bleeding, rates as low as 0.5 mL/min can be detected.[8] An advantage of angiography is its ability to localize the bleeding site, which is important if surgery is required.[9] Additionally, angiography may be helpful in controlling bleeding by arterial embolization or vasopressin infusion. If surgery is anticipated, some surgeons prefer to leave the catheter in place to aid in the intraoperative location of bleeding.

Treatment begins with resuscitation of the patient as described for upper gastrointestinal bleeding. The indication for and order of performance of upper endoscopy, lower endoscopy, angiography, and surgery depend on the preferences of the consulting gastroenterologists and surgeons. Endoscopic laser, heater probe, or bipolar fulguration may be helpful in treating some lesions; however, the recurrence rate is higher than with surgical resection. Surgery should be considered in patients who have received more than 6 units of blood.[10]

POSTOPERATIVE DIARRHEA

Antibiotic-Associated Colitis

It is now well established that patients who have received antibiotics may develop an antibiotic-associated colitis caused by *Clostridium difficile*. Groups at higher risk include women, cancer patients, patients undergoing abdominal surgery, and patients in intensive care units.[11] Nearly all antibiotics and routes of administration have been associated with antibiotic-associated colitis, which may occur as late as 6 weeks after therapy.

Antibiotic-associated colitis typically presents as watery diarrhea and cramping abdominal pain 4 to 9 days after antibiotic therapy, although symptoms may begin within 24 hours. Patients usually have fever, leukocytosis, and abdominal tenderness. The range of severity of symptoms may be quite variable. Occasionally, patients do not have diarrhea but have evidence of toxic megacolon, peritonitis, or perforation. Endoscopy frequently demonstrates the presence of a pseudomembrane. If the colitis is untreated, patients may experience sepsis, shock, and death. Diagnosis is made by detecting the presence of *Clostridium difficile* toxins A and B in the stool.

Both oral vancomycin and metronidazole are effective in treating antibiotic-associated colitis. Because it is less expensive, metronidazole should be used initially and vancomycin reserved for severely ill patients and those who fail to respond to metronidazole. In patients who cannot be treated orally owing to ileus or obstruction, intravenous metronidazole is useful. Alternatively, vancomycin retention enemas can be administered. Patients who do not respond to antibiotic therapy or who have sepsis or toxic megacolon may require colonic resection.

Short Bowel Syndrome

If patients have more than 50% to 70% of their small bowel resected or less than 100 cm of the bowel remains, they will likely suffer malabsorption manifested as diarrhea. Diarrhea results from decreased transit time and incompletely resorbed bile salts passing into the colon. Loss of the ileocecal valve accentuates these problems, worsening diarrhea. Loss of ileum is more significant than an equal loss of jejunum because bile salts are resorbed only by the ileum.

For patients who have undergone resection of a large amount of small bowel, it is helpful to begin enteral feeding with 5% glucose and half-normal saline until fluid balance is maintained. The patient can then be converted to oral feeding, or, if unable to eat, defined formula feeding can be given through a nasoenteric feeding tube. If the latter method is used, feedings initially should be diluted and the concentration gradually increased as tolerated.

Oral feedings should be frequent and small and should be fat restricted. Pharmacologic agents helpful in controlling diarrhea include diphenoxylate (Lomotil), loperamide (Imodium), ranitidine (Zantac), cimetidine (Tagamet), and psyllium hydrophilic mucilloid (Metamucil). If the distal ileum is resected, patients may require monthly injections of vitamin B_{12} to prevent pernicious anemia and vitamin K supplementation to prevent coagulopathy.

MALNUTRITION

Surgeons have long understood that postoperative morbidity and mortality were much lower when patients were in good nutritional condition. However, during the past three decades there has been a dramatic increase in understanding nutritional requirements and administration techniques. In 1968, Dudrick and colleagues demonstrated that total parenteral nutrition could restore weight loss and provide the sole nutritional support for adult patients.[12] These findings promoted an explosion of interest in the nutritional status of patients undergoing surgery by providing an alternative, parenteral avenue to treat nutritionally depleted patients. Today, a multitude of techniques and formulations exist for both enteral and parenteral feeding, providing a spectrum of capabilities, potential complications, and costs. Therefore, proper nutritional support should be initiated after a thoughtful nutritional assessment.

Nutritional Assessment

Malnutrition can be defined as a nutritional deficit associated with an increased risk of morbidity and mortality.[13] The incidence of malnutrition in surgical patients may be as high as 50%.[14] Patients undergoing surgery for malignant disease are the most likely gynecologic patients to be malnourished. However, as the population ages other risk factors for malnutrition increase, and thus many patients undergoing gynecologic surgery for nonmalignant indications may be malnourished as well. This fact is underscored by the recent Joint Commission on Accreditation of Hospitals requirement for nutritional screening.[15] Malnutrition risk factors that may be found in gynecologic patients include malignancy, heart failure, renal disease, infection, or chronic pulmonary disease.

The goal of a nutritional assessment is to identify patients who are at risk for postoperative morbidity resulting from malnutrition. Most nutritional assessment schemes use a combination of weight loss measurements, anthropometric measurements, and laboratory studies.

Weight loss is probably the most commonly used nutritional parameter and is usually the presenting sign of malnutrition. The patient's current weight is compared with the patient's usual weight. Recollected usual weights are nearly always accurate. Alternatively, ideal body weight can be calculated from the following formula.[16]

Ideal weight =
   100 lb for 5 feet + 5 lb/inch over 5 feet

Use of this formula, however, may be misleading, because many patients' usual body weight differs from their calculated ideal body weight. Serial body weight measurements are more reliable, but care must be taken to account for total body water gains and losses. Several studies have suggested an increase in postoperative morbidity with weight loss greater than 10% of usual body weight.[13] Because weight loss alone is not reliable enough to determine nutritional status, it is usually combined with other parameters such as triceps skinfold measurements and serum protein levels.

Triceps skinfold thickness measures the amount of subcutaneous fat and accurately reflects total fat stores. Depletion of fat stores has been correlated with poor outcome.[17] Muscle mass, which is the major source of protein during stressed starvation, can be approximated using measurement of 24-hour urine creatinine levels and a height index. However, muscle mass, when used alone, has not been shown to correlate with morbidity.[18]

Serum protein levels are useful in assessing nutritional status because they reflect the rate of protein synthesis and catabolism. Serum protein synthesis by the liver is decreased when protein intake declines. Therefore, decreased protein intake results in lower circulating serum protein levels in relationship to their half-lives.

Serum albumin has a relatively long half-life (18 days), and significant decreases may not occur for a month after starvation. Because albumin is the major serum protein, it correlates well with the nutritional state and is predictive of mortality.[19] However, its long half-life limits its ability to detect acute changes in nutritional status. Transferrin has a serum half-life of 8 to 10 days, but its synthesis is modulated by iron stores as well as protein intake. Furthermore, serious infection may lower transferrin levels as well. Prealbumin has the shortest half-life (2 to 3 days) and is the protein most rapidly affected by nutritional changes. However, prealbumin has not been shown to be a better predictor of outcome than albumin or transferrin.[20]

Malnutrition decreases cell-mediated immunity, as manifested by reduction in lymphocyte count and delayed cutaneous hypersensitivity. Unfortunately, these parameters are affected by many other conditions frequently found in postoperative patients and are not specific enough for routine use in nutritional assessment.

Multiparameter indices have been used to improve prediction of poor outcome. A model, the Prognostic Nutritional Index, has been validated prospectively in surgical populations.[21] The percent of risk is calculated using the following formula:

$$PNI \ [\% \ risk] = 158 - 16.6 \ [ALB] - 0.78 \ [TSF] - 0.2 \ [TFN] - 5.8 \ [DH]$$

where ALB = serum albumin (g/dL), TSF = triceps skinfold (mm), TFN = transferrin (mg/dL), and DH = delayed skin hypersensitivity (scale 0–2). Patients with values greater than 30% are at high risk for postoperative complications.

Postoperative Nutritional Support

To identify the patient who will benefit from postoperative nutritional support, one must take into account the patient's preoperative nutritional status, the anticipated amount of postoperative nutritional intake, and the patient's underlying disease. It is generally agreed that patients who are malnourished benefit from postoperative nutritional support. Other important factors that may indicate the need for nutritional support include planned chemotherapy, lengthy duration of time without enteral feeding, and hypermetabolic states such as infection.

The ultimate goals of nutritional support are to decrease postoperative morbidity and mortality and prepare the patient for future therapy. To meet these goals, requirements for protein and caloric intake sufficient to maintain an anabolic state should be determined. Certainly it is preferable to prevent nutritional depletion rather than to reverse malnutrition once it has occurred. As a general guideline, patients without oral intake for more than 7 to 10 days should receive nutritional support.

Daily protein requirements for adults range from 1.0 to 1.5 g/kg/d. Patients who are malnourished and those who are hypermetabolic have higher requirements and may require up to 2.0 g/kg/d. Determination of nitrogen balance can be helpful in assessing adequacy of protein intake. In general, nitrogen balance is calculated by subtracting measured urinary losses plus a constant for unmeasured loss from the total nitrogen intake.

Nonprotein caloric requirements can be determined by calculating the resting energy expenditure (REE) and adding the caloric requirements for activity and surgical stress. REE is calculated using the Harris-Benedict equation:

$$REE = 65 + 9.6 \times weight \ (kg) + 1.7 \times height - 4.7 \times age$$

Generally 130% of the REE is given as nonprotein calories. For patients in hypermetabolic states associated with sepsis and fever, underlying malnutrition, or extensive surgery, this may need to be increased to 150%. Nonprotein calories are usually given as carbohydrates and lipids in a 1:1 or 2:1 ratio. When compared with direct measurements of REE by oxygen consumption and carbon dioxide production, the Harris-Benedict equation appears to underestimate caloric requirements. Therefore, it is perhaps easier to provide caloric intake at a rate of 25 to 35 kcal/kg/d because the complications of overnutrition are minimal.

Both enteral and parenteral feeding have been shown to benefit postoperative patients.[22, 23] When these routes are compared, there appears to be no nutritional advantage of one method over another.[24] However, enteral feeding is beneficial in preventing atrophy of gut mucosa. Because of the higher cost and complication rates associated with total parenteral nutrition, it is preferable to use enteral feeding when possible.

Common complications of parenteral nutrition are catheter related and metabolic. Insertion of the central venous catheter may cause pneumothorax in 1% to 2% of patients. Other catheter complications are infection of the catheter or catheter site and venous thrombosis, both of which require removal of the catheter. Metabolic complications include hyperglycemia, electrolyte abnormalities, and azotemia secondary to excessive administration of amino acids. Mild hepatitis, as defined by elevations in serum aspartate aminotransferase and alanine aminotransferase, is common. If elevation of the levels of these liver enzymes becomes greater than twofold or there is an associated elevation in the serum bilirubin level, causes other than parenteral nutrition should be considered.

The most common complications of enteral feeding are diarrhea and colic, but they respond well to decreasing the rate and concentration of the feeding. A more serious complication is aspiration pneumonia. This potentially fatal occurrence can be limited by elevation of the head of the bed and ensuring placement of the feeding tube within the small intestine.

BOWEL OBSTRUCTION

Ileus

Postoperative ileus is familiar to all gynecologic surgeons. After surgery, there is a reduction in the coordinated propulsion of the gastrointestinal tract, resulting in abdominal distention frequently followed by nausea and vomiting. In addition to patient discomfort, this may result in respiratory compromise, wound dehiscence, and anastomotic leakage. Unfortunately, because little is known about the physiologic mechanisms, we cannot predict which patients will develop postoperative, adynamic ileus. There is considerable information concerning return of bowel function and motility after exploratory laparotomy. The stomach remains atonic for 18 to 24 hours, while the small bowel regains motility within a few hours.[25] The colon regains function, based on the passage of flatus, approximately 16 hours after nonabdominal surgery and 48 hours after abdominal surgery. After colonic resection, the colon does not regain function for approximately 110 hours.[26]

Animal studies suggest that adynamic ileus results from sympathetic inhibition initiated by spinal reflexes that are triggered by manipulation of the bowel. It had been widely held that the duration of operation and degree of bowel manipulation were proportional to the duration of ileus. However, in a study that correlated length of operation with duration of ileus, no correlation was found.[26] It was postulated that the afferent reflex pathway may originate in the parietal peritoneum rather than the gut wall. This theory would also explain the prolonged ileus seen in patients with retroperitoneal dissections or hematomas and the absence of ileus in patients undergoing laparoscopy.

The diagnosis of adynamic ileus is made clinically in patients with nausea, vomiting, abdominal distention, abdominal tympany, and the absence of bowel sounds and flatus. Treatment is initiated with institution of bowel rest and repletion of intravascular volume and electrolytes. Nasogastric intubation is helpful to prevent further air swallowing and to control nausea and vomiting. After the passage of flatus the patient's nasogastric tube may be clamped and enteral liquids cautiously given. If enteral feeding is tolerated, the diet is advanced and the nasogastric tube is withdrawn. If postoperative ileus persists for longer than 7 days, mechanical bowel obstruction should be considered.

Postoperative nasogastric intubation has been routinely used to prevent gastric dilatation. Acute gastric dilatation occurs when the stomach becomes overdistended with air and the several liters of bile, gastric juice, pancreatic juice, and succus entericus produced daily (Fig. 18–1). This results in a syndrome of belching and vomiting that leads to increased swallowing of air. The distention stimulates increased secretion of gastrointestinal fluids, and 4 or 5 L may accumulate. Shock may ensue from compression of the diaphragm, which interferes with cardiac and pulmonary function.

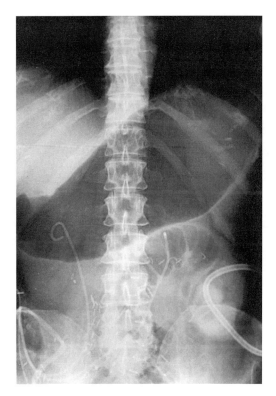

FIGURE 18–1
Acute gastric dilatation after total pelvic exenteration.

Pneumonia and death may result from aspiration of gastric contents. Acute gastric dilatation occurs most frequently after chest trauma and pancreatitis and is uncommon in women or after elective abdominal surgery. Despite the seriousness of acute gastric dilatation, its very rare occurrence probably does not warrent routine postoperative nasogastric intubation.

Small Bowel Obstruction

Nearly all small bowel obstructions occurring in the postoperative period are due to formation of adhesions. In the past, these patients would have undergone immediate reoperation, but more recently a role for nonoperative management has become accepted. Furthermore, the majority of patients treated conservatively have resolution of their obstruction and thus avoid reoperation.[27–29]

Patients with small bowel obstruction usually complain of intermittent nausea and vomiting, loss of appetite, and intermittent colicky pain. The absence of flatus indicates complete obstruction, but flatus may be present in early complete obstruction or partial obstruction. The presence of unremitting pain, fever, leukocytosis, or peritoneal signs such as cough or rebound tenderness suggest bowel strangulation. The degree of abdominal distention is dependent on the level of obstruction and may be unimpressive when the obstruction is proximal.

The diagnosis of obstruction is usually suspected by history and physical examination. Supine and left lateral decubitus abdominal radiographs are often helpful, both for diagnosis and evaluation of conservative therapy. Typical radiographic findings include dilated loops of small bowel with associated air–fluid levels and the absence of colonic gas. However, some colonic gas may be present in early, complete, or partial obstruction. A small amount of barium administered orally may be helpful to discriminate between partial and complete obstruction, although it is not usually necessary because the diagnosis can usually be made from abdominal radiographs and history.

Most patients are candidates for nonoperative management. However, any patient with signs and symptoms of strangulation or sepsis should undergo immediate exploration. When nonoperative management is appropriate, gastrointestinal intubation is instituted. Although data are lacking comparing nasogastric with nasointestinal intubation, most surgeons prefer the latter. Nasogastric intubation is helpful in removing swallowed air and in preventing further distention, whereas nasointestinal intubation decompresses the small bowel, potentially decreasing edema and inflammation. Use of a long tube in patients with obstruction secondary to adhesions has been reported to be successful in two thirds of cases.[27] Disadvantages of the long tube are difficulty in passage into the intestine and a potentially higher tube-associated complication rate.

Patients should be carefully monitored for intestinal strangulation during conservative therapy. The development of leukocytosis, metabolic acidosis, fever, or peritoneal irritation may indicate impending intestinal strangulation. If the signs, symptoms, and radiographic evidence of obstruction have not resolved by 48 hours, nonoperative therapy is unlikely to be successful. Factors associated with success are incomplete obstruction, recurrent obstruction, and passage of the tube beyond the pylorus.[27]

If operative therapy is required, a midline incision offers optimal exposure of the entire abdominal cavity. Care should be given to opening the abdomen especially at the site of the previous incision because this is the most likely site of adhesion. Enterotomy should be avoided because this significantly increases the likelihood of postoperative complications. All adhesions should be lysed and the entire bowel examined for serosal defects. Intraoperative decompression of the bowel should be avoided unless necessary for closure of the abdominal incision.

COLORECTAL COMPLICATIONS

Complications of Colostomy

Minor and major complications after colostomy are common, with incidences reported to be as high as 44% of all cases.[30] Fortunately, most of these complications are minor and require only local care or patient education. Colostomy complications can conveniently be divided into those that occur early and late. Complications occurring early are bleeding, ischemia, infection, and retraction. Those occurring later include stricture, parastomal herniation, and prolapse.

Early postoperative stomal bleeding is usually due to a small bleeding point at the stoma–skin interface. Bleeding is generally minimal and frequently stops spontaneously. A small absorbable suture placed at the point of bleeding is nearly always successful. Heavier parastomal bleeding from a colostomy placed through the rectus muscle may indicate damage to the epigastric vessels. Surgical exploration is usually required to identify the bleeding point and ligate the vessels. Parastomal bleeding after 24 hours is nearly always due to appliance trauma.

Early postoperative bleeding from the stomal lumen is much less common. It most frequently occurs from a nonhemostatic proximal anastomosis or is secondary to stomal necrosis. However, other sources are possible and the patient should be evaluated as for any episode of gastrointestinal bleeding.

Colostomy stomal ischemia is, fortunately, a rare complication often associated with an insufficient fascial defect, stomal tension or torsion, and thick anterior abdominal walls. If the stoma becomes dusky, a glass test tube can be inserted into the stoma to determine the level of ischemia. Ischemia above the level of the faschia can be observed, but ischemia below the fascia mandates exploration and advancement of viable bowel.

Colostomy retraction occurs in patients with thick anterior abdominal walls or when sufficient mobilization of the colon has not been provided. Retraction above the fascia may be carefully observed; however, if retraction occurs to a level below the fascia, revision of the colostomy should be undertaken.

Infection of the stomal site after colostomy has been reported in 3% to 15% of cases.[31–33] Cellulitis of the parastomal skin is the most common infection and is usually treated successfully with broad-spectrum systemic antibiotic therapy and debridement of any necrotic tissue. Abscess formation is much less common and requires drainage and antibiotic therapy. Colostomy infection appears to be more common in patients with unprepared bowel but does not occur more often with placement of the colostomy in the incision.[34] Other predisposing factors are diabetes, chronic corticosteroid use, and immunosuppression. Necrotizing fasciitis is an extremely rare occurrence after colostomy but is often lethal. Signs and symptoms of necrotizing fasciitis include systemic toxicity, a watery, foul-smelling exudate, fever, leukocytosis, and erythematous skin. If necrotizing fasciitis is diagnosed, wide debridement of skin and subcutaneous tissue must be rapidly undertaken in addition to the administration of systemic antibiotics.

Stomal herniation is the most common late complication of colostomy and may be expected in roughly 10% of patients. Large hernias may contain omentum, colon, or small bowel. They are less likely to incarcerate than are small hernias, which usually contain stomal colonic wall. Symptoms of herniation include pain, difficulty with appliance adhesion, and bowel obstruction. Symptomatic hernias are best treated with surgical repair. The principles of repair are similar to those of other hernias, namely, excision of the hernia sac and closure of the fascial defect. Large defects may require relocation of the stoma or supplementation of the fascia with synthetic materials. Stomal binders may be helpful in patients who are not candidates for surgery, but most patients find them uncomfortable.

Stomal prolapse occurs most frequently after creation of loop-type colostomies, particularly transverse loop colostomies. Colostomy closure is the best treatment if feasible. If not possible, then conversion to an end colostomy with resection of the redundant segment and creation of a mucous fistula is the second choice. Nearly all repairs will require some closure of the fascia.

The most frequently observed complications after colostomy closure are anastomotic leakage, bowel obstruction, wound infection, and herniation. It is preferable to delay colostomy closure for 6 to 8 weeks after construction because of increased infectious morbidity associated with early closure. Patients should undergo antibiotic and mechanical bowel preparation before closure to decrease the risk of infection.

Complications of Bowel Resection and Anastomosis

Anastomotic leakage is the most feared and common complication after bowel resection and anastomosis. Colonic anatomoses are much more prone to dihiscence and leakage because of the colon's intrinsic higher bacterial content, thinner muscular wall, and greater distensibility. Anastomoses performed on distal bowel are more likely to leak as compared with anastomoses of proximal bowel. The exact incidence of anastomotic leakage is unclear and varies depending on the diagnostic technique used as well as the site of anastomosis. Radiographically detected leakage may approach 30% to 40%, but clinically detectable leakage ranges from 5% to 15%.[35]

Clinical manifestations of anastomotic leaks usually manifest during the second postoperative week. These clinical manifestations have been conveniently divided into five categories by Moossa and coworkers.[36] A subclinical group is defined by radiographic identification

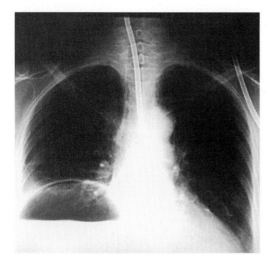

FIGURE 18-2
Chest radiograph demonstrating free air under the right diaphragm caused by a leaking anastomosis.

of leaks that are not clinically detectable and that do not affect the patient's postoperative course. A second group of patients, with clinical evidence of sepsis, have leukocytosis, fever, and tachycardia. The patient generally feels unwell but is usually in good condition initially. Often an ileus is present, but abdominal tenderness is minimal and rebound is absent. This may insidiously progress into a group with diffuse peritonitis that can result in septic shock, cardiovascular collapse, and rapid deterioration. Alternatively, patients can develop localized peritonitis that occurs several days into an uneventful postoperative course. Localized abdominal tenderness is accompanied by fever, leukocytosis, and ileus. Frequently, these patients spontaneously drain feculent material and their condition dramatically improves.

Clinical findings as described earlier lead the surgeon to suspect anastomotic leakage. Definitive preoperative diagnosis, however, is usually made with radiographic studies. An upright or left lateral decubitus radiograph of the abdomen may show free air (Fig. 18-2). The presence of free air in the first postoperative week must be interpreted with caution, however, because air introduced at laparotomy persists for variable periods of time. A single-contrast enema using water-soluble contrast agent such as meglumine diatrizoate (Renografin or Hypaque) demonstrates a leaking anastomosis. Barium sulfate–containing contrast medium should not be used to evaluate an anastomosis because of potential chemical peritonitis. Abdominal-pelvic computed tomographic scans are also useful, especially if localized peritonitis is suspected. They are also helpful to detect leakage into the retroperitoneum (Fig. 18-3). Therapeutic percutaneous computed tomographic guided drainage may obviate the need for a surgical procedure.

Management of anastomotic leakage should be individualized and is dependent primarily on the patient's general condition and the clinical signs and symptoms attributable to the leak. If the patient has signs of sepsis or generalized peritonitis, then expedient surgery is nearly always necessary. Before exploration, the patient should be resuscitated with intravenous hydration, antibiotics, and pressor agents if necessary. If cardiovascular collapse is the presenting sign, then surgery should be undertaken immediately because mortality in this group of patients is very high.[37]

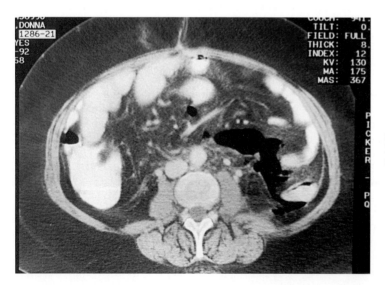

FIGURE 18-3
Pelvic CT scan demonstrating retroperitoneal free air.

At exploration, the entire abdominal cavity should be examined and irrigated. The anastomosis should be externalized if possible. Repair of the anastomotic site is difficult owing to local proteolysis, and continued leakage is likely even when protected by proximal loop diversion. It is preferable to externalize the proximal limb of the anastomosis as an end colostomy or ileostomy with the distal limb as a mucous fistula. If the distal end of the anastomosis is not long enough to externalize, it should be stapled closed. A leaking anastomosis in a segment of mobile bowel can be externalized intact, although this can cause difficulty with appliance application and is also associated with an increase in wound infection. The fascia should be carefully closed and the remainder of the incision left open for delayed primary closure or healing by secondary intention. The placement of drains is controversial and is often reserved for situations in which there are pockets of fluid that should be drained.

Patients with an anastomotic leak who do not exhibit evidence of generalized sepsis have typically walled-off the infection. These patients can be treated more conservatively, allowing time for radiographic study and computed tomographic guided percutaneous drainage of any abscess. The active drainage catheter is left in place, and intravenous antibiotics are continued until drainage is minimal. Complications of this technique include persistence of the abscess and the development of enterocutaneous fistula tracts. Spontaneous fistulization may occur, especially if leakage was not suspected. These patients may have incompletely drained abscess cavities and may benefit from computed tomographic guided drainage. Patients should be reevaluated periodically for repositioning of the catheter to ensure complete drainage of any loculations. Patients who are treated conservatively likely require a lengthy period without enteral feeding, and total parenteral nutrition should be considered.

Postoperative bleeding at the anastomotic site is rare. It is most common after stapled end-to-end anastomosis in which hemostasis cannot be evaluated. If bleeding persists, transanal endoscopy with coagulation of the bleeding point may be helpful. Most small bowel resections performed by gynecologists are undertaken owing to obstruction secondary to ovarian cancer. Complications in this group of patients were similar to those observed after colonic procedures but occurred at a higher rate, which was attributed to the patients' poor

nutritional status.[38] Common complications were wound infection, sepsis, abscess, and fistula.

Strictures occurring after anastomoses of the gastrointestinal tract are relatively common and, depending on the criteria used for diagnosis, occur in 2% to 20% of patients.[39, 40] However, the majority of strictures are asymptomatic. In patients who experience symptoms, resection and reanastomosis are generally required. An exception may be patients with distal strictures after low rectal resection and reanastomosis. Successful treatment by dilatation per rectum has been reported.

Enterocutaneous Fistulas

Enterocutaneous fistulas occurring postoperatively are usually caused by technical complications such as damage to bowel, leaking anastomosis, and bowel obstruction. These complications may be worsened by unhealthy tissue owing to malnutrition, irradiation, infection, inflammation, or chronic metabolic disease. The outcome of enterocutaneous fistulas is greatly dependent on anatomic factors.

Location of the fistula correlates with the amount of fistula output, which in turn influences the spontaneous closure rate and subsequent mortality. Proximal fistulas are associated with high output (>200 mL/d) and provide the most complications and treatment difficulty.[41] Losses from these fistulas cause malnutrition, dehydration, and severe electrolyte deficiencies, which must be carefully and continuously repleted. Because of malnutrition, proximal fistulas result in greater mortality.[42] Sepsis, if present, is also more severe owing to greater intra-abdominal contamination and presence of digestive enzymes. The high concentration of stomach and pancreatic secretions causes more extensive maceration of the skin as well. Conversely, fistulas occurring in the distal ileum or colon have lower output and respond more favorably to nonoperative management.

Fistulas that occur after bowel obstruction or extensive disruption of an anastomosis usually result in end fistulas. In an end fistula, the entire content of the bowel is passed through the fistulous tract. Because of the loss of continuity with the distal bowel segment these fistulas do not spontaneously close and invariably require reoperation. Lateral fistulas exhibit passage of bowel content beyond the fistula opening. In the absence of complication factors, lateral fistulas frequently close with conservative management.

Other anatomic factors important in the assessment of fistulas include distance from the fistula opening to the skin and the number of external drainage sites. Longer fistulous tracts (>2 cm) are less likely to epithelialize and are associated with a higher closure rate. Conversely, fistulas with multiple exits frequently result in large abdominal wall defects and rarely spontaneously close.

Treatment of enterocutaneous fistulas begins with stabilization of the patient. Institution of complete bowel rest should be complemented by parenteral nutrition. Enteral feeding may be used in patients with low output ileal or colonic fistulas. Approximately 4 feet of small bowel proximal to the fistula is required if enteral feeding is contemplated. Anemia and electrolyte abnormalities must be corrected and intravenous volume repleted.

After stabilization, the fistula should be radiographically evaluated. A fistulogram is the most helpful study and is performed by placing a small catheter into the fistula tract and injecting water-soluble contrast medium such as meglumine diatrizoate. The surgeon should be present for the study because much information can be obtained during fluoroscopy, including the location and type of fistula (e.g., end or lateral); the presence of obstruction distal to the fistula; the presence of an abscess cavity adjacent to the fistula; evidence of inflammation or stricturing of adjacent bowel; and the distance from the origin of the fistula to the skin.

All patients should be managed with bowel rest and nutritional supplementation. Early surgery should only be undertaken if sepsis occurs. With conservative therapy, the fistula output should decrease. Gastric secretions can be further decreased using histamine H2 blockers such as ranitidine or cimetidine. The use of somatostatin has been shown to decrease the time to spontaneous closure but has not been proven to increase closure rates.[43] Surgical repair is usually not recommended before 8 weeks.[44] This allows time for nutritional repletion and inflammation to subside. Additionally, mortality and recurrence rates are highest if surgery is performed in the first 6 weeks.[41]

The definitive surgical procedure is resection of the fistulous segment and an end-to-end anastomosis. Direct suturing of the fistula without resection is a less optimal alternative. In patients with prior irradiation or dense adhesions that make dissection unsafe, bypass may be the only reasonable alternative. The abdomen should be incised at a location away from the fistulous tract, preferably as an extension of the prior incision. Care must be given to obtain a secure abdominal wall closure.

Rectovaginal Fistulas

The gynecologist may encounter rectovaginal fistulas after pelvic surgery such as abdominal or vaginal hysterectomy, failed repair of prior obstetric trauma, or pelvic irradiation. The appropriate technique for repair of such fistulas differs depending on their location and etiology. In general, there are four approaches to the repair of rectovaginal fistulas: vaginal, perineal, anal, and abdominal.

Several rectovaginal classification schemes have been developed to guide therapy. Fistulas may be labeled as high, middle, or low depending on their location on the rectovaginal septum. High fistulas enter the vagina at the posterior fornix, connecting with the middle one third of the rectum. Low fistulas enter the vagina at the posterior forchette and the rectum at the dentate line. Middle fistulas are located between the high and low types.

Another system integrates size, location, and cause.[45] Simple rectovaginal fistulas are located in the lower one half of the vagina, are caused by trauma, and are less than 2.5 cm. These fistulas are repaired from the vaginal or perineal approach and do not require a colostomy. Complex fistulas are located in the upper vagina, are caused by pelvic irradiation or bowel disease, and are usually greater than 2.5 cm. These fistulas are usually repaired abdominally and are often protected with a colostomy.

A third classification scheme is based on the anatomy of the rectovaginal septum and perineal body and is used for fistulas caused by obstetric or surgical trauma.[46] The locations of fistulas are divided into three zones: the upper portion of the vagina covered internally by peritoneum; the middle third of the vagina, which is separated from the rectum by a thin fascial layer; and the lower third, where the anal canal and the vagina are separated by the perineal body. In this scheme, surgical repair is influenced by the zone in which the fistula occurs.

The proper timing of rectovaginal fistula repair is critical for success. The repair should not be attempted before inflammation and induration have subsided. It is preferable to evaluate each case on an individual basis rather than waiting a prescribed length of time. Fistulas occurring after obstetric trauma may be repaired rapidly, usually within several months. Excellent results have been reported when repairs were undertaken at 2 to 3 weeks after fistula formation.[47] Conversely, patients with fistulas secondary to radiation damage require a much longer time for resolution of tissue inflammation and induration. Frequently, diversion of the fecal stream to resolve inflammation is necessary before repair of a radiation-related rectovaginal fistula.

Before repair, patients should undergo a thorough mechanical bowel preparation. To improve wound healing, attention should be directed to correction of malnutrition as well as to optimization of any coexisting inflammatory, connective tissue, or metabolic disease. Although of unproven benefit, most surgeons use perioperative intravenous antibiotics.

A vaginal approach is most frequently used for low fistulas. These occur most frequently after obstetric trauma and are usually small. A small Foley urinary catheter passed through the fistula can provide traction and may be helpful with small fistulas. If the fistula is in close proximity to the anal sphincter, it is often easier to convert the fistula into a complete perineal laceration before repair. In patients with failed prior repairs, which are usually due to poor blood supply, the surgeon should give consideration to interposition of healthy tissue into the repair. Use of the bulbocavernosus muscle or fat pad is uncomplicated and highly successful.

Rectovaginal fistulas located high in the vagina are frequently caused by pelvic irradiation or inflammatory bowel disease and are usually approached abdominally. All patients with radiation-induced fistulas must have healthy tissue interposed between the rectum and vagina. Omentum is most frequently used, but some surgeons prefer the rectus, gracilis, or bulbocavernosus muscle. If radiation damage is extensive, proctectomy and primary anastomosis may be required. Omentum wrapped around the anastomosis theoretically provides a new blood supply to the anastomotic line, and interposition between the rectum and vagina isolates small anastomotic leaks. All patients with repairs of radiation-induced rectovaginal fistulas should have a protective colostomy.

Pseudo-Obstruction

Acute colonic pseudo-obstruction (often referred to as Ogilvie's syndrome) is characterized by dilation of the colon in the absence of mechanical obstruction. The cause of the syndrome is unknown, but it may occur postoperatively and is usually self limiting. Patients often present with a distended, tympanitic abdomen, constipation, and minimal abdominal tenderness. If peritoneal signs are present, impending cecal perforation should be suspected.

Abdominal radiographs demonstrate a distended colon, and they should be frequently repeated to prevent perforation. If serial radiographs demonstrate increasing distention or a cecal diameter of 10 to 12 cm, decompression must be accomplished.

Decompression is preferably accomplished during colonoscopy, which is also helpful to exclude a mechanical obstruction. Repeat colonoscopic decompression may be required. Patients who fail successive colonoscopic decompressions require a tube cecostomy.

Complications of Appendectomy

Nearly all complications after appendectomy are associated with appendiceal perforation occurring after acute appendicitis.[48] These patients are usually treated by general surgeons. However, many incidental appendectomies are performed by gynecologists at the time of pelvic surgery. Although it can be argued that an unnecessary appendectomy is in itself a complication, there appears to be no increase in postoperative complications when incidental appendectomy is performed.[49, 50]

REFERENCES

1. Silverstein FE, Gilbert DA, Tedesco FJ, et al. The National ASGE survey on upper gastrointestinal bleeding. Gastrointest Endosc 1981;27:73.
2. Beard K, Walker A, Perera D, et al. NSAIDS and hospitalization for gastroesophageal bleeding in the elderly. Arch Intern Med 1987;147:1621.
3. Hawkey G. NSAIDS and peptic ulcers. Br Med J 1990;300:278.
4. Wara P, Stodkilde H. Bleeding pattern before admission as a guideline for emergency endoscopy. Scand J Gastroenterol 1985;20:72.
5. Allen HM, Block MA, Schuman BM. Gastroduodenal endoscopy: management of acute upper gastrointestinal hemorrhage. Arch Surg 1973;106:450.
6. Nath RL, Sequeira JC, Weitzman AF, et al. Lower gastrointestinal bleeding: diagnostic approach and management conclusions. Am J Surg 1981;141:478.
7. Browder W, Cerise EJ, Litwin MS. Impact of emergency angiography in massive lower gastrointestinal bleeding. Ann Surg 1986;204:530.
8. Koval G, Benner KG, Rosch J, et al. Aggressive angiographic diagnosis in acute lower gastrointestinal hemorrhage. Dig Dis Sci 1987;32:248.
9. Lawrence MA, Hooks VH, Bowden TA. Lower gastro-

intestinal bleeding: a systemic approach to classification and management. Postgrad Med 1989;85:89.

10. Potter GD, Sellin JH. Lower gastrointestinal bleeding. Gastrointest Endosc Clin North Am 1988;17:341.

11. Fekety R, Kim K-H, Brown D, et al. Epidemiology of antibiotic-associated colitis: isolation of *Clostridium difficile* from the hospital environment. Am J Med 1981;70:906.

12. Dudrick SJ, Wilmore DW, Vars HM, Rhoads JE. Long-term total parenteral nutrition with growth, development, and positive nitrogen balance. Surgery 1968;64:134.

13. Smith LC, Mullen JL. Nutritional assessment and indications for nutritional support. Surg Clin North Am 1991;71:449.

14. Bistrian BR, Blackburn GL, Hallowell E, Heddle R. Protein status of general surgical patients. JAMA 1974;230:858.

15. Joint Commission on Accreditation of Hospitals. Joint Commission Accreditation Manual for Hospitals, vol I, section PE.1.3., 1995.

16. Heber D: Nutritional therapy. In: Berek JS, Hacker NF, eds. Practical Gynecologic Oncology, 2nd ed. Baltimore, Williams & Wilkins 1994, p 637.

17. Jeejeebhoy KN, Meguid MM. Assessment of nutritional status in the oncologic patient. Surg Clin North Am 1986;66:1077.

18. Jequier E. Measurement of energy expenditure in clinical nutritional assessment. JPEN 1987;11(suppl):86S.

19. Reinhardt GF, Myscofski JW, Wilkens D, et al. Incidence and mortality of hypoalbuminemic patients in hospitalized veterans. JPEN 1980;4:357.

20. Boraas M, Peterson O, Knox L, et al. Serum proteins and outcome on surgical patients. JPEN 1982;6:585.

21. Buzby GP, Mullen JL, Matthews DC, et al. Prognostic nutritional index in gastrointestinal surgery. Am J Surg 1980;139:160.

22. Collins JP, Oxby CB, Hill GL. Intravenous amino acids and intravenous hyperalimentation as protein-sparing therapy after major surgery: a controlled clinical trial. Lancet 1978;1:788.

23. Askanazi J, Hensle TW, Starker PM, et al. Effect of postoperative nutritional support on length of hospitalization. Ann Surg 1986;203:236.

24. Bower RH, Talamini MA, Sax HC, et al. Postoperative enteral vs. parenteral nutrition. Arch Surg 1986;121:1040.

25. Rothnie NG, Harper RAK, Catchpole BN. Early postoperative gastrointestinal activity. Lancet 1963;2:64.

26. Wilson JP. Postoperative motility of the large intestine in man. Gut 1975;16:689.

27. Wolfson PJ, Bauer JJ, Gelernt IM, et al. Use of the long tube in the management of patients with small-intestinal obstruction due to adhesions. Arch Surg 1985;120:1001.

28. Helmkamp BF, Kimmel J. Conservative management of small bowel obstruction. Am J Obstet Gynecol 1985;152:677.

29. Peetz DJ, Gamelli RL, Pilcher DB. Intestinal intubation in acute mechanical small-bowel obstruction. Arch Surg 1982;117:334.

30. Doberneck RC. Revision and closure of the colostomy. Surg Clin North Am 1991;71:193.

31. Pearl RK, Prasad ML, Orsay CP, et al. Early local complications from intestinal stomas. Arch Surg 1985;120:1145.

32. Miles RM, Greene RS. Review of colostomy in a community hospital. Am Surg 1983;49:182.

33. Mirelman D, Corman ML, Veidenheimer MC, et al. Colostomies: indications and contraindications: Lahey Clinic experience 1963–1974. Dis Colon Rectum 1978;21:172.

34. Porter JA, Salvati EP, Rubin RJ, Eisenstat TE. Complications of colostomies. Dis Colon Rectum 1989;32:299.

35. Daly JM, DeCosse JJ. Complications in surgery of the colon and rectum. Surg Clin North Am 1983;63:1215.

36. Moossa AR, Block GE, Sackier JM. Complications of colorectal operations. In: Moosa AR, Block GE, eds. Operative Colorectal Surgery. Philadelphia, WB Saunders, 1994, p 507.

37. Bunt TJ. Urgent relaparotomy: the high-risk no-choice operation. Surgery 1985;98:555.

38. Clarke-Pearson DL, Chin NO, DeLong ER, et al. Surgical management of intestinal obstruction in ovarian cancer: clinical features, postoperative complications, and survival. Gynecol Oncol 1987;26:11.

39. Griffen FD, Knight CD, Whitaker JM, et al. The double stapling technique for low anterior resection: results, modifications, and observations. Ann Surg 1990; 211:745.

40. Graffner H, Fredlund P, Olsson S-A, et al. Protective colostomy in low anterior resection of the rectum using the EEA stapling instrument. Dis Colon Rectum 1983;26:87.

41. Fazio V, Coutsoftides T, Steiger F. Factors influencing the outcome of treatment of small bowel cutaneous fistulas. World J Surg 1983;7:481.

42. Coutsoftides T, Fazio V. Small intestinal cutaneous fistulas. Surg Gynecol Obstet 1979;149:333.

43. DiCostanzo J, Cano N, Martin J, et al. Treatment of external gastrointestinal fistulas by combination of total parenteral nutrition and somatostatin. JPEN 1987;11:465.

44. Hill G. Operative strategy in the treatment of enterocutaneous fistulas. World J Surg 1983;7:498.

45. Buls JG, Rothenberger DA. Anal and rectovaginal fistulas: repair of the low fistula. In: Kodner IJ, Fry RD, Roe JP, eds. Colon, Rectal and Anal Surgery. St. Louis, CV Mosby, 1985, pp 63–75.

46. Rosenshein NB, Genadry RR, Woodruff JD. An anatomic classification of rectovaginal septal defects. Am J Obstet Gynecol 1980;137:439.

47. Hauth JC, Gilstrap LC III, Ward SC, et al. Early repair of an external sphincter ani muscle and rectal mucosal dehiscence. Obstet Gynecol 1986;67:806.

48. Scher KS, Coil JA. The continuing challenge of perforating appendicitis. Surg Gynecol Obstet 1980;150:535.

49. Westermann C, Mann WJ, Chumas J, et al. Routine appendectomy in extensive gynecologic operations. Surg Gynecol Obstet 1986;162:307.

50. Voitk AJ, Lowry JB. Is incidental appendectomy a safe practice? Can J Surg 1988;31:448.

19

CHAPTER

Eva Chalas

Vascular Access

The gynecologic patient often presents with challenging problems. Among these are major operative procedures requiring central venous or arterial line monitoring, need for prolonged venous access, and management of disease-related effusion or pneumothorax occurring after an attempt to place a central venous catheter. The physician caring for these patients should be able to recognize and accurately diagnose these problems, institute therapeutic intervention, and, when possible, prevent or rapidly identify any complications of therapy. To carry out these tasks effectively, one must be familiar with the clinical course of gynecologic patients undergoing complicated operations and should be knowledgeable with individualized treatment options, proper technique, possible complications, and their treatment.

CENTRAL VENOUS ACCESS

The indications to consider short-term or long-term venous access are many for gynecologic oncology patients. Initially, central venous monitoring is done intraoperatively, followed by intravenous support while awaiting recovery of bowel function postoperatively. Some patients benefit during chemotherapy or for infusion of antibiotics during nadir sepsis. Others may need it for nutritional support, hydration, or administration of agents for pain control. Temporary or permanent lines with peripheral or central access can be chosen based on planned duration of treatment, the osmolality of the infusate, availability of vessels, and patient or physician preference. Each of the options is associated with inherent benefits and risk. Only a well-informed physician can help his or her patients select the best option and diagnose or treat any potential complications.

Venous access lines can be categorized by planned duration of use as temporary or permanent and by site as peripheral and central. Generally, temporary lines are in use for hours or days whereas permanent lines are designed to be used for weeks or longer. A typical case requiring temporary access is a surgical patient during the perioperative period (Table 19–1). These patients require lines that are placed by direct cannulation of the vessel. The procedure can be performed rapidly at the bedside with the use of local anesthesia. The lines must be replaced on a regular basis in accordance with institutional guidelines, which are usually determined by the infection control team. Infectious complications occur more frequently

TABLE 19–1
Indications for Temporary Lines

Hemodynamic monitoring
Poor venous access
Prolonged postoperative ileus
Perioperative nutritional support
Short duration home therapy (e.g., antibiotics)

when such guidelines are not followed. Permanent central lines are well suited for home intravenous therapy or long-term chemotherapy (Table 19–2). These lines exit the skin to be accessed by percutaneous stick with a noncoring needle (e.g., ports) (Figs. 19–1 through 19–3). The rate of infection with port systems is decreased, but the procedure for placement is more complex, is usually performed in the operating room, takes longer to complete, and requires the administration of more local anesthesia. Occasionally, intravenous sedation or general anesthetic is required.

Selection Criteria

The decision to use peripheral or central venous access is made based on many criteria. Peripheral veins such as the brachial or cephalic allow access to the central venous system by advancing the catheter into the subclavian vein. The risk of pneumothorax is low, but the diameter of the catheter is small (e.g., 23 or 18 gauge [1.8F to 5.0F]). Table 19–3 includes the advantages and disadvantages of peripheral versus central venous access. These factors should be carefully considered and an individualized decision made based on indications for use of the access system and the risk–benefit ratio.

Techniques

Central venous access lines are placed under sterile conditions with the surgeons or other properly trained personnel in gowns, gloves, and masks. The selected site is prepared with a sterile scrub.

TABLE 19–2
Indications for Permanent Lines

Long-term nutritional support
Chemotherapy
Supportive care

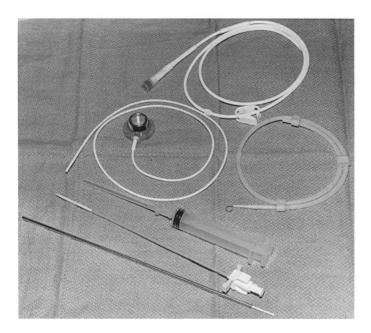

FIGURE 19-1
Permanent lines for venous access. The tunneler is in the forefront, followed by the introducer, the needle and syringe, the port, and the catheter. The sheathed guide wire is to the right of the port.

A peripherally inserted central line catheter can be placed by a trained nurse and may be done at the bedside or even at home if necessary. The patient is placed in a supine position with the arm extended at a 90-degree angle. A tourniquet is applied, and the cephalic or, preferably, the brachial vein is palpated. The sterile site is injected with local anesthesia, and the needle is inserted into the vein with its bevel up. The catheter is then advanced through the introducer 2 to 3 inches, and the tourniquet is released. The catheter is advanced farther, and the introducer is pulled back to be peeled from around the catheter after the needle is removed from the vein. It may be helpful to have the patient turn her head toward the arm as the catheter is advanced to minimize the risk of catheter migration into the neck veins. The catheter is further advanced to its desired position and blood return is confirmed. A sterile dressing is placed after completion of the procedure. A radiograph should be performed to verify line positioning. The advantages of this peripherally

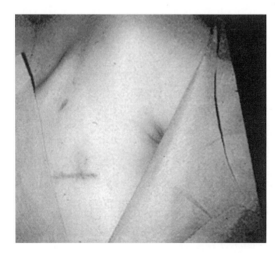

FIGURE 19-2
Side view of the left chest with implanted port. The clavicle can be seen superiorly; the left shoulder and axilla are on the right side of the picture. Access of the port has resulted in some increased pigmentation (just above the port incision).

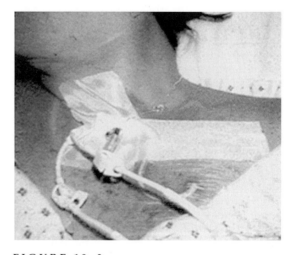

FIGURE 19-3
Permanent catheter shortly after placement in the left subclavian vein. The catheter is dual lumen and is securely taped to prevent inadvertent removal. A transparent dressing is used to allow visualization of the site without manipulation.

TABLE 19–3
Peripheral Versus Central Venous Access

Factor	Peripheral Access	Central Access
Duration of use	Days to weeks	Months to years
Complications	Infrequent	30%–50%
Gauge of line	1.8F to 5.0F	Up to 12.5F
Multilumen	No	Yes
Site discomfort	Some	Rare
Patient acceptance	High	Less

inserted central line catheterization include ease of placement, low cost, and virtually no risk of pneumothorax. However, the peripheral veins must be of adequate caliber and cannot be damaged by previous use.[1]

Alternative low-risk techniques include cutdown of the cephalic, external jugular, or saphenous veins to provide catheterization access of the superior and inferior vena cava, respectively.[2–4] Both permanent catheters and ports can be inserted using these techniques, although the presence of valves may occasionally interfere with central venous placement.

Central venous access can also be achieved by directly inserting the catheter into internal jugular, subclavian, or femoral veins. In the gynecologic oncology patient, the femoral approach is used only as a last resort because of problems related to presence of pelvic tumor, risk of thrombosis, infection, and difficulty in mobility.

The internal jugular approach is often preferred by the anesthesiologist because the neck is easily accessible during pelvic surgery and the risk of pneumothorax is less than when the subclavian vein is used.[5] This is particularly true when the lung is hyperinflated, as would be the case when the patient is anesthetized. The right internal jugular vein is a better choice for cannulation. The right internal jugular vein leads directly into the superior vena cava, the right cupula of the lung is inferior to the left, and there is no concern about injury to the thoracic duct, which empties on the left side.

As previously outlined, the procedure is performed under sterile conditions. The patient is placed into mild Trendelenburg position to distend the venous system and minimize the risk of air embolization. The sternocleidomastoid muscle serves as an important landmark (Fig. 19–4). The most commonly used approach is to place a 1½-inch 22-gauge needle under the lateral head of the muscle at 30 degrees from the skin, away from midline. The needle is advanced while gentle aspiration is applied until the vein is identified. Once the location of the vessel has been identified with a small-gauge needle, a 14-gauge needle is placed in the same manner, through which a guide wire is then advanced. An introducer with a dilator is placed over the guide wire after a 3- to 5-mm incision is made at the skin entry site to facilitate passage. The guide wire and the dilator are then removed and the catheter is advanced through the introducer, which is peeled away when the catheter is in the appropriate position.

The right or left subclavian veins are readily accessible, and placement of a line in this location is associated with freedom of motion of the neck and the extremities. However, the risk of pneumothorax is greater than with cannula-

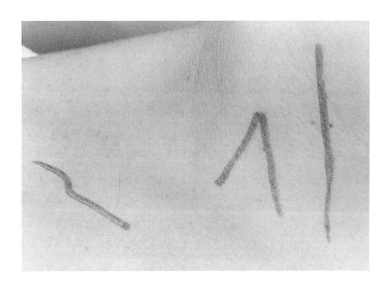

FIGURE 19–4
Skin markings identify the sternocleidomastoid and the inferior notch on the clavicle.

tion of the internal jugular vein. The most commonly used approach is infraclavicular, although a supraclavicular approach is possible. Again, sterile conditions are observed. The patient is placed in mild Trendelenburg position. It may be helpful to place some padding between the shoulder blades to allow displacement of the shoulder posteriorly and inferiorly, but this position may result in narrowing of the space between the clavicle and the ribs in some patients, thus limiting the access to the subclavian vein. Several infraclavicular approaches have been described. One approach relies on identification of an easily visible or, in obese patients, palpable landmark, the inferior notch (see Fig. 19–4). The skin is prepped and draped, and the area is infiltrated with local anesthetic to the periosteum of the clavicle. A 14-gauge needle is then directed under the clavicle at the level of the notch with the bevel up and the needle tip aimed at the sternal notch. Gentle aspiration is applied while the needle is advanced. When venous blood is obtained, the needle is rotated down and the syringe is disconnected. A guide wire is advanced either under fluoroscopy or blindly while an electrocardiographic monitor is observed. When fluoroscopy is not used, the patient's head should be turned toward the surgeon to minimize the risk of advancing the catheter into the internal jugular vein. If the catheter is advanced into the internal jugular vein, the patient may complain of discomfort in the neck or the ipsilateral ear. The appearance of premature atrial contractions is an indication that the guide wire is resting in the right atrium, and it should be pulled back so that the tip is in the superior vena cava. Once the guide wire is in the appropriate position, the introducer and dilator are advanced, followed by the introduction of the catheter as previously described for the internal jugular approach.

Insertion of a permanent catheter or port requires more extensive manipulation. Once the vein of choice has been cannulated with the guide wire and the surgeon is reasonably certain that the catheter can be threaded successfully, the selected port or catheter skin exit site and the tissue in between is infiltrated with local anesthesia. A subcutaneous tunnel is then created, through which the catheter is pulled before the placement into the vein. To minimize the risk of infection, it is recommended that the tunnel be greater than 10 cm long and that the cuff on the catheter be at least 2 cm from the skin exit site.[6] If a port has been selected, it is secured to the fascia of the under-

lying muscle with permanent sutures. In obese patients, it may be helpful to remove some subcutaneous tissue over the port site to facilitate access of the port during future use. To ensure patency of the system, venous return should be confirmed in the operating room before approximation of the skin over the port site and after a suture has been placed at the skin site on a permanent percutaneous catheter. The suture is placed to prevent inadvertent removal of the catheter before fibrosis occurs around the cuff. Placement of a loop in the external tubing with appropriate tape further reduces the risk (see Fig. 19–1).

Complications

There are acute and deleted complications of catheter placement. The most common acute complication of central line placement is pneumothorax, which occurs in 2% to 6% of cases.[3, 4, 7] The risk of this complication is influenced by the vein selected, the technical expertise of the individual inserting the catheter, and patient-related factors such as anatomy and hemodynamic status and vessel scarring. For example, in one study of 297 patients with 355 lines, the 5.6% risk of pneumothorax was incurred only when the subclavian approach was chosen.[3] When a pneumothorax occurs, conservative management is possible in approximately one half of the cases.[4, 7] Other acute complications attributed to central venous catheter placement include vascular perforation, nerve damage, and, rarely, air embolization or embolization of a portion of a catheter.

Later sequelae focus on a number of important issues: infection, thrombosis, and nonfunction. These complications are related to factors intrinsic to the type or location of the catheter, duration of its use, type of maintenance, and patient factors such as susceptibility to infection.

The peripherally inserted central catheter lines are more prone to phlebitis (4%), breakage (5%), and inadvertent dislodgment (3%), even though they are usually used for shorter duration, averaging 20 to 90 days, than the lines placed directly into the central venous system.[8, 9] The short duration of use and a selection bias toward a healthier patient population result in a risk of infection of 1%.[9, 10]

Venous thrombosis occurs in 2% to 10% of cases of central venous catheter use.[4, 7, 11, 12] The risk may be related to the location of the catheter tip. The highest incidence of thrombosis

(28%) was found to occur when a left-sided catheter was used with the tip in the upper part of superior vena cava.[13] Thrombosis of the catheter is more common than thrombosis of the central vein and can often be treated medically. Thrombosis of the catheter does not necessitate the removal of the line. Preventative measures have centered on the use of 1 mg of warfarin daily. In a randomized study, 4 of 42 treated patients had venogram-proven thrombosis 90 days after catheter placement, as compared with 15 of 40 untreated patients.[14] For surveillance, a very sensitive method of detection of thrombi is intravascular ultrasonography, which can detect lesions greater than 1 mm.[15] Therapeutic interventions reported to be successful include intravenous urokinase and recombinant tissue-type plasminogen activator.[16, 17] Instillation of urokinase, 5000 units/mL, according to a protocol that allows for infusion of less than 1 mm to be repeated in 1 hour if repeated aspiration of the catheter fails to demonstrate clearing of the line, was successful 98% of the time.[18]

Infection may occur at the site and usually requires removal of the catheter. With proper maintenance, the risk of this complication is 1% to 2%.[2, 19] Sepsis, with the line as the known or suspected source, occurs in 2.1% to 32% of cases and is clearly dependent on the duration of use, type of expertise in maintenance of the catheter, and the patient's susceptibility to infection.[3, 7, 12, 19, 20] The average duration of use was 6 to 12 months, and the patients were often immunocompromised. The most common organism is *Staphylococcus aureus*. These patients are treated with intravenous antibiotics, and the central line is removed only if this therapy fails. If a multilumen catheter is used, the antibiotics must be infused through all lumina. In one study, results suggested that double-lumen catheters are associated with an increased risk of infection, particularly in younger patients.[21] In another study, performed in an intensive care setting, single-lumen catheters were compared with triple-lumen ones. The lines were changed every 48 hours with a new site selected. The infection rate was identical, and patients with triple-lumen catheter required significantly less peripheral access.[22] Catheters that contain valves for infusion and aspiration and do not require flushing and frequent handling can be selected to minimize the risk of infection.

Nonfunction due to malposition occurs in less than 6% of the patients.[4, 19] Replacement of the line may be necessary, but an attempt at repositioning can be made with the assistance of a radiologist. Migration of the catheters have been reported and if unrecognized can lead to disastrous sequelae.[12, 23] Implantable ports may also become displaced through the skin, causing a dehiscence in up to 1.5% of patients.[11, 12]

Maintenance

To minimize the risk of skin site infection, it is recommended that some basic precautions be observed. Thorough hand washing is imperative. Health care personnel, the patient, and any individuals caring for the line must be properly trained in aseptic technique. The site is cleansed and dressed with antibiotic ointment or povidone-iodine. The dressing is changed biweekly or weekly. Ports requiring continuous access have the noncoring needle replaced on a similar schedule. The catheters are flushed with saline after use, followed by heparin, 100 units/mL. Volumes of less than 5 mL are adequate. Catheters not in use should be flushed biweekly to weekly, and ports should be flushed once per month, although less often for both may be adequate.[11, 24]

ARTERIAL ACCESS

The arterial line provides highly valuable information in patients who are critically ill or are undergoing major operative procedures. The risk of complications is acceptable but is related to duration of use, with thrombosis occurring most frequently. Thus, an intact collateral system must be verified before placement of the line, and the line should be removed as quickly as allowed, based on the clinical course.

An integral part of care of any critically ill or heavily stressed patient is monitoring of vital signs. Cannulation of an artery with placement of an indwelling catheter allows rapid assessment of blood pressure and pulse and provides other clinical information related to the patient's hemodynamic status. For example, blood pressure fluctuations with positive-pressure breathing may indicate hypovolemia.[5] Myocardial contractility is reflected in the upstroke and systemic vascular resistance is reflected in the downslope of the pressure tracing. In addition, the line can be used to obtain arterial blood gases and other hematologic studies rapidly. Medically ill patients undergoing a major operative procedure, those on respiratory support, and hemodynamically unstable patients greatly benefit from such arterial access.

Technique

Although a peripherally accessible artery can be cannulated, the vessel most often chosen is the radial artery. The vessel is easily accessible and has excellent collateral circulation with the ulnar artery. The nondominant hand is selected if possible. An Allen test should be performed to verify the quality of collateral supply by occluding both vessels and having the patient exercise her hand. The palm should become ischemic and appear pale. The compression of the flow to the ulnar artery is relapsed, while the radial artery remains obstructed. The ischemia should resolve with normal color of the palm restored within 5 seconds. If the palm appears pale for more than 15 seconds, cannulation of the radial artery is contraindicated.[5]

Other potential sites include the ulnar, brachial, dorsalis pedis, and lateral plantar arteries. Again, one should check for collateral flow because any arterial catheter may cause thrombosis of the vessel; the arteries in lower extremities do not provide as accurate readings as do the vessels in the arms.

To access the radial artery, one should dorsiflex the hand and secure it in place. The area is prepared with cleansing solution and infiltrated with local anesthesia. The needle with the catheter is then inserted at a 30-degree angle to the skin; this angle is changed to 10 degrees to facilitate advancing the catheter once the vessel is accessed (Fig. 19–5). Teflon catheters are preferred, because they appear less thrombogenic. The catheter is then connected to tubing and a transducer containing heparinized solution.

Complications

The list of potential complications is long, but the most common issues relate to thrombosis. The risk is related to the size and type of the catheter, the diameter of the lumen of the artery, and the duration of dwelling time. Thrombosis occurs in one half of the lines kept in for 2 days.[5] Infusion of 1 to 3 mL of solution containing 1 unit/mL of heparin keeps most lines open, but the thrombosis often occurs after the line has been removed. Infections can lead to pseudoaneurysms and are generally caused by *Staphylococcus aureus*. They are more common in the older, sicker patients because they are also related to duration of use.[25] Other problems include ecchymosis, arteriovenous fistula, ischemia of distal sites, and emboli.

CHEST TUBES

Gynecologic oncology patients may require chest tube placement when disease-related pleural effusions have developed and the patients are symptomatic or when placement of a central venous line resulted in pneumothorax (Fig. 19–6). The tube drains the fluid or air and allows the collapsed lung to reexpand (Fig. 19–7). Although pleural effusions accumulate gradually, the development of a pneumothorax may happen rapidly and could result in tension pneumothorax with mediastinal shift and cardiovascular collapse. Spontaneous pneumothorax can also occur, but an iatrogenic devel-

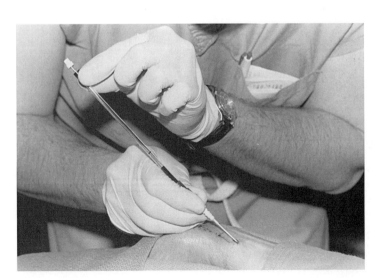

FIGURE 19–5
Placement of an arterial line in the left radial artery.

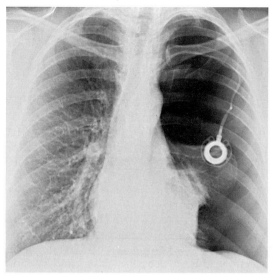

FIGURE 19–6
Massive pneumothorax of the left lung after placement of
a left subclavian port.

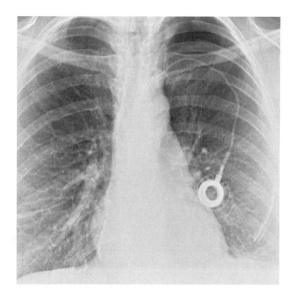

FIGURE 19–7
Residual pneumothorax at the apex of the lung. A chest
tube is visible at the lower right.

opment is far more common in this population.
Absent breath sounds are noted clinically, with
the patient in various stages of compensation
related to the extent of the pneumothorax.
Small lesions can be followed with serial chest
radiographs. Clinically compromised patients
or those with expanding lesions should have a
chest tube placed. Patients with pleural effusions will have diminished breath sounds at
and below the meniscus of the effusate. A chest
radiograph in upright and lateral positions
should be done to rule out loculation of the
fluid, which would decrease the ability to successfully drain it.

Technique

The patient is in supine position, prepped, and
draped. A size 36F Silastic tube or a so-called
pigtail catheter is placed on the surgical field
(Fig. 19–8). A minor suture set is used, the fifth
intercostal space is identified, and the area over
the sixth rib is infiltrated with local anesthesia.
For chest tube placement, an incision is made
superior to the rib through the skin and muscle, thus avoiding the intercostal vessels that
run inferior to the rib. A clamp is then used to
bluntly enter the pleural space and place the
chest tube to rest with its tip up toward the
clavicle. The chest tube is connected to suction
because negative pressure must be maintained
at all times. A suture is placed at the skin site
to secure the tube and prevent air leakage. If a
pigtail catheter has been selected, it is introduced through a sheath that encases a slim
trocar (Fig. 19–9). The trocar is introduced first;
and when the pleural space is entered, the
trocar is removed and the catheter is advanced

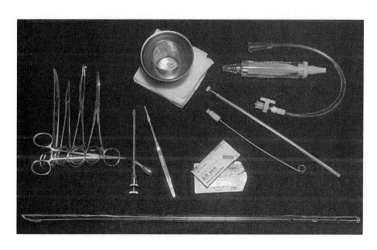

FIGURE 19–8
Minor tray set with chest tube, pigtail
catheter, and accessories.

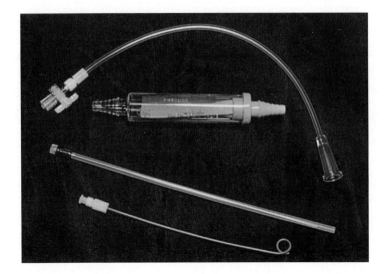

FIGURE 19-9
Close-up view of the pigtail catheter with a sheathed trocar, valve, and tubing with a stopcock.

through the sheath. The catheter is then secured as previously described. These catheters are well tolerated and effective.[26]

The decision to remove the tube or catheter depends on the reexpansion of the lung and the ability to tolerate lack of negative pressure. If a pneumothorax does not recur after 8 to 12 hours off suction, the tube is removed and a repeat radiograph is performed. In case of pleural effusion, the amount of daily drainage should ideally be less than 100 mL. The patient may benefit from pleurodesis, which will frequently prevent fluid reaccumulation. Bleomycin, 60 units in 60 mL, tetracycline powder, talc, and other agents have been used to incite an intense inflammatory response in the pleura and result in adhesion formation, thus obliterating potential space for effusions. The patient must remain supine and move from side to side to promote even distribution of the fluid. Analgesics should be provided liberally, because the inflammation results in pleuritic pain. The fluid should be drained with suction after several hours, and the pleura should be kept in proximity for 24 hours. Repeat radiographs should be performed; if fluid had reaccumulated, the tube can be repositioned and the procedure can be repeated. Otherwise, the tube is removed.

Complications

Chest tube insertion is associated with potentially life-threatening complications and should be performed by individuals comfortable with the technique and capable of managing any resulting problems. Injury to any intrathoracic and even upper abdominal structure can occur, because the procedure is performed without direct visualization. Empyema, unilateral pulmonary edema, bronchopleural fistula, hemothorax, Horner's syndrome, and shock have all been described.[27, 28] Thus, careful observation with clinical examination and chest radiographs is advisable.

REFERENCES

1. Rountree D. The PIC catheter: A different approach. Am J Nurs 1991;91:22–26.
2. Perry EP, Nash JR, Klidjian AM. Direct cephalic vein cannulation for safe subclavian access. J R Coll Surg Edinb 1990;35:218–220.
3. Henriques HF, Karmy-Jones R, Knoli SM, et al. Avoiding complications of long-term venous access. Am Surg 1993;59:555–558.
4. Nelson BE, Mayer AR, Tseng PC, et al. Experience with the totally implanted port in patients with gynecologic malignancies. Gynecol Oncol 1994;53:98–102.
5. Kaplan JA. Hemodynamic monitoring. In: Kaplan JA, ed. Cardiac Anesthesia, 2nd ed. Philadelphia, WB Saunders, 1987.
6. Hayward SR, Ledgerwood AM, Lucas DE. The fate of 100 prolonged venous access devices. Am Surg 1990;56:515–519.
7. Barrios CH, Zuke JE, Blaes B, et al. Evaluation of an implantable venous access system in a general oncology population. Oncology 1992;49:474–478.
8. Masoorli S, Angeles T. PICC lines: The latest home care challenge. RN 1990;53:44–50.
9. Markel S, Reynen K. Impact of patient care: 2652 days in the alternative setting. J Intravenous Nurs 1990; 13:347–351.
10. Graham DR, Kelsermans MM, Klemm LW, et al. Infectious complications among patients receiving home intravenous therapy with peripheral, central or peripherally placed central venous catheters. Am J Med 1991;91(suppl 3B):95S–100S.
11. Freytes CO, Reid P, Smith KL. Long-term experience with totally implanted catheter system in cancer patients. J Surg Oncol 1990;45:99–102.
12. Koonings PP, Given FT. Long term experience with

a totally implantable catheter system in gynecologic oncology patients. J Am Coll Surg 1994;178:165–166.

13. Puel V, Caudry M, Le Metayer P, et al. Superior vena cava thrombosis related to catheter malposition in cancer chemotherapy given through implanted ports. Cancer 1993;72:2248–2252.

14. Bern MM, Lokish JJ, Wallach SR, et al. Very low doses of warfarin can prevent thrombosis in central venous catheters. Ann Intern Med 1990;112:423–428.

15. Bolz K, Aadahl P, Mangersnes J, et al. Intravascular ultrasonographic assessment of thrombus formation on central venous catheters. Acta Radiol 1993;34:162–167.

16. Greenberg S, Kosinski R, Daniels J. Treatment of superior vena cava thrombosis with recombinant tissue type plasminogen activator. Chest 1991;99:1298–1301.

17. Theriault RL, Buzdar A. Acute superior vena caval thrombosis after central venous catheter removal: successful treatment with thrombolytic therapy. Mod Pediatr Oncol 1990;18:77–80.

18. Lawson M, Bottino JC, Hurtubise MR, et al. The use of urokinase to restore the patency of occluded central venous catheters. Am J Intravenous Ther Clin Nutrition 1982;41:29–31.

19. Broadwater JR, Henderson MA, Bell JL, et al. Outpatient percutaneous central venous access in cancer patients. Am J Surg 1990;160:676–680.

20. Gleeson NC, Fiorica JV, Mark JE, et al. Externalized groshong catheters and hickman ports for central venous access in gynecologic oncology patients. Gynecol Oncol 1993;51:372–376.

21. Keung Y, Watkins K, Chen S, et al. Comparative study of infectious complications of different types of chronic central venous access devices. Cancer 1994;73:2832–2837.

22. Farkas J, Liu N, Bleriot J, et al. Single versus triple lumen central catheter related sepsis: a prospective randomized study in a critically ill population. Am J Med 1992;93:277–282.

23. Manheimer F, Aranda CP, Smith RL. Necrotizing pneumonitis caused by 5-fluorouracil infusion. Cancer 1992;70:554–556.

24. Kelly C, Dumenko L, McGregor E, et al. A change of flushing protocols of central venous catheters. Oncol Nurs Forum 1992;19:599–602.

25. Falk PS, Scuderi PE, Sherertz RJ, et al. Infected radial artery pseudoaneurysms occurring after percutaneous cannulation. Chest 1992;101:490–495.

26. Van Le L, Parker LA, DeMars LR, et al. Pleural effusions: outpatient management with pigtail catheter chest tubes. Gynecol Oncol 1994;54:215–217.

27. Resnick DK. Delayed pulmonary perforation: a rare complication of tube thoracostomy. Chest 1993;103:311–313.

28. Gerard PS, Kaldawi E, Litani V, et al. Right-sided pneumothorax: a result of a left sided chest tube. Chest 1993;103:1602–1603.

20

Laurie S. Swaim

Postoperative Neuropathy

Neuropathies occurring after gynecologic procedures have gained little attention in the literature. This is most likely because many postoperative neuropathies are undiagnosed and self-limited. However, certain postoperative neuropathies such as those affecting the femoral and iliohypogastric nerves can result in significant patient discomfort and impairment. Neuropathies occurring after gynecologic surgery can be subdivided into two general groups: (1) those related to patient position and (2) those related to surgical trauma. Neuropathies occurring after aberrant patient positioning include femoral, sciatic and peroneal, and brachial plexus injury. Those occurring secondary to surgical trauma include obturator, iliohypogastric, ilioinguinal, and, possibly, pudendal neuropathies (Table 20–1).

Abnormal nerve conduction can result from transection, stretch, or angulation of the nerve; ischemia resulting in anoxia; and mechanical compression of the nerve. Neuropathies are classified into three basic categories. The first is neurapraxia, which is associated with conduction loss without structural changes to the axon or the neural structures. The nerve remains in continuity; however, there is focal demyelination. Neurapraxia is the mildest form of neuropathy and may result from transient loss of blood flow and anoxia or from mechanical factors that result in displaced axoplasm. Axonotmesis refers to the loss of continuity of axons but the connective tissue supporting elements remain intact. This leads to wallerian degeneration. The nerve regenerates 1 to 3 mm per day, and months to years are required for recovery. Neurotmesis describes both axonal and connective tissue damage. Here, less chance of regeneration exists secondary to loss of connective tissue support, which may result in a poorly organized repair. Sequelae of nerve damage may be varied and can include loss of sensation, pain, and weakness. Nerve entrapment is secondary to pressure, stretch, angulation, and friction. The significance of the neuropathy is influenced by contributing factors such as age and by systemic disease such as diabetes mellitus.

NEUROPATHIES RELATED TO PATIENT POSITION

Femoral Neuropathy

Postoperative femoral neuropathy was first described in 1822 by Descartes. There have been more than 80 case reports since the 1800s, but the actual occurrence is probably much higher than appreciated. Many of these cases have minimal symptomatology, are of limited duration, and may go unrecognized by both the patient and her surgeon. Kvist-Poulsen and Borel[1] found a frequency of 11.6% in their study of 147 patients. A more recent study by Goldman and coworkers in 1985,[2] revealed an incidence of 7.45% in over 3000 patients undergoing pelvic surgery when a self-retaining abdominal wall retractor was used.

ANATOMY

The femoral nerve is derived from the dorsal rami of the second, third, and fourth lumbar

TABLE 20–1
Comparison of Postoperative Neuropathies

Nerve	Mechanism of Injury	Symptoms	Signs	Diagnosis	Treatment
Femoral	Self-retaining retractor	Pain over anterior hip Knee joint instability Numbness over anteromedial thigh	Absent patellar reflex Unable to raise thigh while supine Decreased sensation anteromedial thigh and medial leg	Physical exam/ electromyography	Physical therapy
Sciatic/ peroneal	Stretch/ pressure	Lower limb and foot numbness	Unable to evert foot Decreased sensation lower leg	Physical exam/ electromyography	Physical therapy
Iliohypo-gastric	Entrapment	Lower quadrant pain ± radiation to groin	Point tenderness 3 cm medial to anterior-superior iliac spine	Nerve block	Nerve block or surgical reexploration
Obturator	Transection	Decreased sensation anteromedial thigh	Adductor weakness	Electromyography/ nerve block	Epineural repair if transection

nerves, which fuse in the psoas muscle and emerge at its distal lateral border. It then lies in a groove as it travels distally between the psoas and iliacus muscles and travels under the inguinal ligament lateral to the femoral artery. The nerve then divides into muscular and sensory branches. The muscular branches supply the quadriceps, iliacus, sartorius, and pectineus muscles. The sensory branches of the femoral nerve include the anterior femoral cutaneous nerve, the medial femoral cutaneous nerve, and the long saphenous nerve supplying the anterior medial thigh and the medial surface of the leg over the tibia to the medial malleolus. The intrapelvic segment of the femoral nerve receives its blood supply from one small artery from the iliac ramus of the iliolumbar artery, as well as some collateral supply from the deep circumflex iliac artery. The right intrapelvic femoral artery receives more collateral supply than does the left, and there are more anastomotic branches from the fourth and fifth lumbar arteries on the right. The extrapelvic segment of the femoral nerve is supplied by the lateral circumflex artery.

FUNCTION

The femoral nerve and the muscles that it innervates are responsible for hip flexion and knee extension. The nerve also assists with hip adduction and outward rotation of the thigh. Sensory branches of the nerve provide input from the anterior medial thigh and tibial surface of the leg to the medial malleolus.

SIGNS AND SYMPTOMS

Onset of femoral neuropathy usually occurs in the immediate postoperative period, commonly noted on postoperative day 1 or 2. The patient typically complains of instability of the knee, citing that her "knee gives out" when she attempts to walk. Other complaints include pain over the anterior hip and numbness over the anterior medial thigh, leg, and, sometimes, foot. Sinclair and Pratt[3] also reported that there is occasional pain in the knee. The patient also will report there is no pain sensation in the area of numbness. A classic finding is that the patient is unable to climb stairs. A patient with a total femoral nerve palsy walks well on a flat surface and is able to stand without support but often falls on her first attempt to walk and may find walking backward easier than walking forward.

On physical examination, the patellar reflex is absent and there is decreased sensation to touch and pain over the anteromedial aspect of the thigh and the medial aspect of the leg. The patient is unable to raise the leg while supine and has difficulty extending the knee. There may be decreased ability to adduct and rotate the thigh externally.

ETIOLOGY

Early attempts to determine the etiology of femoral neuropathy included consideration of anesthetic and psychiatric involvement, as well as intraoperative complications. Postoperative femoral neuropathy occurs after various intraabdominal and intrapelvic procedures and is most common after an abdominal hysterectomy. Winkleman,[4] in his review of six cases, was the first to implicate self-retaining retractors as a possible cause of postoperative femoral neuropathy. Vosburgh and Finn[5] agreed, citing ischemia of the nerve secondary to compression or traction. Cadaver studies to determine the anatomic relationship of the retractor blades to the femoral nerve revealed compression of the femoral nerve 4 cm proximal to the inguinal ligament, as well as compression of the psoas muscle against the lateral pelvic sidewall. McDaniel and associates[6] cited constant pressure from a self-retaining retractor and suggested that any type of self-retaining retractor could be responsible. Fourteen autopsy dissections performed by Rosenblum and colleagues[7] demonstrated direct pressure of the lateral blades of the self-retaining retractor on the psoas muscle and in close proximity to the femoral nerve. They found that the type of incision, of hysterectomy technique, and of pelvic pathology were not contributing factors in the development of postoperative femoral neuropathy.

The Pfannenstiel incision has been presumed to be more likely related to the development of a femoral neuropathy than a vertical incision. However, femoral neuropathy after vertical incisions has been reported.[2, 8, 9] A Pfannenstiel incision allows the lateral blades of a self-retaining retractor to be in more intimate contact with the psoas muscle and therefore the femoral nerve. A thin body habitus was believed to contribute in the same manner, and Goldman and coworkers[2] suspect that this subgroup of patients may be more prone to this neuropathy. Georgy[8] hypothesized that the body habitus was the most important etiologic finding. However, of 17 patients with a postoperative femoral neuropathy, none were underweight and 6 were overweight.[1]

In a case report of femoral neuropathy after

a vaginal hysterectomy, it was speculated that femoral neuropathy was secondary to nerve entrapment as a result of angulation of the nerve while in the dorsal lithotomy position.[10] The same investigator believed that an operating time greater than 2 hours also played a role in the development of the neuropathy. Cadaveric dissections performed by Hopper and Baker[11] revealed that Heaney retractors placed vaginally are not in close proximity to the femoral nerve.

In reports involving patients undergoing microsurgery, a long operating room time, wide incision, and continuous downward pressure of the retractor by the operator's hand have been implicated.[12]

In the largest study to date and the only study with a control group, Goldman and coworkers[2] studied postoperative femoral neuropathies. The first group consisted of 3786 patients between the years of 1970 and 1974 who underwent pelvic surgery with a self-retaining retractor. The second group consisted of 2965 patients who underwent pelvic surgery between the years of 1980 and 1984 without the use of a self-retaining retractor. The incidence of postoperative femoral neuropathy was 7.45% in the self-retaining retractor group and 0.7% in the hand-held retractor group. Hand-held retractors do not produce a constant downward pressure on the lateral pelvic sidewall or the psoas muscle as do self-retaining retractors. Walsh and Walsh[13] have cited the poor blood supply of the intrapelvic femoral nerve as an explanation for the development of postoperative neuropathy after local compressive forces are applied. Because hand-held retractors result in only intermittent pressure in the area, this could allow reperfusion of the femoral nerve when downward pressure is minimal.

OUTCOME

Total recovery is the rule, although rare patients are reported who have incomplete recovery and quadriceps atrophy. The timing of recovery is varied, ranging from the early postoperative period to 6 months. Most patients recover in 1 to 6 months,[1, 6] and many investigators report excellent functional recovery of patients after femoral neuropathy.[7–9]

PREVENTION

Several preventative measures have been suggested. Because it seems likely that femoral neuropathy results from direct compression of

the nerve or the tissue surrounding the nerve, most preventative measures involve manipulation of the self-retaining retractor. McDaniel and associates[6] first recommended placing a folded laparotomy pack under the lateral blades to form a cushion, and they also recommended using the smallest possible lateral blades. The notion was later criticized by Georgy[8] because he speculated that the laparotomy pack could result in compression of the vasa vasorum. McDaniel and associates[6] proposed avoiding overextension of the Pfannenstiel incision to prevent close contact of the lateral blades with the pelvic sidewall. Rosenblum and colleagues[7] suggested careful placement of the self-retaining retractor such that it results in minimal pressure on the psoas muscle. They also mentioned periodic assessment of the femoral pulses, suggesting that if the femoral pulses distal to the placement of the retractor were absent then the femoral nerve was also compressed. However, the presence of femoral artery pulsation does not preclude compression of the femoral nerve.

Georgy[8] modified his self-retaining retractor by changing its 3.4-inch lateral blades to 1.7 inches, in an effort to decrease the risk of femoral nerve compression. Meldrum[12] suggests avoidance of the O'Connor-O'Sullivan retractor, especially during long operative procedures. He also recommends estimating the retractor pressure by palpating below the blades with downward pressure on the surface of the retractor.

Other suggestions include careful determination of the relationship of the lateral blades of the self-retaining retractor to the psoas muscle repeatedly during the operation[1] and frequent release of the retractor during the operation. Goldman and coworkers[2] advised using a hand-held retractor and reported excellent exposure with the use of steep Trendelenberg positioning and deep anesthesia.

TREATMENT

Treatment should begin early in the diagnosis of the neuropathy. The majority of individuals with femoral neuropathy recover without therapy. Therapeutic modalities available include heat, electric stimulation, and physical therapy with gait training and active exercise. Electromyography has been suggested for follow-up in these patients.

SUMMARY

Femoral neuropathy probably occurs more commonly than is recognized. Because the femoral nerve supplies large and bulky muscles rapid recovery is promoted and many cases are not recognized. However, femoral neuropathy is important to recognize as a complication of gynecologic surgery. The patient often complains of weakness in the knee, pain over the anterior hip, and decreased sensation of the anteromedial aspect of the thigh and medial leg. The hallmark is the inability of the patient to climb stairs. It seems likely that the self-retaining retractor is responsible for the majority of postoperative femoral neuropathies in gynecologic surgery. However, no one self-retaining retractor can be implicated. Femoral neuropathies may occur more commonly after Pfannenstiel incision but are encountered in patients with vertical midline incisions as well. A thin body habitus may play a contributing role in the development of this neuropathy.

Therefore, it seems prudent in all gynecologic laparotomies, to avoid excessive pressure of lateral blades of the self-retaining retractor on the lateral pelvic sidewall, and to release the self-retaining retractor in operative cases lasting more than 2 hours. In the event that a patient develops the classic signs and symptoms of a femoral neuropathy, prompt physiotherapy is recommended and full recovery is anticipated.

Sciatic and Peroneal Neuropathy

The sciatic nerve is derived from the fourth and fifth lumbar and the first, second, and third sacral nerve roots. The nerve traverses the sciatic notch and then lies between the greater trochanter and the ischial tuberosity, behind the gluteus maximus. The nerve then descends in the posterior thigh between the adductor magnus and the biceps muscle. Division of the nerve into lateral popliteal (peroneal) and medial popliteal (tibial) branches usually occurs at two thirds of the distance from the hip to the knee.

The sciatic nerve and its divisions supply the skin of the leg, the hamstrings, and the muscles of the lower leg and foot. The peroneal nerve descends to the head of the fibula and winds around the neck of the fibula, where it divides into the deep peroneal and superficial peroneal (musculocutaneous) nerves. The muscular branches of the peroneal nerve supply the extensor hallucis longus, extensor digitorum longus, peroneus tertius, extensor digitorum brevis, peroneus longus, and peroneus brevis. The cutaneous branches supply the posterior leg

and lateral foot. The tibial nerve innervates the muscles of the calf.

Injury to the sciatic trunk results in compromised hamstring function and inability to flex the knee. The peroneal division of the sciatic nerve appears to be more prone to intraoperative injury than the tibial division. This is thought to be because the peroneal division is well fixed at two points along its length (the sciatic notch and the fibular head). The peroneal nerve therefore is more susceptible to stretch injury than the tibial nerve, which is not fixed distally.[14-16] Peroneal nerve palsy results in lateral foot numbness, footdrop, and inability to extend the toes and evert the foot.[16] Tibial nerve injury is characterized by absence of the ankle jerk.

INCIDENCE

Reports of injury to the sciatic nerve from gynecologic procedures are rare. Burkhart and Daly[16] encountered five sciatic and peroneal neuropathies after more than 2000 gynecologic procedures. McQuarrie and colleagues[17] reported four cases of sciatic neuropathy occurring in 1000 patients after vaginal surgery, and Batres and Barclay[14] reported two additional cases in 1983. Hoffman and associates[15] described three cases (two sciatic, one peroneal) occurring in 377 patients undergoing radical pelvic surgery for gynecologic malignancies.

ETIOLOGY

Putative mechanisms of sciatic and peroneal nerve injury include stretching of the nerve, direct pressure on the peroneal nerve at the fibular head, and hyperflexion of the back. Direct intraoperative trauma to the nerve is also possible when managing hemorrhage during radical pelvic operations. Because the sciatic nerve is fixed at two points it is susceptible to stretch injury. The sciatic nerve can tolerate 1.5 inches of stretching without injury.[18] Excess stretching can be caused by hip hyperflexion and knee extension, as well as by lateral rotation of the thigh. The lithotomy position predisposes the patient to sciatic nerve injury, and improper placement of the stirrups and the patient can lead to this neuropathy. Stirrups placed too high can result in hip flexion and knee extension. The patient's body habitus may play a role, because heavier thighs and legs tend to externally rotate when "candy cane" stirrups are used. Surgical assistants leaning on the medial thigh or knee will enhance external rotation. Mild stretch injuries probably result from transient ischemia, whereas severe stretch results in vascular injury and necrosis of the nerve. The peroneal division can be directly injured by pressure from a stirrup or hard object at the fibular head.[17]

Back hyperflexion can result in disk herniation and possible trauma to the sciatic nerve.[14] This is more likely in a patient whose buttocks are too far off the edge of the table.[17] Hoffman and associates[15] reported two cases of sciatic nerve palsy after radical pelvic operations complicated by intraoperative hemorrhage. One case required mattress sutures in the area of the sacroiliac fossa, and in the second a pressure pack was placed in the region of the hypogastric vein for 3 days and extensive leg edema developed. Although no controlled studies have been performed, reports in the literature favor improper patient positioning in the operating room as the major etiology of this neuropathy. Thirteen of 15 case reports since 1965 have occurred in patients undergoing surgery in the lithotomy position. Batres and Barclay[14] suggest that because of the rarity of the lesion a predisposing factor may exist. Branching of the sciatic nerve into its two main trunks is variable, and certain anatomic variations may predispose individual nerves to stretch injury.

SYMPTOMS AND MANAGEMENT

Initially the patient complains of lower limb numbness. Early onset of symptoms is common in many patients with this neuropathy, with 11 of 15 patients noting numbness within 24 hours of surgery. Sciatic nerve injury can occur anywhere along its length; thus, combined sciatic and peroneal palsy has been reported.[16] The patient may then display a steppage gait and is unable to evert the foot. The diagnosis is confirmed by electromyography or nerve conduction studies.

Physical therapy, foot braces, and nerve stimulation have been reported for the treatment of sciatic or peroneal neuropathy. The majority of the reviewed patients underwent some form of therapy; therefore, the natural history of these lesions occurring after gynecologic surgery is unknown. The majority of patients achieve full recovery in 3 to 6 months[14, 16, 17]; indeed the only patients with serious long-term sequelae were those with neuropathy developing after complicated and/or extensive pelvic surgery.[15]

PREVENTION

Sciatic neuropathy, although rare, is probably best prevented by meticulous attention to patient positioning. To decrease manipulation of the patient, her position on the operating room table should be as close to the final position needed for surgery before intubation. Sudden shift or jerking movements of the extremities should be avoided. Both legs are to be positioned simultaneously by two operators. Tightening of the stirrups before leg placement may avoid sudden leg extension and subsequent sciatic nerve stretching. The patient should be positioned so that minimal tension is placed on the sciatic nerve. Tension is least when the knee and hip are flexed and the hip is mildly externally rotated. Maximal tension occurs when the hip is flexed, the knee is extended, and the hip is externally rotated. Assistants should avoid leaning on the patient's legs. Firm objects against the fibular head should be padded. The patient's back should be flat, with the buttocks at the edge of the table.

SUMMARY

Sciatic neuropathy is an extremely rare occurrence after gynecologic surgery. The nerve is stretched with improper patient positioning in the operating room. Patients complain of lateral foot and leg numbness and may have associated footdrop as well as loss of calf muscle and hamstring function depending on the level of the injury to the nerve. Most often symptoms arise early in the postoperative period and with physical therapy abate within 6 months.

Brachial Plexus Neuropathy

Postoperative brachial plexus neuropathy has been reported after first rib resection, median sternotomy, liver transplantation, tonsillectomy and adenoidectomy, appendectomy, total vaginal hysterectomy, and pelviscopy.[19–22] Dawson and Krarup[20] state that the brachial plexus is the most susceptible nerve group to intraoperative position injuries. Nevertheless, brachial plexus injuries are rare, occurring with a frequency of less than 0.2%.

The most commonly recognized cause of this neuropathy is stretch or compression resulting from intraoperative upper extremity position.[20, 22] However, some investigators speculate that the true cause is unclear, citing brachial plexus palsy occurring in awake patients and the long latency between surgery and onset of symptoms in some patients.[19] When considering patient position, an upper plexus injury results from arm abduction and lower plexus injuries are more common with the arm at the side. Issues of patient positioning specifically related to gynecology focus on shoulder braces used during pelviscopic procedures requiring steep Trendelenburg positioning. Here, the humeral head may be forced into and stretch nerves leaving the plexus.[22]

Patients complain of arm, shoulder, or scapular pain that may persist for days to years. Others report painless upper extremity weakness as the most common finding. The majority of patients recover spontaneously.

NEUROPATHIES RELATED TO SURGICAL TRAUMA

Obturator Neuropathy

ANATOMY

The obturator nerve is derived from the anterior divisions of the second, third, and fourth lumbar nerves; pierces the psoas muscle; and then travels along its medial border. It is then found along the lateral pelvic sidewall before its entrance into the obturator foramen, where it divides into anterior and posterior branches. The obturator nerve does not give off any branches in the pelvis. Eight to 10% of individuals possess an accessory obturator nerve that is derived from either L2–3 or L3–4 and lies on the pectineus muscle.[23] The anterior division of the nerve distributes an articular branch to the knee and supplies the skin of the anteromedial thigh and the gracilis, adductor longus, and sometimes the adductor brevis muscles of the thigh. The posterior division of the nerve also innervates the adductor longus and adductor brevis and the obturator externus muscles. Additionally, the division gives rise to an articular branch to the hip.

INCIDENCE

The frequency of obturator neuropathy is unknown, but its occurrence is thought to be rare. Only a few reports of postoperative obturator neuropathy have been published. Incidences of 0.5% to 0.7% have been reported after pelvic lymphadenectomy in patients with prostatic carcinoma.[24] No comparative reports appear to be available in the gynecologic literature.

ETIOLOGY

The exact cause of postoperative obturator neuropathy is unknown. Obturator neuropathy has been reported in conjunction with obstetric injury, endometriosis, total hip replacement, and radical pelvic surgery.[25–28] Tumors, hematomas, and obturator hernias have also been implicated. Mechanisms of injury during pelvic surgery include complete transection of the nerve, electrocautery, and surgical clips.[24] Extensive postoperative scarring around the area of the obturator nerve has also been cited as a possible cause of this neuropathy.[27]

SIGNS AND SYMPTOMS

Patients reportedly complain of decreased pain sensation in the upper anteromedial thigh. One patient experienced intense pruritus and burning along the cutaneous distribution of the obturator nerve.[27] Adductor weakness is usually present and the patients may demonstrate a characteristic "waddling" gait.

DIAGNOSIS

Electromyography may be useful; however, the electromyogram is sometimes normal in the early stages of nerve embarrassment. Nerve block using lidocaine has been suggested as both a diagnostic and therapeutic procedure for neuropathies unrelated to complete transection.[27] Case reports reveal that a few patients have experienced relief of symptoms for a period of months after nerve block.

TREATMENT

As stated earlier, a nerve block with a local anesthetic may provide some short-term relief. When nerve transection is recognized during surgery, epineural repair has been advocated.[28] Although very little is known about this neuropathy the existing literature suggests that individuals with obturator nerve damage may recover without therapy over a period of months to years. Physical therapy is initiated to enhance adductor strength.

SUMMARY

Scant information is available regarding obturator neuropathies, especially as they relate to gynecologic procedures. Obturator neuropathy should be considered in any individual who complains of numbness of the medial thigh or who demonstrates a gait disturbance. These symptoms occurring postoperatively would probably be more likely secondary to femoral neuropathy, but obturator nerve involvement should be included in the differential diagnosis. Physical examination alone should enable the practitioner to pinpoint the nerve involved because individuals with obturator neuropathy should have a normal patellar reflex. Neurosurgical consultation should be obtained to assess the patient for epineural repair in the event that obturator transection is recognized intraoperatively. Nerve block with a local anesthetic can aid in the diagnosis and may offer some temporary relief of symptoms.

Iliohypogastric and Ilioinguinal Nerve Entrapment

ANATOMY

The iliohypogastric and ilioinguinal nerves supply sensory innervation to the lower anterior abdominal wall and medial groin. The iliohypogastric nerve also divides and innervates some of the skin of the buttock. These are branches of L1 and may receive fibers from T12.[29–31] The ilioinguinal and iliohypogastric nerve may share a common trunk or be given off separately at their origin from the spinal roots. The iliohypogastric nerve becomes superficial to the transversus abdominus muscle at the midpoint between the iliac crest and the twelfth rib. It then lies between the transversus abdominus and internal oblique muscles and pierces the internal oblique 3 cm medial to the anterior-superior iliac spine. The iliohypogastric nerve then curves parallel to the inguinal ligament and in cadaver studies is found to be approximately 4 cm cephalad to the inguinal ligament.[32]

The ilioinguinal nerve becomes superficial to the transversus abdominus much closer to the iliac crest than the iliohypogastric and pierces the internal oblique 1 to 2 cm more medially than the iliohypogastric nerve. The ilioinguinal nerve then enters the inguinal canal.[32] The genitofemoral nerve, also derived from L1 as well as L2, supplies the skin of the medial groin as well as the medial thigh. Clinically it may be difficult to differentiate lesions of the genitofemoral nerve from the iliohypogastric nerve.

ETIOLOGY

Ilioinguinal and iliohypogastric nerve injury and subsequent symptoms may be the result of direct intraoperative trauma in the form of transection, or entrapment may occur from inadvertent stapling or suturing of the nerve. Cicatrix formation can also cause tethering of tissues that could place nerves under tension. Neuroma formation might also be etiologic in cases where no discernible causes are evident.[31–34] The iliohypogastric nerve may become entrapped or damaged during Pfannenstiel incision formation and repair, and for this reason Mandelkow and Loeweneck[32] suggest performing this incision 5 cm above the inguinal ligament.

INCIDENCE

The incidence of iliohypogastric nerve damage after gynecologic surgery is essentially unknown. The paucity of reports in the literature point to either the rarity of this lesion or the lack of symptoms occurring after iliohypogastric entrapment. Hahn[34] reported 46 cases in 150,000 women, and Sippo and associates[33] reported 9 cases over a time period of 16 months. Although generally regarded as a result of surgical injury or lower quadrant trauma,[31] "spontaneous" cases of iliohypogastric nerve entrapment have been reported, which has led some investigators to consider this lesion as a cause of chronic pelvic and abdominal pain in some women.[34]

Ilioinguinal nerve entrapment is considerably more common than iliohypogastric nerve entrapment. The well-known occurrence of this lesion after inguinal herniorrhaphy has led surgeons to perform careful and meticulous dissection of the ilioinguinal nerve during this procedure. Because the ilioinguinal and iliohypogastric nerves are closely related anatomically, damage to either nerve is possible during gynecologic procedures using the Pfannenstiel incision and are more likely if the incision is carried into the internal oblique muscle.[33] Ilioinguinal nerve entrapment has also been reported after needle suspension procedures for urinary incontinence.[35]

SYMPTOMS AND DIAGNOSIS

Patients with iliohypogastric nerve entrapment present with pain that has been described as sharp and burning.[20, 31, 33] Sometimes the pain is noted to radiate to the groin[31] and may not present until years after the initial insult.[20, 31, 33] Over time the discomfort changes character from sharp to dull.[33] Patients with ilioinguinal nerve entrapment may complain of sharp or burning pain radiating to the labia.[35] Activity such as walking and hip extension exacerbate the symptoms, and hip flexion offers some relief. Some investigators have noted that the patient does not have specific complaints of sensory loss in the groin.[34] Point tenderness may be evident at an area approximately 3 cm medial to the anterior-superior iliac spine.[32] Liszka and colleagues[36] speculate that point tenderness is more likely associated with a neuroma and not entrapment.

The diagnosis is confirmed by nerve block. Local anesthetic is injected lateral to the area of point tenderness, approximately 1 inch medial and 1 inch inferior to the anterior-superior iliac spine, with continual injection toward the pubic tubercle in a fan-like manner.[33] With this technique, Sippo and associates[33] were able to affect a positive diagnosis and short-term relief in 100% of their patients.

TREATMENT

Although nerve block has been suggested for the long-term relief of pain from ilioinguinal or iliohypogastric nerve entrapment, only 55% of patients improved with this therapy in one study,[33] and others point out that symptoms return after a short period of time.[34] Hahn[34] cites dissection and rerouting of the nerve, crushing the nerve, transcutaneous electrical nerve stimulation, acupuncture, paravertebral block, rhizotomy, and biofeedback as possible therapeutic modalities. Both segmental nerve resection and nerve transection have been described, with 80% of patients noting improvement in one study.[34] However, randomized trials for the treatment of iliohypogastric entrapment are lacking and would presumably be difficult to perform because of the rarity of the syndrome. Pain secondary to ilioinguinal entrapment after needle suspension procedures can be treated by removing the suture and replacing it medial to the pubic tubercle.[35]

PREVENTION

Although the incidence of these neuropathies is rare, the pain suffered by patients with iliohypogastric neuropathy can be significant. Prevention of iliohypogastric nerve entrapment would be ideal; however, iliohypogastric nerve identification is not routine during pelvic surgery. However, it seems prudent to avoid vastly lateral fascial incisions when performing a Pfannenstiel incision and to make the incision 5 cm above the inguinal ligament if possible. Furthermore, avoiding incorporation of muscle during the repair of the fascial incision may help to decrease the incidence of entrapment.

One series reported an incidence of 1 in 57 cases of ilioinguinal nerve entrapment occurring after needle suspension procedures. Placement of sutures medial to the pubic tubercle may avoid this occurrence.

SUMMARY

Both symptomatic ilioinguinal and iliohypogastric nerve entrapment syndromes are rarely reported in relation to gynecologic surgery. The true incidence is probably higher than that reflected by the literature. Patients often complain of decreased sensation at one or both lateral borders of a Pfannenstiel incision. These entrapment syndromes should be considered in the differential diagnosis of any patient complaining of lower quadrant pain, especially if the pain is stabbing, burning, and radiating to the groin. Symptoms may not present until years after the procedure, and even some spontaneous cases have been reported. Diagnosis is made by local anesthetic nerve block, which may have to be repeated for accurate diagnosis. If the patient does not acquire adequate long-term relief from this procedure, exploration and nerve transection may be required.

Postoperative Urinary Dysfunction

Postoperative urinary dysfunction after gynecologic surgery is a common occurrence.[37, 38] However, long-term postoperative urinary symptoms are rare. Chronic sequelae, including stress urinary incontinence, bladder hypotonia or hypertonia, and decreased sensation probably do not occur after a total abdominal hysterectomy or total vaginal hysterectomy.[38, 39] Radical hysterectomy, however, may cause prolonged urinary symptoms that have been reported to occur with a frequency of 20% to 80%. These abnormalities are diverse and include stress urinary incontinence, urge incontinence, decreased sensation, and hypertonic or hypotonic bladder dysfunction.[40]

A neurologic etiology for postoperative urinary pathology has been suggested by many investigators. Both pelvic nerve damage as well as pudendal neuropathy have been implicated. Innervation of the bladder and urethra is derived from the sacral plexus. The nerves then pass along the lateral pelvic sidewall, dip underneath the uterine artery, and are located approximately 1 cm inferolateral to the cervix. They then fan out over the upper vagina, bladder, and lower ureter. The pudendal nerve supplies somatic innervation to the periurethral levator ani muscle.

Investigators have hypothesized that postoperative urinary dysfunction after radical hysterectomy may be secondary to significant dissection occurring in areas with a high density of nerves that innervate the bladder and urethra. Pathologic specimens after radical hysterectomy have been shown to contain numerous nerve fibers. The type of radical hysterectomy has not been shown to effect the incidence of postoperative urinary voiding difficulties.[40]

The association of the pudendal nerve with postoperative urinary dysfunction is somewhat speculative. Although pudendal nerve injury occurs after vaginal delivery, its incidence after routine gynecologic procedures is not well delineated. Pudendal nerve motor latencies are increased in women with stress urinary incontinence and pelvic floor prolapse. For this reason, individual investigators have hypothesized that pudendal nerve damage may be operative in individuals experiencing stress urinary incontinence as a postoperative complication. Indeed, in a study by Benson and McClellan,[41] pudendal nerve motor latencies were found to be increased preoperatively in women undergoing abdominal or vaginal repair for prolapse and stress urinary incontinence. Postoperative pudendal nerve motor latencies were significantly prolonged in the group undergoing a total vaginal hysterectomy and sacrospinous ligament fixation versus those undergoing total abdominal hysterectomy and sacral colpopexy. Unfortunately Benson and McClellan did not report the incidence of stress urinary incontinence or urinary tract symptomatology occurring in these women postoperatively.

Routine abdominal gynecologic procedures with the exception of radical hysterectomy most likely do not result in significant neurologic damage predisposing to postoperative urinary tract dysfunction. However, it is possible that significant vaginal dissection may cause interruption of pelvic or pudendal nerves, as evidenced by increased pudendal nerve motor latency. More studies are needed to prove a definite cause-and-effect relationship.

REFERENCES

1. Kvist-Poulsen H, Borel J. Iatrogenic femoral neuropathy subsequent to abdominal hysterectomy: incidence and prevention. Obstet Gynecol 1982;60:516.
2. Goldman JA, Feldberg D, Dicker D, et al. Femoral neuropathy subsequent to abdominal hysterectomy: a comparative study. Eur J Obstet Gynecol Reprod Biol 1985;20:385.
3. Sinclair RH, Pratt JH. Femoral neuropathy after pelvic operation. Am J Obstet Gynecol 1972;112:404.
4. Winkelman NW. Femoral nerve complication after pelvic surgery: a report of six cases. Am J Obstet Gynecol 1958;75:1063.
5. Vosburgh LF, Finn WF. Femoral nerve impairment subsequent to hysterectomy. Am J Obstet Gynecol 1961;82:931.
6. McDaniel GC, Kirkley WH, Gilbert JC. Femoral nerve injury associated with the Pfannenstiel incision and abdominal retractors. Am J Obstet Gynecol 1963;87:381.
7. Rosenblum J, Schwarz GA, Bendler E. Femoral neuropathy: a neurological complication of hysterectomy. JAMA 1966;195:409.
8. Georgy FM. Femoral neuropathy following abdominal hysterectomy. Am J Obstet Gynecol 1975;123:819.
9. Kenrick M. Femoral nerve injuries following pelvic surgery: diagnosis and treatment. South Med J 1963;56:152.
10. Roblee MA. Femoral neuropathy from the lithotomy position: case report and new leg holder for prevention. Am J Obstet Gynecol 1967;97:871.
11. Hopper CL, Baker JB. Bilateral femoral neuropathy complicating vaginal hysterectomy. Obstet Gynecol 1968;32:543.
12. Meldrum DR. Femoral nerve compression injury and tubal microsurgery. Fertil Steril 1979;32:345.
13. Walsh C, Walsh A. Postoperative femoral neuropathy. Surg Gynecol Obstet 1992;174:255.
14. Batres F, Barclay DL. Sciatic nerve injury during gynecologic procedures using the lithotomy position. Obstet Gynecol 1983;62:92S.
15. Hoffman MS, Roberts WS, Cavanagh D. Neuropathies associated with radical pelvic surgery for gynecologic cancer. Gynecol Oncol 1988;31:462.
16. Burkhart FL, Daly JW. Sciatic and peroneal nerve injury: a complication of vaginal operations. Obstet Gynecol 1966;28:99.
17. McQuarrie HG, Harris JW, Ellsworth HS, et al. Sciatic neuropathy complicating vaginal hysterectomy. Am J Obstet Gynecol 1972;113:223.
18. Sunderland S. The relative susceptibility to injury of the medial and lateral popliteal divisions of the sciatic nerve. Br J Surg 1953;41:300.
19. Malamut RI, Marques W, England JD, et al. Postsurgical idiopathic brachial neuritis. Muscle Nerve 1994;17:320.
20. Dawson DM, Krarup C. Perioperative nerve lesions. Arch Neurol 1989;46:1358.
21. Moreno E, Gómez SR, Gonzalez I, et al. Neurologic complication in liver transplantation. Acta Neurol Scand 1993;87:25.
22. Romanowski L, Reich H, McGlynn F. Brachial plexus neuropathies after advanced laparoscopic surgery. Fertil Steril 1993;60:729.
23. Hollinshead WH, Rosse C. Buttock, thigh and hip joint. In: Smith MK, ed. Textbook of Anatomy, 4th ed. Philadelphia, Harper & Row, 1985, p 386.
24. Fishman J, Moran M, Carey R. Obturator neuropathy after laparoscopic pelvic lymphadenectomy. Urology 1993;42:198.
25. Warfield CA. Obturator neuropathy after forceps delivery. Obstet Gynecol 1984;64S:47S.
26. Redwine D, Sharpe D. Endometriosis of the obturator nerve. J Reprod Med 1990;35:434.
27. Crews D, Dohlman L. Obturator neuropathy after multiple genitourinary procedures. Urology 1987;29:504.

28. Vasilev S. Obturator nerve injury: a review of management options. Gynecol Oncol 1994;53:152.
29. Hollinshead WH, Rosse C. The abdomen in general. In: Smith MK, ed. Textbook of Anatomy, 4th ed. Philadelphia, Harper & Row, 1985, p 591.
30. Hollinshead WH, Rosse C. The posterior abdominal wall and associated organs. In: Smith MK, ed. Textbook of Anatomy. Philadelphia, Harper & Row, 1985, p 694.
31. Starling JR, Harms BA, Schroeder ME, et al. Diagnosis and treatment of genitofemoral and ilioinguinal entrapment neuralgia. Surgery 1987;102:581.
32. Mandelkow H, Loeweneck H. The iliohypogastric and ilioinguinal nerves. Surg Radiol Anat 1988;10:145.
33. Sippo WC, Captain MC, Burghardt A, et al. Nerve entrapment after Pfannenstiel incision. Am J Obstet Gynecol 1987;157:420.
34. Hahn L. Clinical findings and results of operative treatment in ilioinguinal nerve entrapment syndrome. Br J Obstet Gynecol 1989;96:1080.
35. Miyazaki F, Shook G. Ilioinguinal nerve entrapment during needle suspension for stress incontinence. Obstet Gynecol 1992;80:246.
36. Liszka TG, Dellon AL, Manson PN. Iliohypogastric nerve entrapment following abdominoplasty. Plast Reconstr Surg 1994;93:181.
37. Jequier AM. Urinary symptoms and total hysterectomy. Br J Urol 1976;48:437.
38. Smith PH, Ballantyne B. The neuroanatomical basis for denervation of the urinary bladder following major pelvic surgery. Br J Surg 1968;55:929.
39. Mundy AR. An anatomical explanation for bladder dysfunction following rectal and uterine surgery. Br J Urol 1982;54:501.
40. Scotti RJ, Bergman A, Bhatia NN, et al. Urodynamic changes in urethrovesical function after radical hysterectomy. Obstet Gynecol 1986;68:111.
41. Benson JT, McClellan E. The effect of vaginal dissection on the pudendal nerve. Obstet Gyncol 1993;82:387.

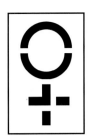

Index

■ ■ ■ ■ ■ ■ ■ ■

Note: Page numbers in *italics* refer to illustrations;
page numbers followed by t refer to tables.

ISBN 0-7216-5881-4

90038